Current Concepts in Dental Implantology - From Science to Clinical Research

Edited by Dragana Gabrić and Marko Vuletić

Published in London, United Kingdom

Current Concepts in Dental Implantology - From Science to Clinical Research
http://dx.doi.org/10.5772/intechopen.94961
Edited by Dragana Gabrić and Marko Vuletić

Contributors
Joy-anne N. Oliver, Olanrewaju Akande, Melanie Ecker, Gaurav Gupta, Petrică Vizureanu, Mădălina Simona Bălţatu, Andrei Victor Sandu, Dragos Cristian Achitei, Dumitru Doru Burduhos Nergis, Manuela Cristina Perju, Deeksha Gupta, Charles D. Schlesinger, Ahmad Al Jaghsi, Leandro Díez Suárez, Marko Blašković, Dorotea Blaskovic, Abdulqadir Rampurawala, Amol Patil, Fares Kablan, Dragana Rakasevic, Dragana Gabrić, Sergio Alexandre Gehrke, Dubravka Knezović Zlatarić, Robert Ćelić, Hrvoje Pezo, Sukumaran Anil, Sara Gibreel, Hasaan Gassim Mohamed, Amartya Raj Suraj, Ivica Pelivan, Amer Shatta, Gopathy Sridevi, Seshadri Srividya

First published in London, United Kingdom, 2022 by IntechOpen
IntechOpen is the global imprint of INTECHOPEN LIMITED, registered in England and Wales, registration number: 11086078, 5 Princes Gate Court, London, SW7 2QJ, United Kingdom
Printed in Croatia

British Library Cataloguing-in-Publication Data
A catalogue record for this book is available from the British Library

Additional hard and PDF copies can be obtained from orders@intechopen.com

Current Concepts in Dental Implantology - From Science to Clinical Research
Edited by Dragana Gabrić and Marko Vuletić
p. cm.

This title is part of the Dentistry Book Series, Volume 11
Topic: Prosthodontics and Implant Dentistry
Series Editor: Sergio Alexandre Gehrke
Topic Editor: Wen Lin Chai
Associate Topic Editor: Ghee Seong Lim

Print ISBN 978-1-83969-863-7
Online ISBN 978-1-83969-864-4
eBook (PDF) ISBN 978-1-83969-865-1
ISSN 2631-6218

For EU product safety concerns:
IN TECH d.o.o., Prolaz Marije Krucifikse Kozulić 3, 51000 Rijeka, Croatia,
info@intechopen.com or visit our website at intechopen.com.

IntechOpen Book Series

Dentistry

Volume 11

Aims and Scope of the Series

This book series will offer a comprehensive overview of recent research trends as well as clinical applications within different specialties of dentistry. Topics will include overviews of the health of the oral cavity, from prevention and care to different treatments for the rehabilitation of problems that may affect the organs and/or tissues present. The different areas of dentistry will be explored, with the aim of disseminating knowledge and providing readers with new tools for the comprehensive treatment of their patients with greater safety and with current techniques. Ongoing issues, recent advances, and future diagnostic approaches and therapeutic strategies will also be discussed. This series of books will focus on various aspects of the properties and results obtained by the various treatments available, whether preventive or curative.

Meet the Series Editor

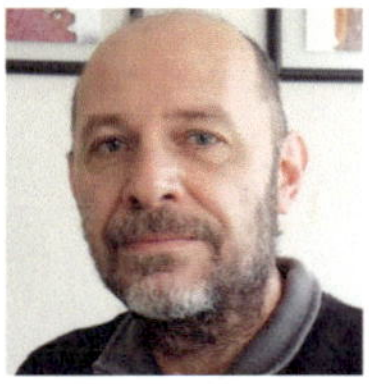

Dr. Sergio Alexandre Gehrke is a doctorate holder in two fields. The first is a Ph.D. in Cellular and Molecular Biology from the Pontificia Catholic University, Porto Alegre, Brazil, in 2010 and the other is an International Ph.D. in Bioengineering from the Universidad Miguel Hernandez, Elche/Alicante, Spain, obtained in 2020. In 2018, he completed a postdoctoral fellowship in Materials Engineering in the NUCLEMAT of the Pontificia Catholic University, Porto Alegre, Brazil. He is currently the Director of the Postgraduate Program in Implantology of the Bioface/UCAM/PgO (Montevideo, Uruguay), Director of the Cathedra of Biotechnology of the Catholic University of Murcia (Murcia, Spain), an Extraordinary Full Professor of the Catholic University of Murcia (Murcia, Spain) as well as the Director of the private center of research Biotecnos – Technology and Science (Montevideo, Uruguay). Applied biomaterials, cellular and molecular biology, and dental implants are among his research interests. He has published several original papers in renowned journals. In addition, he is also a Collaborating Professor in several Postgraduate programs at different universities all over the world.

Meet the Volume Editors

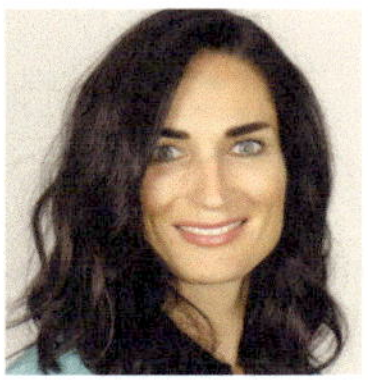

Dragana Gabrić, DMD, Ph.D., is an associate professor and a scientific advisor at the Department of Oral Surgery, School of Dental Medicine, University of Zagreb, and also a specialist in oral surgery, at the Clinical Department of Oral Surgery, University Dental Clinic, University Hospital Center Zagreb Croatia. She is head of the Reference Center for Dental Implantology, Ministry of Health of the Republic of Croatia. Dr. Gabrić is the author and coauthor of many cited scientific and professional papers and reviews as well as twenty-six book chapters. She has been an invited speaker at many international scientific and professional courses, congresses, and universities. She is a Member of the Croatian Chamber of Dental Medicine, Croatian Society of Oral Surgeons, Croatian Association for Dental Implantology, Croatian Medical Association, Laser and Health Academy, Croatian Association for Minimally Invasive Dental Medicine, and Croatian Society for Maxillofacial and Plastic and Reconstructive Surgery of the Face and Neck. Dr. Gabrić holds one registered patent.

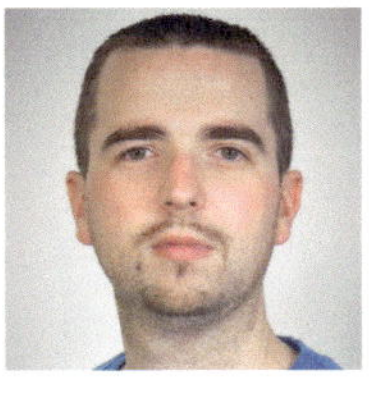

Marko Vuletić, DMD, Ph.D., is a scientific associate at the Department of Oral Surgery, School of Dental Medicine, University of Zagreb and he is a specialist in oral surgery at the Clinical Department of Oral Surgery, University Dental Clinic, University Hospital Center Zagreb, Croatia. He is the author and co-author of many cited scientific papers and reviews and two book chapters. He is an active participant in many national and international scientific and professional courses and congresses. He has been an invited speaker at a few scientific and professional congresses. Dr. Vuletić is a Member of the Croatian Chamber of Dental Medicine, Croatian Society of Oral Surgeons, Croatian Association for Dental Implantology, Croatian Medical Association, and Croatian Society for Maxillofacial, Plastic and Reconstructive Surgery of the Face and Neck. He is a pioneering researcher in methods and quality of life in children with clefts.

Contents

Preface

Our love and passion for dentistry as well as a desire to share what we have learned over the years as clinicians, teachers, and researchers helped us in collaboration with colleagues from different countries to write this international text based on current concepts in dental implantology. The procedures presented herein are technically demanding and not intended for the novice; these procedures require a great deal of skill, training, and experience to perform.

This book is divided into four sections with seventeen chapters that discuss modern scientific and clinical methods used in today's dental implantology. Topics include osseointegration and basic science in dental implantology, current trends and biomaterials of clinical relevance, advanced clinical techniques, peri-implantitis, and prosthodontic trends in dental implantology. This book provides a better understanding of the scientific approach to basic concepts in dental implantology and presents the results of many clinical studies.

I am thankful to all my national and international colleagues for their excellent contributions. I would also like to extend my gratitude to my co-editor Dr. Marko Vuletić for assisting me in compiling and reviewing the chapters and managing all other details of the publication process.

I sincerely hope this book will be of use to all clinicians who practice this fascinating discipline, and that all readers will enjoy seeing the results of our professional journey in this challenging field and enjoy reading this book as much as we enjoyed composing it.

Dragana Gabrić, DDM, Ph.D.
Professor,
Department of Oral Surgery,
School of Dental Medicine,
University of Zagreb,
Zagreb, Croatia

Clinical Department of Oral Surgery,
Clinical Hospital Center Zagreb,
University Dental Clinic,
Zagreb, Croatia

Marko Vuletić, DDM, Ph.D.
Department of Oral Surgery,
School of Dental Medicine,
University of Zagreb,
Zagreb, Croatia

Clinical Department of Oral Surgery,
Clinical Hospital Center Zagreb,
University Dental Clinic,
Zagreb, Croatia

Section 1

Osseointegration and Basic Science in Dental Implantology

Chapter 1

Characteristics of Implant Systems That Can Accelerate and Improve the Osseointegration Process

Sergio Alexandre Gehrke

Abstract

The research and development of new implant models modifying the micro and macro design has increased significantly in the last decades. With the advancement of knowledge about the biological behavior of these materials when implanted in living tissue, a great search for morphological changes at macrogeometric, microgeometric and even nanogeometric levels was started, to accelerate the process of osseointegration of implants, reducing the time for the rehabilitation treatment. This chapter will seek to demonstrate, through scientific evidence, the potential effect of the morphological characteristics of implants on osseointegration. Modifications in the surface treatment of implants will be discussed to improve the osseointegration process in terms of quality and time reduction, changes in the surgical technique used for the osteotomy of the implant installation site, and macrogeometric changes in the shape of the implant body.

Keywords: implant design, implant microgeometry, implant macrogeometry, rapid osseointegration, titanium implants

1. Introduction

Dental implants have become a predictable and safe form of treatment for the replacement of missing teeth. Surely, implants have revolutionized dentistry practice in worldwide, enabling the rehabilitation of patients who have lost single teeth to patients with loss of all teeth. Thus, various types of treatments made possible by improving the quality of life and patient satisfaction. Among these treatments that had the greatest representation, we can mention: the cases of totally edentulous people, who could receive implants to improve the fixation of removable dentures or even receive fixed dentures; patients with partial losses with a lack of posterior pillars (teeth) who had to wear removable dentures and could receive fixed dentures; and patients who had unit losses where it was possible to rehabilitate them without wearing out natural healthy teeth.

Since its diffusion by Branemark in the 60s [1, 2], dental implants have been the object of many studies and, consequently, have undergone several changes. However, the base material for its manufacture, titanium, continues to be used due to its excellent biological and mechanical characteristics. Surgical techniques have also undergone several advances and modifications. Initially, a waiting time for the beginning of the rehabilitation procedures of 6 months was recommended, with implants installed in the bone tissue and covered by mucosa during this waiting period for osseointegration. With the advancement of knowledge, it was proposed that for implants installed in the mandible, the waiting time could be less than in the maxilla, due to the difference in density between the two anatomical sectors. However, Gehrke and Tavares da Silva Neto [3], showed in a clinical study that the evolution of osseointegration is the same in the 2 types of bone (maxilla and mandible) and that the implants could be loaded in both arches with the same waiting time, as long as these sites who received implants were in adequate condition. On the other hand, new techniques aiming to speed up the treatment time and provide greater comfort to patients, such as post-extraction implants (immediate), immediate loading on the implants, implants with simultaneous bone regeneration, among others, were proposals and studied and, currently, are widely used.

Different changes at nano-, micro- and macro-structural levels have been researched and proposed with the aim of improving and/or accelerating the processes involved in the osseointegration of dental implants. Such possibilities became possible with the evolution of scientific knowledge about the events involved in the healing process of peri-implant tissues after implant insertion. In this sense, several types of surface treatment have been proposed in order to promote a physical–chemical stimulation capable of accelerating the initial phases of bone neoformation on the implant [4, 5]. Among the main methods used to produce surface roughness of implants are the addition processes (e.g., titanium plasma spray, hydroxyapatite coating) and subtraction processes (e.g., acid etching, microparticle blasting, laser). Among all of them, the most used procedure currently by most of the world industry is the subtraction methods, as they have shown good results and are less costly. On the other hand, the addition of ions (e.g., Calcium, Magnesium, hydroxyapatite) on these surfaces at nano- and/or micrometric levels has shown good results for the osseointegration.

Initially, the implants had a cylindrical macrogeometry, being later proposed implants with macrogeometry with conical designs. Tapered shaped implants had advantages over cylindrical ones, especially regarding the surgical process, where they were shown to generate less trauma to the bone tissue resulting from the drilling process used for this type of implant. In addition to this change in the body of the implant body, changes in the shape of the turns, which were initially triangular and with little depth, received other shapes, such as trapezoidal, square, and with greater depth and distance in the thread pitch. Also, changes in the cervical portion of the implants, which are in contact with the cortical bone, have been proposed. Among these changes, we can mention the presence of smooth (polished) surfaces, treated (rough) surfaces and the presence of micro-turns. Regarding the prosthetic connections, the implants had several alterations, being proposed different models of fittings, always with the intention of improving the stability of the rehabilitation in the long term. **Figure 1** shows different types of implants and designs proposed in recent decades.

More recently, with scientific evidence that the installation of implants with less compression of the bone tissue could benefit and accelerate the osseointegration process, new macrogeometric models of implants were proposed. In this sense, it was shown that the presence of free spaces of bone tissue or the presence of uncompressed fragments can facilitate the cellular work of phagocytosis and bone matrix neoformation, as shown schematically in the **Figure 2**. This type of condition, creating a space

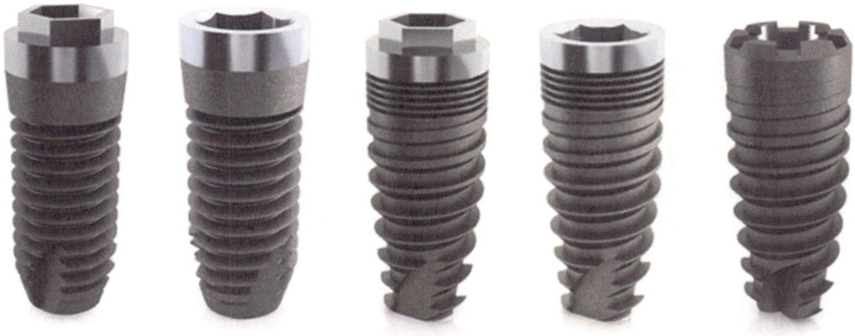

Figure 1.
Available dental implants with different design and connections. (courtesy of Implacil De Bortoli company, Brazil).

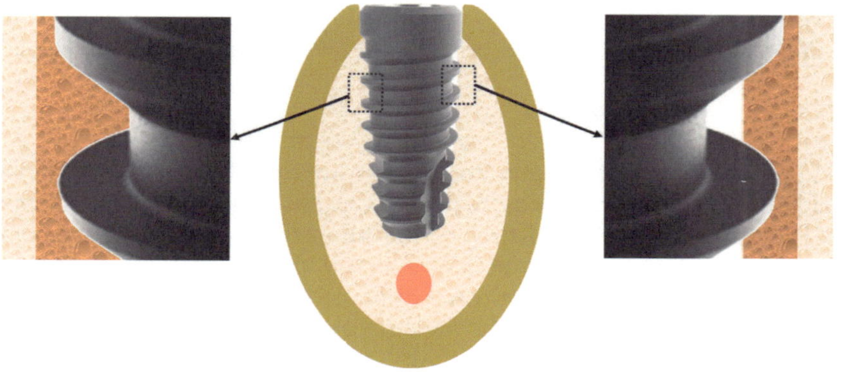

Figure 2.
Schematic image depicting the installation of an implant in a conventional technique (left) causing bone compression over an extensive area, and the implant insertion with spaces between the bone and the implant (right) decreasing bone compression area.

between the bone tissue and the implant, is achieved through a modification in the surgical technique, that is, in the relationship between the diameter of the last reamer used and the diameter of the implant to be inserted into the bone. Thus, in this chapter we will describe and discuss some advances resulting from these changes in the structure of dental implants during the last decades.

2. Characteristics of implants, proposed changes and results obtained

2.1 Surface treatments

The first dental implants were developed without any type of surface treatment, they were carried out by a machining process, which resulted in implants with a smooth surface. For a long time, this implant was conceived as the gold standard. Experimental studies comparing smooth and rough surfaces demonstrate a better biological response to the latter. With the evolution of implantology, changes in implant surfaces began to be carried out in order to improve osseointegration [6].

The processes of changes in the surface of implants can be carried out by the addition method, when some type of material is added to the layer by means of plasma spray coating, or subtraction, when part of this surface layer is removed by physical and/or chemical processes, such as abrasion by blasting or acid etching [7]. The texturing of the implant surface can influence the osseointegration process both in cell differentiation, after implant placement, and in the amount of calcified bone matrix [7, 8]. Thakral et al. [9], reported that texturing techniques in dental implants can influence the establishment of osseointegration, both for cell differentiation, after implant insertion, and for calcified bone matrix. Also, according to Wennerberg and Albrektsson [10], the treated surfaces result in greater bone/implant contact (BIC), compared to smooth implants. Thus, implants with textured surfaces are indicated for sites with a lower BIC at the end of surgery. On the other hand, Att et al. [11], state that bone is indistinctly deposited on porous or smooth surfaces. Therefore, porosity would not be a necessary condition for bone apposition to occur.

Regarding the initial stability of the implants, the surface treatment of the implants does not change the initial stability values of the implants, as shown in studies comparing the insertion torque and stability analysis by resonance frequency using implants with the same design with and without surface treatment [12, 13].

2.1.1 Machined surfaces (smooth)

Machined implants with an untreated surface are considered to have a smooth surface. Machined implants with an untreated surface are considered to have a smooth surface. However, they have small grooves that allow the bone mineralization process towards the implant, but they do not have an osteoinductive surface. This type of surface is considered anisotropic, which is responsible for promoting the cell adhesion process and the production of the protein matrix. The machined implant has a surface roughness between 0.5 μm and 1 μm. This smooth surface is formed a surficial microgroove, resulting from the machining process, produced by the passage of the cutting tool. This type of surface does not receive chemical or mechanical treatment, presenting only the micromorphology of the machining process [9]. **Figure 3** shows representative images of a smooth surface at different magnifications.

2.1.2 Surfaces textured by the plasma spray process

Plasma spray is the type of plasma spray treatment that has been most used, which is elaborated with the ionized flame of a gas heated between 10000°C and 30000°C,

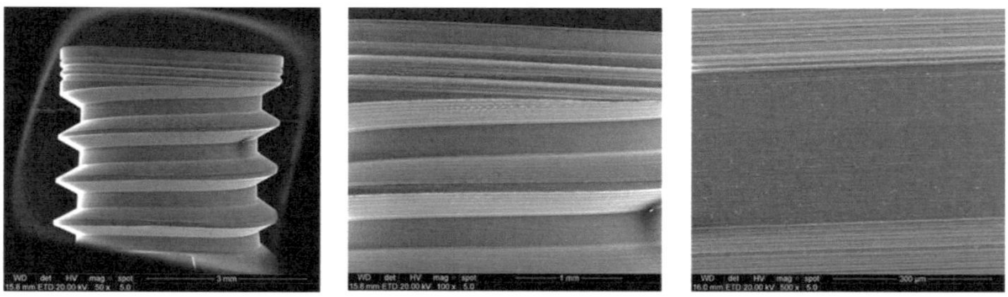

Figure 3.
Representative SEM images with different magnifications of the surface micro grooves resulting from the machining process, produced by the passage of the cutting tool.

and the particles are launched at high speed against the implant body. Upon contact, these particles cool and solidify. Plasma spray is used to apply and incorporate Ti (titanium) and HA (hydroxyapatite) onto the implant surface [14].

Titanium plasma spray is formed by coating the implant with ionized gases by thermal spraying with titanium plasma spray. In this method, the ionized flame of a gas is launched against the implant wall at an elevated temperature between 10000°C and 30000°C. With this change, there is an acceleration of blood absorption, due to the effect on the wettability of this surface, there is an increase in the surface contact area, promoting better osseointegration [14, 15]. The titanium particle is fused on the surface, forming a ~ 50 μm thick layer, with the resulting coating being between 10 μm and 40 μm, increasing the surface of the implant. Herrero-Climent et al. [16], carried out a comparative study between plasma spray titanium (TPS) and titanium oxide blasted surfaces, demonstrating that the TPS surface presented a unique pattern of bone matrix formation when compared to the titanium oxide blasted surface.

Meanwhile, the treatment for coating with apatite nucleation occurs through three stages: alkaline treatment, thermal treatment, and immersion in a synthetic solution equivalent to blood plasma. This layer is obtained by spraying the plasma spray of hydroxyapatite onto the implant surface [15]. Roughness depends on the size of the particles, their adhesion, the speed and distance at which they were launched against the implant [14]. According to De Groot et al. [17], hydroxyapatite plasma spray implants have already been studied and considered to have a high potential for osseointegration. Other authors showed that titanium implants coated with plasma spray of hydroxyapatite had greater amounts of bone at the bone/implant interface when compared to implants with smooth surface [18, 19].

2.1.3 Laser surface treatment

In this type of surface treatment, the implant's surface is modified by irradiation by means of laser beams, producing erosions and a rough surface. It is considered a clean treatment as it does not interact with any external material during the surface modification process, in which the laser beam acts as a physical means in the treatment of this surface [15]. Studies have shown that this method can stimulate adequate osseointegration to implants [20, 21]. In addition, laser treatment has the advantage that oriented, regular micro-grooves with different depths can be created at defined points on the surface [14]. Roughness sizes depend on the pulse intensity of the emitting source [9]. This type of surface has been extensively studied by Ricci et al. [22], showing that micro sulci can modulate cell organization and, consequently, positively influence the osseointegration process.

2.1.4 Surface blasting by micro particles

This type of treatment for the implant surface is blasting with microparticles of some abrasive material (e.g., aluminum oxide or titanium oxide), which promotes irregular surface depressions. Ideally, there should be no adhesion of particles to the implant (residues), which should be removed during the cleaning and decontamination processes. Obviously, the roughness caused depends on the size of the microparticles used, the time and pressure used in the process [9, 14, 15, 21]. In **Figure 4** it is possible to observe the result of the treatment of a surface using only the sandblasting with aluminum oxide particles. However, the roughness produced has sharp edges and several non-uniform irregularities, which can make contact and cell organization difficult and, consequently, have an opposite effect to what is expected for an adequate osseointegration. Currently, this type of isolated treatment is little used by the industry.

Moreover, SEM (scanning electron microscopy) analysis of implants subjected to microparticle blasting, in this case aluminum oxide (Al_2O_3), show residues from the manufacturing process that can contaminate the implant surface (**Figure 5**), which would be harmful to osseointegration, as they would compete with calcium for bone formation. On the other hand, the use of titanium oxide in place of alumina can be an alternative to avoid these undesirable effects on the implant surface [23–25].

In this sense, Gehrke and Collaborators, comparing implants blasted with aluminum oxide and titanium oxide, demonstrated that the residual particles from blasting can interfere in the osseointegration process in these places where they are present [23]. Moreover, in other studies using in vitro and in vivo tests, were demonstrated an excellent biologic response of the surfaces treated by sandblasting with microparticles of titanium oxide [24], with minimal risk of contamination by the residual debris from the blasting procedure [25].

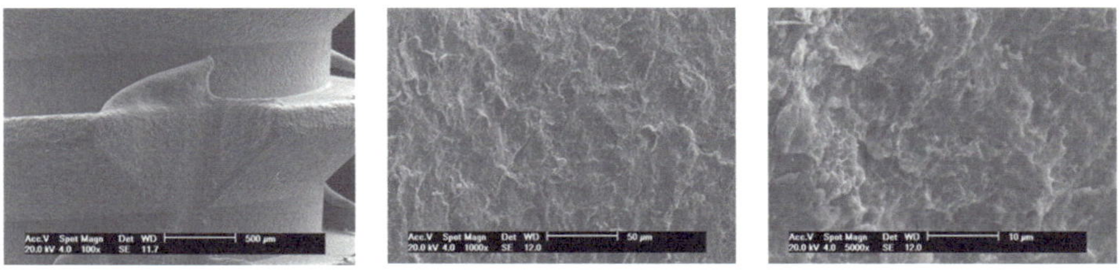

Figure 4.
SEM images of a surface treated by sandblasting with aluminum oxide, where we can observe in higher magnifications the presence of sharp edges and other deformations resulting from this surface treatment process.

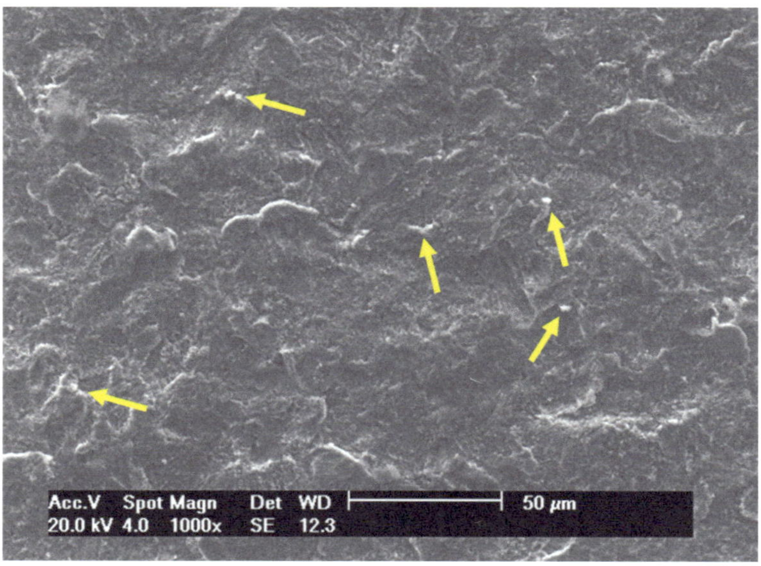

Figure 5.
SEM image showing some locations, among several in the same sample, with the presence of residual microparticles on a blast-treated surface. This surface continued to show the presence of residues even after the washing and decontamination process.

2.1.5 Surface blast treatment followed by acid etching

As described above, the sandblasting process, which can be done by different particles (e.g., aluminum oxide or titanium oxide) and different sizes (150–500 μm), creates deep, amorphous roughness and can leave sharp edges sharp on the surface of the implants. Therefore, acid etching was used after the blasting process, leaving a much more regular surface, and eliminating (rounding) the peaks left by the first process. This union between the 2 types of treatment was called and patented as SLA surface (Sandblasted, large grit, acid-etched implant surface) by the Straumann Company. For the treatment of SLA Straumann surface implants, blasting with coarse-grained aluminum oxide (250–500 μm) is initially performed, producing macro-roughness in the implant, followed by an acid etching (HCl/H2SO4), which is responsible for the microroughness on this surface [6]. However, this treatment model is used by several companies, with variation both in the blasting process and in the acid etching process.

In this sense, comparing 2 different models of implant surface blasting with aluminum oxide and titanium oxide and subsequent etching by different acids in scanning microscopy images, we can observe that the texture of the surfaces has a different morphology between them, as shown in images in **Figure 6.**

To accelerate and improve the osseointegration process of this type of SLA surface, the processing means were modified, being made under nitrogen atmosphere and later stored in isotonic NaCl (sodium chloride), this surface being called SLActive. Thus, these implants could provide a more active osseointegration process than other implants [26] and, consequently, could be loaded with a reduced waiting time. In this new technique, the surface is hydroxylated, and this chemical change improves the surface structures, which are ideal for protein adsorption and to promote immediate implant intent into bone tissue. The SLActive surface was developed to optimize implant stability in less time and reduce treatment risks in the early stages [27]. Rupp et al. [27], demonstrated that the SLActive and SLA surfaces did not show apparent differences when both had the same topography, however, statistically significant differences were observed within two or four weeks of BIC repair (bone/implant contact). This demonstrates that the changes were not a consequence of the topography, but that they were probably due to changes in the chemical structures made on the surface. Oates et al. [28] demonstrated that accelerated bone formation can influence

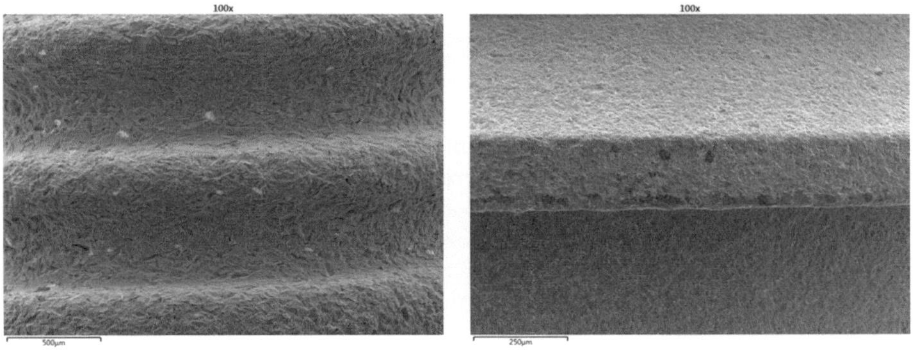

Figure 6.
Images obtained by SEM at 100x magnification, showing 2 different models of implant surface sandblasting: (a) with aluminum oxide and (b) with titanium oxide. Both received further conditioning by different acids. We can observe that the surface texture has a different morphology between them.

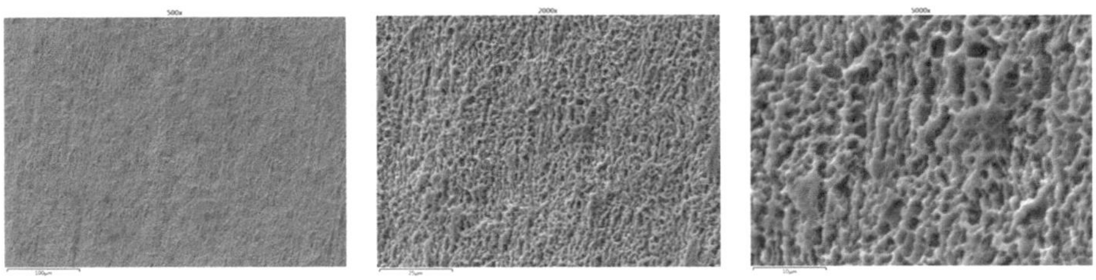

Figure 7.
SEM images at different magnifications of an acid-etched implant surface.

implant stability. Also, in that same study, the authors observed that the transition time from primary stability to secondary stability was two weeks for SLActive surface and four weeks for SLA.

2.1.6 Acid conditioning treatment

The surface treatment by conditioning through acids is made by immersing the implant in an acidic substance, which causes erosion on this surface. Acid concentration, time and temperature are determining factors of the surface microstructure. On the smooth surface, the most used process is the double acid attack, carried out with sulfuric acid and hydrochloride [29]. This surface treatment process provides a very uniform morphology, however, with less depth of ripple compared to SLA-type surfaces. An advantage of this type of treatment is that it supposedly does not leave residues of contaminants in your process. In **Figure 7** we can see an implant surface treated by acid etching.

2.1.7 Anodized surfaces

In the case of nanotextured surfaces, treated with anodizing, they receive an extra layer of titanium dioxide. Thus, these surfaces are obtained using the implant as an anode, activating ions, and applying an electrical potential, which generates charge and ion transfer reactions. Controlled, the electric field will guide the oxidation process that takes place on the implant and results in an increase in the thickness of the titanium oxide (TiO_2) layer. With the increase of this titanium oxide layer and the addition of other elements, such as phosphate (PO_4), there is a potentialization of osseointegration [9].

Corrosion resistance and biocompatibility are related to the presence of a non-reactive oxide layer, which prevents the formation of fibrous tissue around the implant and creates a direct contact with the bone tissue [21, 27]. Implants with this surface treatment are less dependent on chemical composition, as the resulting process is defined by a complementary increase in bone-implant contact [30]. This type of surface treatment has become well known in the implantology field for being used in implants from the Nobel Biocare company (Sweden). **Figure 8** shows images obtained by SEM of the surface of an anodized implant.

2.1.8 Biomimetic surfaces

Abe et al. [31], presented a procedure that allowed to cover the implant surface with a uniform layer of HA similar to the biological layer, up to 15 μm thick, called the biomimetic method. This type of surface treatment consists of the heterogeneous

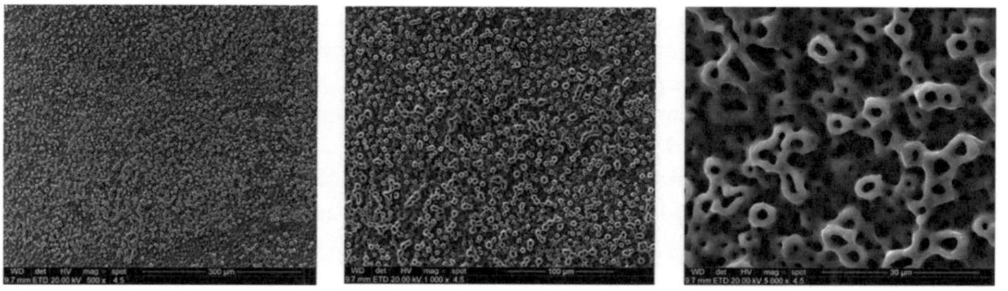

Figure 8.
SEM images with different magnifications of an implant surface treated by the anodized method.

precipitation of calcium phosphate under physiological conditions of temperature and pH on the dental implant, using a solution of ions similar to blood plasma with a view to deposition of the apatite layer. Once the molecules are integrated into the material structure, they are gradually released, thus being able to increase bone conductivity and enhance bone formation around the implant [32]. Currently, calcium phosphate is one of the main biomaterials for bone tissue replacement and regeneration, as its main characteristics are similar to the mineral phase of bone tissue, excellent biocompatibility, bioactivity, absence of toxicity, degradation rates variables and osteoconductivity [32]. Another advantage of this surface treatment is that biologically active molecules, such as osteogenic agents, can be precipitated as inorganic components to form a matrix with both osteoinductive (growth factors) and osteoconductive (calcium phosphate layer) properties [21, 27]. **Figure 9** shows SEM images of an implant surface treated by the biomimetic method.

Studies on this type of surface have shown greater contact between bone and implant on surfaces with biomimetic calcium phosphate coatings than on untreated surfaces [21]. Huang et al. [33], investigated the effects of chemical and nanotopographic modifications in the initial stages of osseointegration, and the results showed a greater removal torque and greater bone apposition for implants with chemical nanotopographic modifications. Recently, we presented in a study of adhesion, cell growth and in vitro mineralization using a surface with deposition of hydroxyapatite nanoparticles showed a superior result to the control group [23]. Furthermore, our group studied the deposition of calcium–magnesium on the surface of implants, where an acceleration and improvement in the osseointegration of implants inserted in rabbit tibiae was observed histomorphometrically, compared to implants with surface treated by blasting with titanium oxide and conditioning acid.

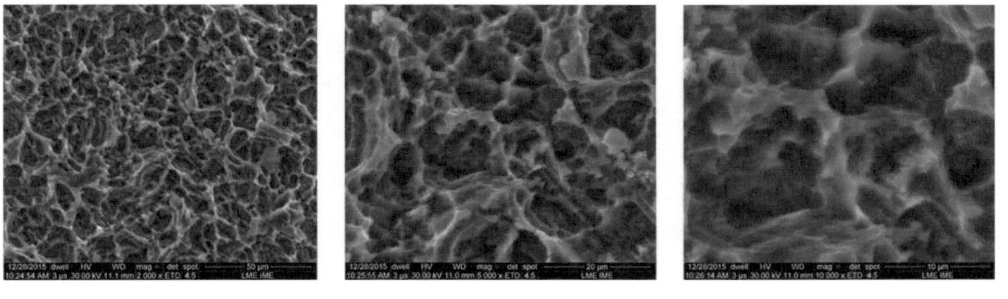

Figure 9.
SEM images at different magnifications showing an implant surface treated by the biomimetic method.

In conclusion, we can say that the main results of surface treatments with the aim of improving osseointegration were to accelerate the osseointegration time, allowing the anticipated loading of implants. On the other hand, osseointegration occurs on the surfaces of dental implants, regardless of whether these are treated or not. Surface treatments improve the result of osseointegration, especially in the initial stages, benefiting a bone apposition with qualitative and quantitative density. Despite the results presented, the dental literature is not unanimous as to the best type of surface treatment.

2.2 Implant body shape

Bone density and quality, surgical technique and implant body geometry are factors to be considered to obtain a shorter period of osseointegration, thus enabling a reduction in treatment time [34]. The relationship between these factors will determine the initial stability of the implant, defined as the absence of movement after its surgical insertion [35–38]. According to some studies [34, 39, 40], the success of implants is dependent on the initial stability achieved, as this is a prerequisite for bone cell differentiation and osseointegration [41]. The shape of the implant has been one of the most contested variables among engineers and researchers, as it can directly influence the biomechanics of the implant inserted into bone tissue [42].

Regarding the implant body shapes most frequently found on the world market, we have cylindrical, semi-tapered and tapered implants, as shown schematically in **Figure 10**. Currently, most implant manufacturing companies use the last two implant designs mentioned above (semi-tapered or tapered). Initially, tapered implant designs were introduced in implant dentistry with the main advantage of producing better initial stability compared to cylindrical implants. Later, several studies were developed and published comparing the tapered with the cylindrical implant designs [43–45]. Recently, new discoveries about the advantages of these designs were observed, such as and, mainly, the lesser surgical trauma during the drilling procedures and insertion of these implants in the bone tissue [46].

Other authors have shown that the use of implants with a conical design can increase stability in low-density bone, since results demonstrated greater contact osteogenesis with this type of design [45]. However, the difference in this stability between implants with different designs has not been sufficiently investigated, with

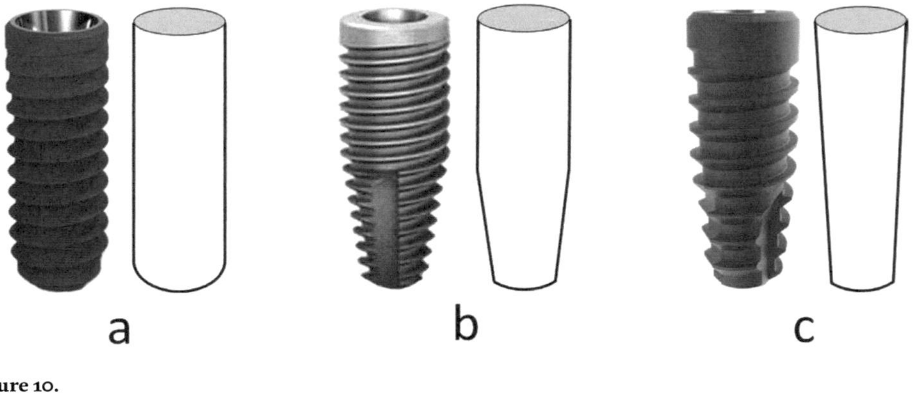

Figure 10.
Representative images of 3 implant designs: (a) cylindrical implant, (b) semi-tapered implant and (c) tapered implant.

disagreements about the fact that the tapered implant shows higher values of initial stability when compared to the cylindrical implant [47] or not cylindrical [48].

For years, companies have sought to commercialize the tapered shape in order to combine the advantages of the two designs, considering that a tapered implant creates a basis for adequate primary stability, by allowing the gradual expansion of thin bone crests and determining a minimum of possible stress at the interface with the surrounding bone [49]. In addition, tapered implants can be used in different clinical situations, being installed with less damage to the bone bed, but their installation in the lower arch has not been widespread, as it is strongly recommended for areas with low density bone or bone beds after dental extractions [50].

2.3 Shape of the implant threads

During the last decades, different implant macrogeometries have been proposed and marketed, with variation in different points, such as body design, cervical and apical design, threads design, among others. As for the thread design, these can be found with square, V-shaped, trapezoidal and inverted trapezoidal shapes [45]. **Figure 11** demonstrates different implant coil designs presented and marketed by different implant companies.

For some authors, implants with narrow pattern threads increase the surface area, leading to a more favorable stress distribution, and achieving higher primary stability values [51, 52]. In addition, stresses are more sensitive to thread pitch in cancellous bone than in cortical bone [53]. However, considering that the ideal implant should provide a balance between compression and traction forces, minimizing the generation of shear force, the square shape was designed to reduce such force at the bone-interface. Implant and increase the stability of the implant [53]. Thread depth, thickness, angle, end and helical angle are some of the various geometric patterns that determine the functional surface of the thread and affect the distribution of biomechanical loads on implants [7].

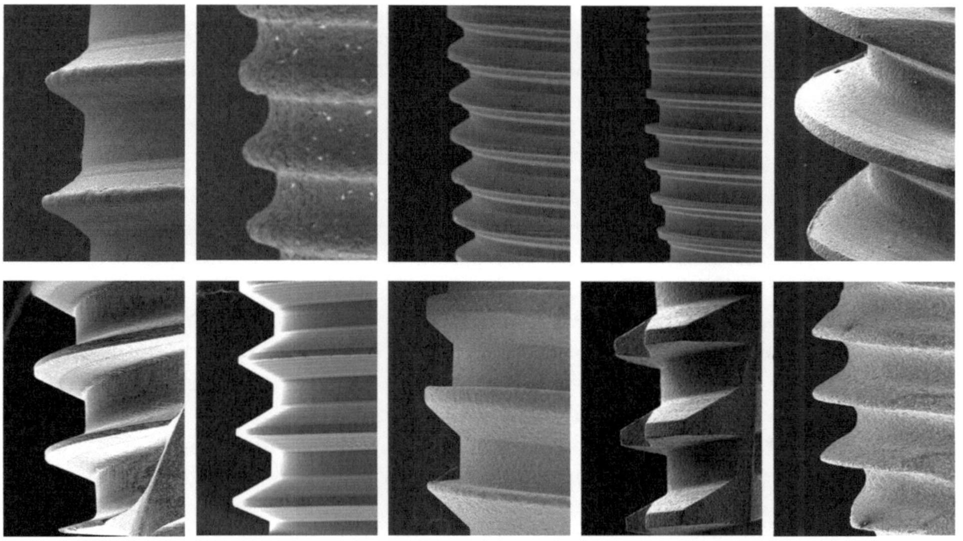

Figure 11.
Images of different designs of implant threads produced and marketed.

Transforming shear forces into resistance forces at the bone interface is the proposal to incorporate threads into the body of implants [54, 55]. This is why most implants are currently threaded, as non-threaded implants essentially result in shear forces at the bone-implant interface [26, 56–58]. Kohn et al. [59], demonstrated that the tension is more concentrated in the area of contact between the bone and the crest of the thread and that this tension decreases from the crest to its most basal portion. It has been proposed that threads, due to their shapes, would generate heterogeneous stress fields within the "physiological overload zone", thus promoting new bone formation [60], which would justify the formation of bone in intimate contact with the crest of the threads. However, it should be noted that the threads have different shapes, therefore different distributions of forces and biological responses, which will be discussed below.

The functional surface area per unit of implant length can be modified by varying 3 parameters of the thread geometry: pitch, shape and depth [61]. The shape of the thread is a very important feature of its general geometry. The shape of the thread can change the direction of occlusal loading of the prosthesis to different directions in the bone. Under axial loads, a triangular thread is comparable to a trapezoidal thread when the face angles are similar, which are usually 30 degrees [62]. It has been suggested that a square thread design reduces the shear force component, transferring the axial force that falls on the prosthesis to the implant body in a more axial fashion, favoring bone compression [63]. This would be particularly important for the bone crest region, where, according to Lum [64], most occlusal forces are distributed. Therefore, implant design considerations that reduce the development of shear forces at the bone-implant interface can improve long-term success, particularly in low-density bones [65]. The original Bränemark implant, introduced in 1965, had triangular threads, to be installed in place with threaded osteotomy16. The initial design has been modified over the years to allow for a simpler and more efficient installation, as well as a better distribution of loads. Albrektsson et al. [66], recommend that the top of the threads be rounded to relieve stress concentration.

The thread pitch is defined as the number of threads per unit of length in the same axial plane and on the same side of the axis of the implant body [61]. The smaller the pitch, the greater the number of threads in the implant body, and therefore the greater surface area. So, if the magnitude of force is increased or bone density is reduced, the thread pitch can be reduced to increase the functional surface area, thus improving the stress distribution. Ease of surgical insertion is also associated with the number of threads. The smaller the number of threads, the easier the implant insertion. In denser bones, however, a smaller number of threads is more favorable, since the hard bone offers greater resistance during insertion of a threaded implant [61]. Another important factor to be discussed is the difference between the final milling dimension proposed by the manufacturer and the implant body. Usually, the dimension of the last reamer used for the osteotomy corresponds to the diameter of the implant body. Thus, the deeper the turns, the greater this difference will be, causing a greater insertion of the implant (threads) into the bone tissue. **Figure 12** schematically shows the difference between the cutter and the implant in two different thread models.

Other concept is the "double-thread" and "triple-thread" implants has been recently introduced [63]. These implants have been associated with faster threading in the surgical alveolus and with an increase in primary stability, as they require a higher insertion torque, and are indicated for cases of low density bone [67]. However, the number of threads, their depth and the total surface area are exactly the same regardless of the number of threads, whether single, double or triple.

DOI: http://dx.doi.org/10.5772/intechopen.99937

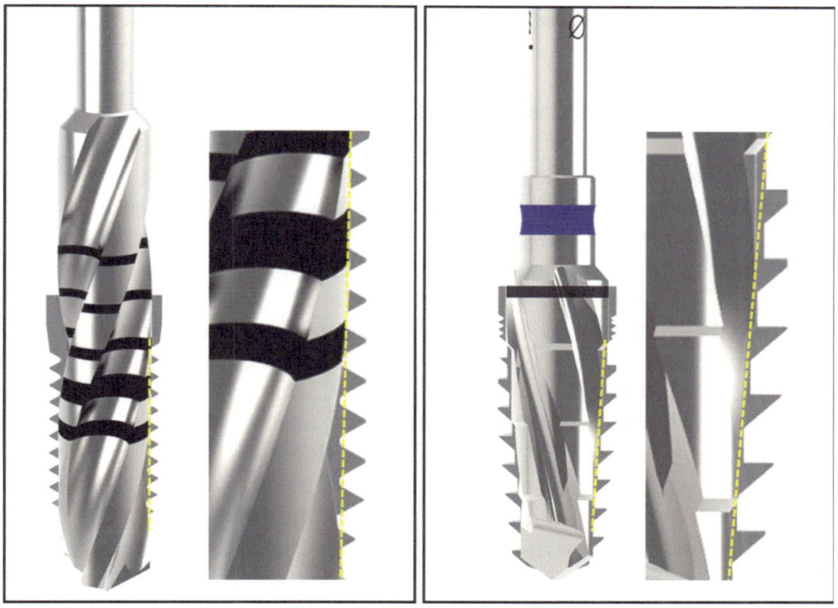

Figure 12.
Schematic images of the difference between the final reamer used for the osteotomy of each implant model and the thread depth that would be introduced into the bone tissue.

Instead of using a single instrument to make a 0.6 mm thread for each turn on the device, 2 or 3 instruments make 2 or 3 turns at the same time. These 2 or 3 devices are independent, starting 180° apart from each other and are also 0.6 mm threaded apart. In other words, a single thread contours the implant body 0.6 mm apart and the double thread 1.2 mm apart, on the same surface area. This technique allows installation of the implant in half the time [63].

The triangular thread shape has a 10 times greater shear over the bone than a square thread and is similar to the trapezoidal thread [61]. Square threads have an optimized surface area, which is great for transmitting intrusive and compressive loads, resulting in less bone tension. Trapezoidal threads are optimized to resist tensile loads [68]. Implants with reverse trapezoidal threads have fewer and shallower threads [63].

Another advance in the shape of threads has been the introduction of round shapes, which are said to induce osseocompression [63]. A round-shaped design has shown, in histological observations in animals, the formation of lamellar bone by osseocompression [69]. This allows the bone to be shaped and compacted circumferentially.

Thread depth refers to the distance between the largest and smallest diameter of the thread. Traditional implants offer a uniform thread depth, however this can be varied along the length of the implant in order to provide a functional surface area in the most intense stress regions (such as the alveolar bone crest region) [61]. Regarding the quality and percentage of osseointegration, Steigenga et al. [70], analyzed the effect of 3 types of threads (triangular, square and trapezoidal) through histomorphometric and reverse torque analyses. They found a significantly higher reverse feel and percentage of bone-to-implant contact for implants with square threads. No significant difference was found between the tests for implants with triangular and trapezoidal threads, corroborating the results of other studies with different methodologies [61, 62, 70]. It should be considered that the different shapes of the threads cause different distributions of forces and biological responses [56, 57, 59, 60, 62, 71, 72].

2.4 New implant macrogeometries

Modifications in the morphology and roughness of the implant surface were initially attempted not only to accelerate the host's response to the implant, but also to increase the level of mechanical locking between the bone and the implant surface, thus improving initial stability and subsequent dissipation loads during the functional requirements of the system [72]. Numerous studies based on histological tests have shown that surface texturing, created by different processes, leads to greater contact between bone and implant compared to the machined surface [6, 10, 73], which is a desirable answer to improve the overall biomechanics of the system, as show in the Section 2.1 of the present chapter. However, recently, new implant designs have been developed that seek, mainly, to accelerate and improve the quality of osseointegration through the concept of decreasing bone tissue compression during implant installation.

In most implant systems, osteotomy is recommended using the last drill with a diameter slightly smaller than the diameter of the implant, so that it can be inserted with a high degree of torque. Obviously, the more undersized the site that will receive the implant, the greater the insertion torque. However, studies have shown that high levels of torque can cause high compression of bone tissue, which can lead to extensive bone remodeling over time [74]. Several other studies have shown that, depending on the implant insertion torque and the physiological tolerance limit, microfractures or compression osteonecrosis may occur [75–77].

In this sense, it was recently proposed in some studies that approximating the osteotomy diameter with the diameter of the implant that will be implanted can facilitate and improve osseointegration [77, 78]. This fact was demonstrated in other animal studies, in which implants that were installed with high torque had a certain amount of necrotic bone inside the threads of the implants, while in samples where a perforation with a diameter closer to the diameter of the implant, greater new bone formation [78]. In this case, the free space created within the implant threads, resulting from the diameter-drill-implant relationship, was called healing chambers (**Figure 13**).

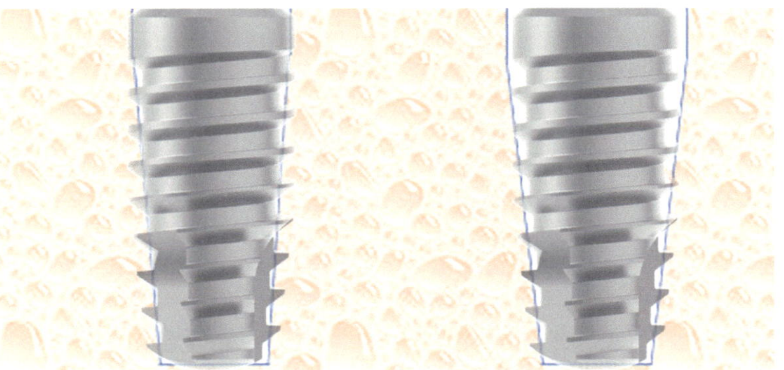

Figure 13.
Schematic images of the relationship between the osteotomy (blue lines) and the implant diameter inserted. In the left image the regular osteotomy and in the right image the oversized osteotomy generating the healing chambers.

In order to reduce the compression during insertion of the implant into bone tissue, two new implant models were recently launched on the world market, the BLX Straumann model (Basel, Switzerland) and the Maestro Implacil De Bortoli model (São Paulo, Brazil), that are presented in the **Figure 14**.

The first model (BLX Straumann implant) has technical recommendations to avoid bone compression, that during the execution of movements for insertion, whenever the torque of 35 N is reached, the professional must perform anti-rotational turns movements (removal torque) and then go back to inserting, repeating this movement whenever necessary. Thus, with a torque value below 35 N, bone tissue compression would be low, facilitating the osseointegration process. While in the second model described (Maestro Implacil implant), healing chambers were created in the implant body, which consist of small circular cavities 0.2 mm deep by 0.5 mm in diameter, as shown in **Figure 15**. With the presence of these healing chambers, bone tissue decompression occurs automatically during its insertion, not

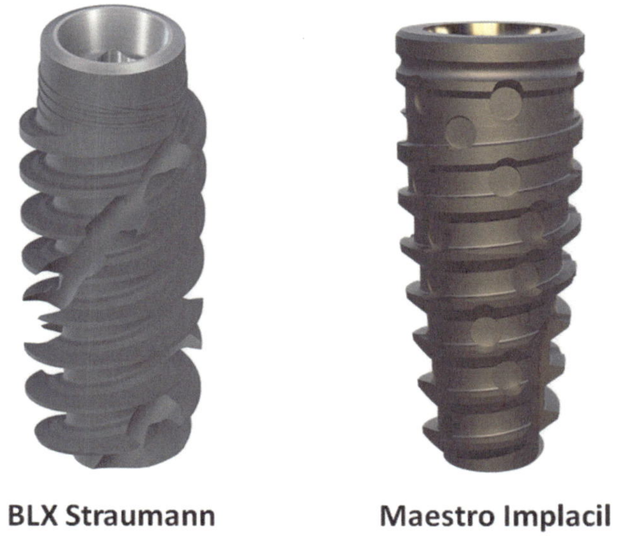

Figure 14.
Image of both implant models recently launched on the world market that were developed to reduce bone compression during the insertion process.

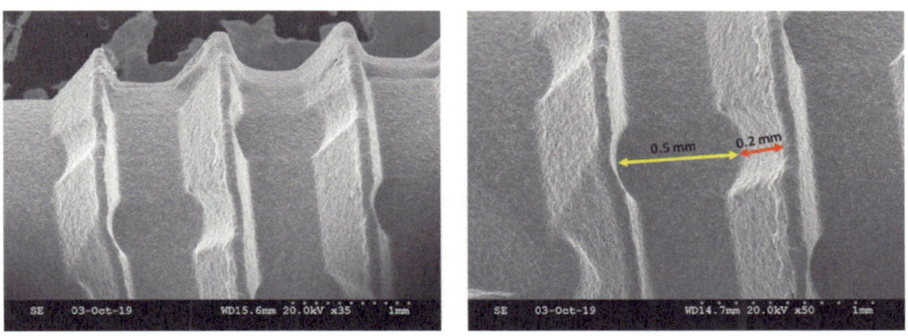

Figure 15.
SEM image of the healing chambers that were created in the implant body, which consist of small circular cavities 0.2 mm deep by 0.5 mm in diameter.

requiring any additional maneuvers. As reported in our studies of this new implant macrogeometries, this implant model has a reduced insertion torque compared to the model that does not feature healing chambers but did not show lower initial stability values measured by resonance frequency [12, 79–81].

3. Conclusions

Within the exposed in this chapter, we can conclude that there is no implant with ideal characteristics, whether from a nano-, micro- or macrogeometric point of view. However, great advances in the knowledge of biological processes involving implant osseointegration have been discovered in recent years, which allowed a better understanding of these events. Undoubtedly, the new macrogeometric designs, based on the biological concept of minimizing surgical trauma, brought important advances in terms of accelerating the osseointegration process and, mainly, being able to benefit patients with systemic and/or local weaknesses that could negatively interfere in the process of implant osseointegration.

Conflict of interest

The authors declare no conflict of interest.

Author details

Sergio Alexandre Gehrke[1,2]

1 Department of Research, Biotecnos – Technology and Science, Montevideo, Uruguay

2 Department of Biotechnology, Catholic University of Murcia (UCAM), Murcia, Spain

*Address all correspondence to: sergio.gehrke@hotmail.com

References

[1] Branemark PI, Adell R, Breine U, Hansson BO, Lindström J, Ohlsson A. Intra-osseous anchorage of dental prostheses. I. Experimental studies. Scand J Plast Reconstr Surg. 1969;3:81-100. doi: 10.3109/02844316909036699.

[2] Albrektsson T, Branemark PI, Hansson HA, Lindstrom J. Osseointegrated titanium implants. Requirements for ensuring a long-lasting, direct bone-to-implant anchorage in man. Acta Orthop Scand 1981; 52(2):155-170. doi: 10.3109/17453678108991776.

[3] Gehrke SA, Tavares da Silva Neto U. Does the time of osseointegration in the maxilla and mandible differ? J Craniofac Surg. 2014;25(6):2117-2120. doi: 10.1097/SCS.0000000000001067.

[4] Elias CN, Oshida JHC, Limad M. Relationship between surface properties, roughness, wettability and morphology of titanium and dental implant removal torque. J Mech Behav Biomed Mater 2008; 1(3):234-242. doi: 10.1016/j.jmbbm.2007.12.002.

[5] Zhao G, Schwartz Z, Wieland M, Rupp F, Geis-Gerstorfer J, Cochran DL, Boyan BD. High surface energy enhances cell response to titanium substrate microstructure. J Biomed Mater Res A 2005; 74:49-58. doi: 10.1002/jbm.a.30320.

[6] Novaes AB, Souza SL, Barros RR, Pereira KK, Iezzi G, Piattelli A. Influence of implant surfaces on osseointegration. Braz Dent J 2010; 21:471-481. doi: 10.1590/s0103-64402010000600001.

[7] Misch CE. Implant design considerations for the posterior regions of the mouth. Imp Dent 1999; 8:376-385. doi: 10.1097/00008505-199904000-00008.

[8] Tsujita H, Nishizaki H, Miyake A, Takao S, Komasa S. Effect of Plasma Treatment on Titanium Surface on the Tissue Surrounding Implant Material. Int J Mol Sci. 2021;22(13):6931. doi: 10.3390/ijms22136931.

[9] Thakral G, Thakral R, Sharma N, Seth J, Vashisht P. Nanosurface – the future of implants. J Clin Diagn Res 2014;8(5):ZE07-ZE10. doi: 10.7860/JCDR/2014/8764.4355.

[10] Wennerberg A, Albrektsson T. Effects of titanium surface topography on bone integration: a systematic review. Clin Oral Impl Res 2009; 20(4):172-184. doi: 10.1111/j.1600-0501.2009.01775.x.

[11] Att W, Yamada M, Ogawa T. Effect of titanium surface characteristics on the behavior and function of oral fibroblasts. Int J Oral Maxillofac Implants 2009; 24(3):419-431.

[12] Gehrke SA, Pérez-Díaz L, Mazón P, De Aza PN. Biomechanical Effects of a New Macrogeometry Design of Dental Implants: An In Vitro Experimental Analysis. J Funct Biomater. 2019;10(4):47. doi: 10.3390/jfb10040047.

[13] Gehrke SA, Cavalcanti de Lima JH, Rodriguez F, Calvo-Guirado JL, Aramburú Júnior J, Pérez-Díaz L, Mazón P, Aragoneses JM, De Aza PN. Microgrooves and Microrugosities in Titanium Implant Surfaces: An In Vitro and In Vivo Evaluation. Materials (Basel). 2019;12(8):1287. doi: 10.3390/ma12081287.

[14] Galli S, Jimbo R, Andersson M, Bryington M, Albrektsson T. Surface characterization and clinical review of two commercially available implants. Implant Dent 2013; 22(5):507-518. doi: 10.1097/ID.0b013e318294308f.

[15] Naves MM, Menezes HH, Magalhães D, Ferreira JA, Ribeiro SF, de Mello JD, Costa HL. Effect of Macrogeometry on the Surface Topography of Dental Implants. Int J Oral Maxillofac Implants 2015; 30(4):789-99. doi: 10.11607/jomi.3934.

[16] Herrero-Climent M, Lázaro P, Vicente Rios J, Lluch S, Marqués M, Guillem-Martí J, Gil FJ. Influence of acid-etching after grit-blasted on osseointegration of titanium dental implants: in vitro and in vivo studies. J Mater Sci Mater Med 2013; 24(8):2047-2055. doi: 10.1007/s10856-013-4935-0.

[17] De Groot K, Geesink R, Klein CPA. Plasma sprayed coatings of hydroxylapatite. J Biomed Mat Res 1987; 21(12):1375-1381. doi: 10.1002/jbm.820211203.

[18] Park EJ, Song YH, Hwang MJ, Song HJ, Park YJ. Surface Characterization and Osteoconductivity Evaluation of Micro/ Nano Surface Formed on Titanium Using Anodic Oxidation Combined with H2O2 Etching and Hydrothermal Treatment. J Nanosci Nanotechnol 2015; 15(8):6133-6136. doi: 10.1166/jnn.2015.10469.

[19] Yan J, Sun JF, Chu PK, Han Y, Zhang YM. Bone integration capability of a series of strontium-containing hydroxyapatite coatings formed by micro-arc oxidation. J Biomed Mater Res A 2013; 101(9):2465-2480. doi: 10.1002/jbm.a.34548.

[20] Berardi D, De Benedittis S, Scoccia A, Perfetti G, Conti P. New laser-treated implant surfaces: a histologic and histomorphometric pilot study in rabbits. Clin Invest Med 2011; 34(4):E202. doi: 10.25011/cim.v34i4.15361.

[21] Colombo JS, Satoshi S, Okazaki J, Crean SJ, Sloan AJ, Waddington RJ. In vivo monitoring of the bone healing process around different titanium alloy implant surfaces placed into fresh extraction sockets. J Dent 2012; 40(4):338-346. doi: 10.1016/j.jdent.2012.01.010.

[22] Ricci JL, Grew JC, Alexander H. Connective-tissue responses to defined biomaterial surfaces. I. Growth of rat fibroblast and bone marrow cell colonies on microgrooved substrates. J Biomed Mater Res A. 2008;85(2):313-325. doi: 10.1002/jbm.a.31379.

[23] Gehrke SA, Ramírez-Fernandez MP, Granero Marín JM, Barbosa Salles M, Del Fabbro M, Calvo Guirado JL. A comparative evaluation between aluminium and titanium dioxide microparticles for blasting the surface titanium dental implants: an experimental study in rabbits. Clin Oral Implants Res. 2018;29(7):802-807. doi: 10.1111/clr.12973.

[24] Gehrke SA, Taschieri S, Del Fabbro M, Coelho PG. Positive Biomechanical Effects of Titanium Oxide for Sandblasting Implant Surface as an Alternative to Aluminium Oxide. J Oral Implantol. 2015;41(5):515-522. doi: 10.1563/AAID-JOI-D-13-00019.

[25] Gehrke SA, Zizzari VL, Iaculli F, Mortellaro C, Tetè S, Piattelli A. Relationship between the surface energy and the histologic results of different titanium surfaces. J Craniofac Surg. 2014;25(3):863-867. doi: 10.1097/SCS.0000000000000873.

[26] Klein MO, Bijelic A, Ziebart T, Koch F, Kämmerer PW, Wieland M, Konerding MA, Al-Nawas B. Submicron scale-structured hydrophilic titanium surfaces promote early osteogenic gene response for cell adhesion and cell differentiation. Clin Implant Dent Relat Res 2013; 15(2):166-175. doi: 10.1111/j.1708-8208.2011.00339.x.

[27] Rupp F, Gittens RA, Scheideler L, Marmur A, Boyan BD, Schwartz Z, Geis-Gerstorfer J. A review on the wettability of dental implant surfaces I: theoretical and experimental aspects. Acta Biomater 2014 ; 10(7):2894-2906. doi: 10.1016/j.actbio.2014.02.040.

[28] Oates TW, Valderrama P, Bischof M, Nedir R, Jones A, Simpson J, Toutenburg H, Cochran DL. Enhanced implant stability with a chemically modified SLA surface: a randomized pilot study. Int J Oral Maxillofac Implants 2007; 22(5):755-760.

[29] Schlee M, Pradies G, Mehmke WU, Beneytout A, Stamm M, Meda RG, Kamm T, Poiroux F, Weinlich F, del Canto Pingarron M, Crichton E, Poulet JB, Bousquet P. Prospective, Multicenter Evaluation of Trabecular Metal-Enhanced Titanium Dental Implants Placed in Routine Dental Practices: 1-Year Interim Report From the Development Period (2010 to 2011). Clin Implant Dent Relat Res 2015; 17(6):1141-1153. doi: 10.1111/cid.12232.

[30] Meirelles L, Currie F, Jacobsson M, Albrektsson T, Wennerberg A. The effect of chemical and nanotopographical modifications on the early stages of osseointegration. Int J Oral Maxillofac Implants. 2008 Jul-Aug;23(4):641-647.

[31] Abe Y, Kokubo T, Yamamuro T. Apatite coating on ceramics, metals and polymers utilizing a biological process. J Mater Sci Mat Med 1990; 1:233-238.

[32] Kurtz SM, Kocagöz S, Arnholt C, Huet R, Ueno M, Walter WL. Advances in zirconia toughened alumina biomaterials for total joint replacement. J Mech Behav Biomed Mater 2014; 31:107-116. doi: 10.1016/j.jmbbm.2013.03.022

[33] Huang Y, He J, Gan L, Liu X, Wu Y, Wu F, Gu ZW. Osteoconductivity and osteoinductivity of porous hydroxyapatite coatings deposited by liquid precursor plasma spraying: in vivo biological response study. Biomed Mater 2014; 9(6):065007. doi: 10.1088/1748-6041/9/6/065007.

[34] Suer BT, Yaman Z, Buyuksarac B. Correlation of Fractal Dimension Values with Implant Insertion Torque and Resonance Frequency Values at Implant Recipient Sites. Int J Oral Maxillofac Implants. 2016;31(1):55-62. doi: 10.11607/jomi.3965.

[35] Wilson TG Jr, Miller RJ, Trushkowsky R, Dard M. Tapered Implants in Dentistry: Revitalizing Concepts with Technology: A Review. Adv Dent Res. 2016;28(1):4-9. doi: 10.1177/0022034516628868.

[36] Bahat O, Sullivan RM. Parameters for successful implant integration revisited part I: immediate loading considered in light of the original prerequisites for osseointegration. Clin Implant Dent Relat Res. 2010;12 Suppl 1:e2-12. doi: 10.1111/j.1708-8208.2010.00279.x.

[37] Romanos GE, Ciornei G, Jucan A, Malmstrom H, Gupta B. In vitro assessment of primary stability of Straumann® implant designs. Clin Implant Dent Relat Res. 2014;16(1):89-95. doi: 10.1111/j.1708-8208.2012.00464.x.

[38] Xu C, Wei Z, Liu N, Sun F, Chen H, Lin T, Zhang B, Tang T, Lu E. The effect of implant shape and screw pitch on microdamage in mandibular bone. Clin Implant Dent Relat Res. 2015;17(2):365-372. doi: 10.1111/cid.12100.

[39] Chong L, Khocht A, Suzuki JB, Gaughan J. Effect of implant design on initial stability of tapered implants. J Oral Implantol. 2009;35(3):130-135. doi: 10.1563/1548-1336-35.3.130.

[40] Rozé J, Babu S, Saffarzadeh A, Gayet-Delacroix M, Hoornaert A, Layrolle P. Correlating implant stability to bone structure. Clin Oral Implants Res. 2009;20(10):1140-1145. doi: 10.1111/j.1600-0501.2009.01745.x.

[41] Khayat PG, Milliez SN. Prospective clinical evaluation of 835 multithreaded tapered screw-vent implants: results after two years of functional loading. J Oral Implantol. 2007;33(4):225-231. doi: 10.1563/1548-1336(2007)33[225:PCEOMT]2.0.CO;2.

[42] Ormianer Z, Palti A. Long-term clinical evaluation of tapered multi-threaded implants: results and influences of potential risk factors. J Oral Implantol. 2006;32(6):300-307. doi: 10.1563/0.830.1.

[43] Waechter J, Madruga MM, Carmo Filho LCD, Leite FRM, Schinestsck AR, Faot F. Comparison between tapered and cylindrical implants in the posterior regions of the mandible: A prospective, randomized, split-mouth clinical trial focusing on implant stability changes during early healing. Clin Implant Dent Relat Res. 2017;19(4):733-741. doi: 10.1111/cid.12501.

[44] Cochran D, Stavropoulos A, Obrecht M, Pippenger B, Dard M. A Comparison of Tapered and Nontapered Implants in the Minipig. Int J Oral Maxillofac Implants. 2016;31(6):1341-1347. doi: 10.11607/jomi.4712.

[45] Wilson TG Jr, Miller RJ, Trushkowsky R, Dard M. Tapered Implants in Dentistry: Revitalizing Concepts with Technology: A Review. Adv Dent Res. 2016;28(1):4-9. doi: 10.1177/0022034516628868.

[46] Gehrke SA, Treichel TLE, Aramburú Júnior J, de Aza PN, Prados-Frutos JC. Effects of the technique and drill design used during the osteotomy on the thermal and histological stimulation. Sci Rep. 2020;10(1):20737. doi: 10.1038/s41598-020-77762-z.

[47] Torroella-Saura G, Mareque-Bueno J, Cabratosa-Termes J, Hernández-Alfaro F, Ferrés-Padró E, Calvo-Guirado JL. Effect of implant design in immediate loading. A randomized, controlled, split-mouth, prospective clinical trial. Clin Oral Implants Res. 2015;26(3):240-244. doi: 10.1111/clr.12506.

[48] Sakoh J, Wahlmann U, Stender E, Nat R, Al-Nawas B, Wagner W. Primary stability of a conical implant and a hybrid, cylindric screw-type implant in vitro. Int J Oral Maxillofac Implants. 2006;21(4):560-566.

[49] Dos Santos MV, Elias CN, Cavalcanti Lima JH. The effects of superficial roughness and design on the primary stability of dental implants. Clin Implant Dent Relat Res. 2011;13(3):215-223. doi: 10.1111/j.1708-8208.2009.00202.x.

[50] Schiegnitz E, Al-Nawas B, Tegner A, Sagheb K, Berres M, Kämmerer PW, Wagner W. Clinical and Radiological Long-Term Outcome of a Tapered Implant System with Special Emphasis on the Influence of Augmentation Procedures. Clin Implant Dent Relat Res. 2016;18(4):810-820. doi: 10.1111/cid.12338.

[51] Brinley CL, Behrents R, Kim KB, Condoor S, Kyung HM, Buschang PH. Pitch and longitudinal fluting effects on the primary stability of miniscrew implants. Angle Orthod. 2009;79(6):1156-1161. doi: 10.2319/103108-554R.1.

[52] Orsini E, Salgarello S, Bubalo M, Lazic Z, Trire A, Martini D, Franchi M, Ruggeri A. Histomorphometric evaluation of implant design as a key factor in peri-implant bone response: a

preliminary study in a dog model. Minerva Stomatol. 2009;58(6):263-275.

[53] Abuhussein H, Pagni G, Rebaudi A, Wang HL. The effect of thread pattern upon implant osseointegration. Clin Oral Implants Res. 2010;21(2):129-136. doi: 10.1111/j.1600-0501.2009.01800.x.

[54] Richter EJ, Jovanovic SA, Spiekermann H. Rein implantatgetragene Brucken – eine alternative zur verbundbrucke? Zeitschrift fur Zahnarztliche Implantologie. 1990;6:137-144.

[55] Albrektsson T. On long-term maintenance of the osseointegrated response. Aust Prosthodont J. 1993;7 Suppl:15-24. PMID: 8054223.

[56] Block CM, Tillmanns HW, Meffert RM. Histologic evaluation of the LaminOss osteocompressive dental screw: a pilot study. Compend Contin Educ Dent. 1997;18:676-685.

[57] Carlsson L, Röstlund T, Albrektsson B, Albrektsson T. Removal torques for polished and rough titanium implants. Int J Oral Maxillofac Implants. 1988;3(1):21-24.

[58] Dietrich U, Lippold R, Dirmeier TH, Behneke N, Wagner W. Statistische Ergebnisse zur Implantatprognose am Beispiel von 2017 IMZ-implantaten unterschiedlicher Indikation det letzen 13 Jahre. Zeitschrift fur Zahnarztliche Implantologie. 1993;9:9-18.

[59] Ko CC, Kohn DH, Hollister SJ. Micromechanics of implant/tissue interfaces. J Oral Implantol. 1992;18(3):220-230.

[60] Wiskot HW, Belser UC. Lack of integration of smooth titanium surfaces: a working hypothesis based on strains generated in the surrounding bone. Clin Oral Implants Res. 1999;10(6):429-444. doi: 10.1034/j.1600-0501.1999.100601.x.

[61] Misch CE. Contemporary Implant Dentistry. 2nd ed. St. Louis: Mosby; 2000.

[62] Misch CE, Qu Z, Bidez MW. Mechanical properties of trabecular bone in the human mandible: implications for dental implant treatment planning and surgical placement. J Oral Maxillofac Surg. 1999;57(6):700-708. doi: 10.1016/s0278-2391(99)90437-8.

[63] Steigenga JT, Al-Shammari KF, Nociti FH, Misch CE, Wang HL. Dental implant design and its relationship to long-term implant success. Implant Dent. 2003;12(4):306-317. doi: 10.1097/01.id.0000091140.76130.a1.

[64] Lum LB. A biomechanical rationale for the use of short implants. J Oral Implantol. 1991;17:126-131.

[65] Bumgardner JD, Boring JG, Cooper RC Jr, Gao C, Givaruangsawat S, Gilbert JA, Misch CM, Steflik DE. Preliminary evaluation of a new dental implant design in canine models. Implant Dent. 2000;9(3):252-260. doi: 10.1097/00008505-200009030-00011.

[66] Albretksson T. On long-term maintenance of the osseointegrated response. Aust Prosthodont J. 1993;7(Suppl.):15-24.

[67] Sykaras R, Iacopino AM, Marker VA, Triplett RG, Woody RD. Implant materials, designs, and surface topographies: their effect on osseointegration. A literature review. Int J Oral Maxillofac Implants. 2000;15(5):675-690.

[68] Misch CE, Bidez MW, Sharawy M. A bioengineered implant for a predetermined bone cellular response to

loading forces. A literature review and case report. J Periodontol. 2001;72(9):1276-1286. doi: 10.1902/jop.2000.72.9.1276.

[69] Valen M, Locante WM. LaminOss immediate-load implants: I. Introducing osteocompression in dentistry. J Oral Implantol. 2000;26(3):177-184. doi: 10.1563/1548-1336(2000)026<0177:LIIII O>2.3.CO;2.

[70] Steigenga J, Al-Shammari K, Misch C, Nociti FH Jr, Wang HL. Effects of implant thread geometry on percentage of osseointegration and resistance to reverse torque in the tibia of rabbits. J Periodontol. 2004;75(9):1233-1241. doi: 10.1902/jop.2004.75.9.1233.

[71] Branemark PI, Hansson BO, Adell R, Breine U, Lindström J, Hallén O, Ohman A. Osseointegrated implants in the treatment of the edentulous jaw. Experience from a 10-year period. Scand J Plast Reconstr Surg Suppl. 1977;16:1-132.

[72] Textor M, Sittig C, Frauchiger V, Tosatti S, Brunette DM. Properties and biological significance of natural oxide films on titanium and its alloys. In: Brunette DM, Tengvall P, Textor M, Thomsen P, editors. Titanium in Medicine. Berlin: Springer. 2001:171-230.

[73] Wennerberg A, Albrektsson T, Andersson B, Krol JJ. A histomorphometric and removal torque study of screw-shaped titanium implants with three different surface topographies. Clin Oral Implants Res 1995;6:24-30. doi: 10.1034/j.1600-0501.1995.060103.x.

[74] Marin C, Bonfante E, Granato R, Neiva R, Gil LF, Marão HF, Suzuki M, Coelho PG. The Effect of Osteotomy Dimension on Implant Insertion Torque, Healing Mode, and Osseointegration Indicators: A Study in Dogs. Implant Dent 2016;25:739-743. doi: 10.1097/ID.0000000000000476.

[75] Cha JY, Pereira MD, Smith AA, Houschyar KS, Yin X, Mouraret S, Brunski JB, Helms JA. Multiscale Analyses of the Bone-implant Interface. J Dent Res 2015;94:482-490. doi: 10.1177/0022034514566029.

[76] Bashutski JD, D'Silva NJ, Wang HL. Implant compression necrosis: current understanding and case report. J Periodontol 2009;80:700-704. doi: 10.1902/jop.2009.080581.

[77] Tabassum A, Meijer GJ, Walboomers XF, Jansen JA. Evaluation of primary and secondary stability of titanium implants using different surgical techniques. Clin Oral Implants Res 2014;25:487-492. doi: 10.1111/clr.12180.

[78] Jimbo R, Tovar N, Anchieta RB, Machado LS, Marin C, Teixeira HS, Coelho PG. The combined effects of undersized drilling and implant macrogeometry on bone healing around dental implants: an experimental study. Int J Oral Maxillof Surg 2014;43:1269-1275. doi: 10.1016/j.ijom.2014.03.017.

[79] Gehrke SA, Tumedei M, Aramburú Júnior J, Treichel TLE, Kolerman R, Lepore S, Piattelli A, Iezzi G. Histological and Histomorphometrical Evaluation of a New Implant Macrogeometry. A Sheep Study. Int J Environ Res Public Health. 2020;17(10):3477. doi: 10.3390/ijerph17103477.

[80] Gehrke SA, Aramburú J Júnior, Pérez-Díaz L, do Prado TD, Dedavid BA, Mazon P, N De Aza P. Can changes in implant macrogeometry accelerate the osseointegration process?: An in vivo experimental biomechanical and histological evaluations. PLoS One.

2020;15(5):e0233304. doi: 10.1371/journal.pone.0233304.

[81] Gehrke SA, Aramburú Júnior J, Pérez-Díaz L, Eirles Treichel TL, Dedavid BA, De Aza PN, Prados-Frutos JC. New Implant Macrogeometry to Improve and Accelerate the Osseointegration: An In Vivo Experimental Study. Appl Sci 2019;9,3181.

Chapter 2

Osseointegration of Dental Implants and Osteoporosis

Sara Gibreel, Hasaan Gassim Mohamed, Amartya Raj Suraj and Sukumaran Anil

Abstract

Osteoporosis is a disease characterized by low bone mass and microarchitectural deterioration of bone tissue, leading to enhanced bone fragility and susceptibility to fractures. Osteoporosis also results in loss of bone mineral density throughout the body, including the maxilla and mandible. Successful osseointegration of dental implants is attributed to their ability to integrate well with bone. The influence of bone quality on dental implant osseointegration has been discussed in several studies, and higher rates of dental implant failure have been reported in patients with low bone quality and an inadequate bone volume. Osteoporosis represents a risk factor for osseointegration, and this relationship may be derived from the association of the disease with a deficiency in bone formation. This condition would compromise the healing capacity and the apposition of bone at the implant interface. Currently, there is no clear consensus regarding dental implant treatment in osteoporotic individuals. Studies have revealed contradictory reports regarding the success and failure of dental implants in patients with osteoporosis. Antiresorptive agents have been widely used to treat osteoporosis. Dental implant placement in patients on bisphosphonate therapy may trigger osteonecrosis of the bone. Hence, it is important to analyze factors that have to be taken into consideration prior to implant therapy in patients with osteoporosis and those undergoing treatment. This chapter outlines dental implant osseointegration under osteoporotic conditions. The possible effect of bisphosphonate therapy on dental implant survival will also be discussed based on the current literature.

Keywords: osteoporosis, osteopenia, bisphosphonates, osseointegration, implant, bone mineral density, risk factors

1. Introduction

Osteoporosis is a systemic skeletal disease that deteriorates bone mass and strength and affects the microarchitecture of bone, thus increasing bone turnover and bone fragility [1]. Osteoporosis is categorized into primary and secondary types. Primary osteoporosis is considered decreased bone density attributed to aging, post-menopausal conditions and idiopathic osteoporosis. Secondary osteoporosis occurs in patients with predisposing factors, such as other endocrinopathies and a history of using some drugs. Osteoporotic bone is characterized by a decreased thickness, deranged trabecular structure, reduced mineral content, as well as an increased carbonate-to-phosphate ratio [2]. The reduction in osteoid formation is attributed to the absence of or a deficit in pre-osteoblast differentiation into osteoblasts or a reduction in the number of osteoprogenitor cells and defects in their proliferation and differentiation [3].

Dental implant placement has become a common and frequent option for tooth replacement. The success of dental implants largely depends on their osseointegration. Factors that interfere with osseointegration act as potential threats to implant survival. Osteoporosis is considered a questionable condition in dental implant placement since it affects the jaw bones, and bisphosphonates (BPs) are the first line of therapy [4–6]. Local and systemic factors can influence the osseointegration. The implant surface and the bone are the main interacting entities, and changes to these affect the healing and osseointegration of the implant. It is recognized that any compromise in the bone quality and quantity adversely affects the osseointegration. A microrough implant surface results in better osseointegration than a smooth implant surface. The relationship between osteoporosis and bone formation around implants is still unclear [7, 8]. Osteoporosis in the elderly, especially in postmenopausal women, is significantly correlated with tooth loss [9]. In fractures, delayed bone healing occurs due to low bone density, poor bone quality and osseous microstructural changes [10]. The endosseous implant healing mechanism is similar to that of bone fracture healing; hence, it is reasonable to assume that dental implant survival may be negatively affected by osteoporosis [11]. Animal studies have shown a relatively low rate of osseointegration in an osteoporotic environment [12, 13]. While most of these experimental studies were carried out on long bones rather than jaw bones, [14] studies of experimentally induced osteoporosis in the mandible failed to show a significant difference in peri-implant bone formation [15–18].

2. Pathophysiology of osteoporosis

Osteoporosis is a condition characterized by decreased bone mineral density and deteriorated bone microarchitecture and hence compromised bone quality. Osteoporosis can be classified into primary and secondary types. Primary osteoporosis can also be subclassified as type I and type II osteoporosis [17]. Type I osteoporosis occurs primarily due to the loss of trabecular bone, leading to distal forearm and vertebral body fractures. Type II osteoporosis is also known as senile osteoporosis and mainly occurs in men and women over the age of 70 years due to the loss of cortical and trabecular bone. Osteoporosis may also result from genetic and endocrine disorders, hypogonadal states, deficiencies, drug-induced and inflammatory states, and hematologic and neoplastic disorders as secondary causes. Estrogen deficiency is thought to be critical in the pathogenesis of postmenopausal osteoporosis. In the postmenopausal period, the bone structure changes due to estrogen deficiency, and osteoporosis can occur as a result of an imbalance in bone remodeling leading to enhanced bone resorption [3].

Osteoporosis leads to bone demineralization, which begins to manifest clinically in the fourth and fifth decades of life. Modifiable and nonmodifiable risk factors are responsible for osteoporosis [19]. Nonmodifiable risk factors include age, sex, genetic factors and early menopause, while modifiable risk factors include inadequate calcium consumption, lack of exercise, and behavioral factors, such as smoking and alcoholism. Other factors that can contribute to the development of osteoporosis

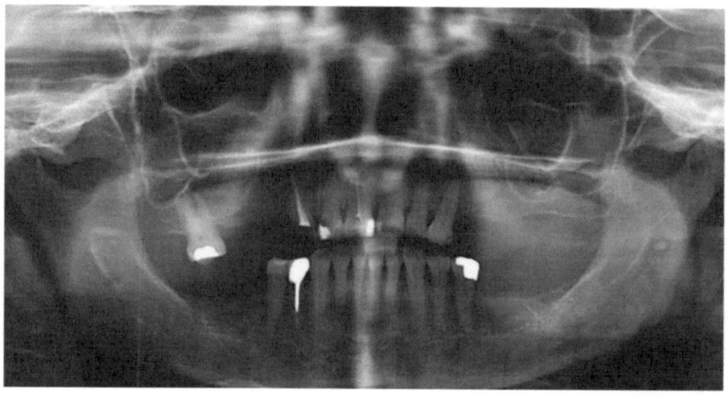

Figure 1.
Orthopantomogram of a 65-year-old patient with osteoporosis. Note the area of low bone density, alveolar bone loss and tooth loss.

include certain endocrine diseases, such as hyperparathyroidism, chronic renal and hepatic disease, malabsorption, and the use of certain drugs, such as oral glucocorticoids [18, 19].

The role of estrogen in the development of osteoporosis is well documented. Studies have shown that sex steroids, particularly estrogen, are important in developing peak bone mass and that estrogen deficiency is an important determinant of bone loss in both sexes [20, 21]. Estrogen can directly and/or indirectly affect osteoclasts, osteoblasts and osteocytes. It has been firmly established that these cells express functional estrogen receptors, [22] and studies have clearly demonstrated that estrogen can induce osteoclast apoptosis through the osteoclast-specific deletion of estrogen receptors. This can reduce osteoclast apoptosis and increase the osteoclast lifespan, which results in decreased trabecular bone mass (**Figure 1**) [23, 24]. Aging and estrogen deficiency may lead to an impairment in bone formation involving oxidative stress. Estrogen deficiency can also lead to a marked increase in NF-kB activity in osteoblasts. In osteoporotic patients, estrogen treatment induces the expression of sclerostin, a potent inhibitor of bone formation [25]. As sclerostin is expressed by osteocytes, estrogen also affects osteocytes. Estrogen deficiency may enhance the rate of bone loss by stimulating the synthesis of several inflammatory cytokines that regulate osteoclast generation, such as IL-1, IL-2, IL-6, and prostaglandin E [26].

A recent study among Swedish women showed a previous history of fracture and low bone mineral density as important factors that can lead to an increased rate of hip and fragility fractures among them [27]. Another study conducted in the United States revealed that several factors, such as age, self-reported health, weight, height, self-reported physical activity, history of fracture after the age of 50, parental hip fracture, smoking, use of corticosteroids, and treated diabetes, may be early indicators of hip fractures [28]. Factors associated with an increased risk for osteoporosis in men include glucocorticoid treatment, hypogonadism, excessive alcohol consumption, anticonvulsant use, osteomalacia, severe hyperthyroidism, and bone marrow neoplasia [29].

3. Dental implants and osteoporosis

Osteoporosis causes a range of skeletal changes that may impact the feasibility of dental implant placement. Greater alveolar ridge resorption, altered trabecular patterns in the anterior maxilla and posterior mandible, erosion of the inferior border of the mandible and increased resorption and thinning of the inferior mandibular cortical margin have been reported among osteoporotic individuals [30, 31]. Subjects with osteoporosis show a decreased number and thickness of trabecular plates as a characteristic feature of the disease. There have also been anecdotal reports that the incidence of maxillofacial fractures during the placement of endosseous implants is increased in patients with osteoporosis [32]. Additionally, bone changes evident on panoramic radiographs can be correlated with general osteoporosis, and dental radiography can serve as both a reliable indicator of bone loss in osteoporosis and a useful tool for diagnosing skeletal osteoporosis [33].

The osseointegration of an implant is a wound healing process that depends upon the quality, quantity, and healing capacity of the host bone and various other systemic conditions. Osseointegration is based on intimate bone-implant contact achieved during healing. Thus, any condition affecting bone quality or quantity or microarchitectural changes in bone structure, including a reduction in the cancellous bone volume and bone-implant contact, could theoretically have a negative impact on the survival and function of an endosseous implant [34]. There are relatively few absolute contraindications to rehabilitation with dental implants, including a recent myocardial infarction or cerebrovascular accident, history of valvular prosthesis placement, immune suppression, bleeding issues, active treatment of malignancy, drug abuse, psychiatric illness, and intravenous BP treatment [35]. Some relative contraindications and conditions that may unfavorably impact the outcomes of dental implant placement discussed in the literature include adolescence, aging, osteoporosis, smoking, diabetes, positive IL-1 genotype, human immunodeficiency virus infection, cardiovascular disease and hypothyroidism [36–38]. Controversy about the importance and effects of osteoporosis in dental therapy has continued [39].

In a study of implant placement in patients diagnosed with osteoporosis, Friberg et al. [40] found a success rate of 97% for the maxilla and 97.3% for the mandible on follow-up. Most studies have shown that it is feasible to place implants in subjects with osteoporosis, with success rates similar to those in healthy subjects, even in cases of poor bone quality during or after placement [4, 41–44].

4. Osteoporosis in implant Osseointegration

The osseointegration of an implant can be affected by the characteristics of the implant, the surgical procedure, and patient-dependent variables that can affect the quantity and quality of bone (**Table 1**). Osteoporosis, characterized by bone loss, microstructural alterations and a reduced bone regeneration capacity, has been considered a potential contraindication to or risk factor for dental implant placement. It has been established that osteoporosis affects the jaw in the same manner as other bones of the skeleton and thus may also alter the metabolic microenvironment of bone around the implant [56]. Bone is constantly metabolized throughout life by bone-resorbing osteoclasts and bone-forming osteoblasts. Osteocytes play an active role in modulating the process of bone metabolism through the lacunocanalicular system [57, 58]. Studies in osteoporotic animal models have shown altered osseointegration, especially in trabecular bone, which resulted in a significant reduction in bone-implant contact [59–61].

Elucidation of the role of osteocytes in peri-implant bone remodeling will help clarify the dynamics of bone metabolism following osseointegration. Since osteocytes

Author (year)	Study type/sample size	Follow-up period	Result/outcome
Becker et al. (2000) [45]	Retrospective case–control 49 cases, 49 controls, 5 osteoporosis, 7 osteoporosis	3.9 years	No association between dual-energy X-ray absorptiometry values or diagnosis of osteoporosis and implant loss
Friberg et al. (2001) [40]	Retrospective cohort 13 cases of osteoporosis	3.4 years	Successful implantation in osteoporosis provided adapted bone technique used and increased healing time allowed
von Wowern and Gotfredsen (2001) [46]	Retrospective cohort, 7 cases of osteoporosis, 11 controls	5 years	Mandibular osteoporosis a risk factor for peri-implant bone loss
Amorim et al. (2007) [47]	Retrospective case–control 19 cases of osteoporosis, 20 controls	9 months	No difference in implant survival between the two groups
Amorim et al. (2007) [47]	Prospective, 19 cases of osteoporosis, 20 controls	9 months	Failure in 1 (2.56%) case of osteoporosis, 0 controls
Alsaadi et al. (2008) [48]	Retrospective study,187 total, 29 cases of osteoporosis	2 years	Failure in 0 cases of osteoporosis and 14 controls
Alsaadi et al. (2008) [49]	Retrospective, 19 cases of osteoporosis, 393 controls	2 years	Failure in 9 (13.24%) cases of osteoporosis and 92 (6.3%) controls
Holahan et al. (2008) [50]	Retrospective,94 controls, 57 cases of osteopenia, 41 cases of osteoporosis	10 years	No difference between controls and cases; equal implant survival in all groups.
Dvorak et al. (2011) [51]	Cross-sectional,46 cases of osteoporosis, 16 cases of osteopenia, 115 controls	6 ± 4 years	Failure in 6 (13%) cases of osteoporosis, 3 (18.75%) cases of osteopenia, and 15 (13%) controls
de Souza et al. (2013) [52]	Retrospective, 6 cases of osteoporosis, 186 controls	1 year	Failure in 12 (50%) cases of osteoporosis and 203 (29%) controls
Famili and Zavoral (2015) [53]	Case–control study, 30 patients	2 years	No difference: 100% survival
Siebert et al. (2015) [54]	Prospective study, 24 patients	1 year	100% implant survival
Temmerman et al. (2017) [55]	Prospective study, 48 patients	1 year	100% implant survival

Table 1.
Studies evaluating the outcome of dental implants among subjects with osteoporosis.

are the terminal cells of osteoblasts, understanding the relationship between osteocytes and implants will also shed light on the relationship between osteoblasts and implants in early bone formation. Research on the influence of estrogen deficiency and its treatment with alendronate and estrogen on bone density around osseointegrated implants in rats has shown that estrogen deprivation has a negative effect only on trabecular bone and that treatment with estrogen and alendronate can effectively prevent bone loss around osseointegrated implants [62]. Histological studies in humans have also shown the osseointegration of implants retrieved from osteoporotic individuals [63, 64]. A histological study that evaluated the bone-implant contact of failed implants after retrieval showed no differences between implants originating from patients with and without osteoporosis [41]. The most important complication of implant placement in osteoporotic patients is bisphosphonate-related osteonecrosis of the jaw (BRONJ), that interferes with osseointegration. BPs act by inhibiting and inducing the apoptosis of osteoclasts, increasing collagen synthesis and inhibiting osteoblast proliferation. A systematic review showed that the placement of dental implants in osteoporotic patients who used oral BPs for less than five years did not develop BRONJ and that most adverse effects were related to the intravenous administration of BPs [65].

5. Dental implants and bisphosphonate therapy

Bisphosphonates are widely prescribed for the management of osteoporosis. They are pyrophosphate analogs containing a phosphate-carbon-phosphate bond, which is stable against chemical and enzymatic hydrolysis. BPs strongly bind to hydroxyapatite (HA) crystals and potently inhibit osteoclast-mediated bone resorption while minimally inhibiting osteoblast activity [66]. BPs are used for increasing or maintaining bone mass and reducing excessive bone turnover [67]. By inhibiting osteoclast-mediated bone resorption, BPs contribute to an increase in bone mineral density as well as a decrease in the risk of fracture [68, 69]. Two routes of administration are commonly used: oral and intravenous. BPs act almost exclusively on bone when administered at physiological doses because of their specific affinity to bone; they are deposited both in newly formed bone and in proximity to osteoclasts. The half-life of BPs in the circulation is quite short, ranging from thirty minutes to two hours [70]. However, once incorporated into bone tissue, they can persist for up to 10 years, depending on the skeletal turnover time [71]. Oral BPs are commonly used in the treatment of osteoporosis, Paget's disease, and osteogenesis imperfecta, whereas intravenous BPs are used in the treatment of osteolytic tumors, hypercalcemia of malignancy, multiple myeloma, bone metastases from solid tumors, and other tumors [72, 73]. The most common oral BPs are alendronate (Fosamax), risedronate (Actonel), and ibandronate (Boniva).

There have been conflicting reports regarding installation of dental implants in patients undergoing bisphosphonate therapy [74, 75]. Experimental studies have shown a positive effect of BPs on peri-implant bone in experimental animals [76, 77]. Although some studies have reported that BPs have no effect on implant stability, [78] a few other reports have suggested that BPs may have a negative impact on osseointegration. Additionally, osteointegration failure has been reported in patients on BP therapy [79–81]. Current guidelines indicate that implant placement may be avoided if the patient has a serious bone disease or is on high doses of BPs. Osteoporotic patients on lower doses need to provide fully informed consent before proceeding with treatment, and patients with existing implants on BP therapy should be regularly monitored. Increased bone density around the implant may also occur. If bone pain or loss of integrity occurs, the superstructure should be removed, and the implant should be left submerged [82]. In such cases, bone surgery must be avoided because the bone is exceedingly dense, and avascular necrosis may occur (**Figure 2**).

The chances of developing osteonecrosis depend on the potency and duration of BP exposure [84–86]. BRONJ is a condition characterized by nonhealing exposed necrotic bone in the mandible or maxilla persisting for more than 8 weeks in a patient who has taken or is currently taking a BP and who has no history of radiation therapy of the

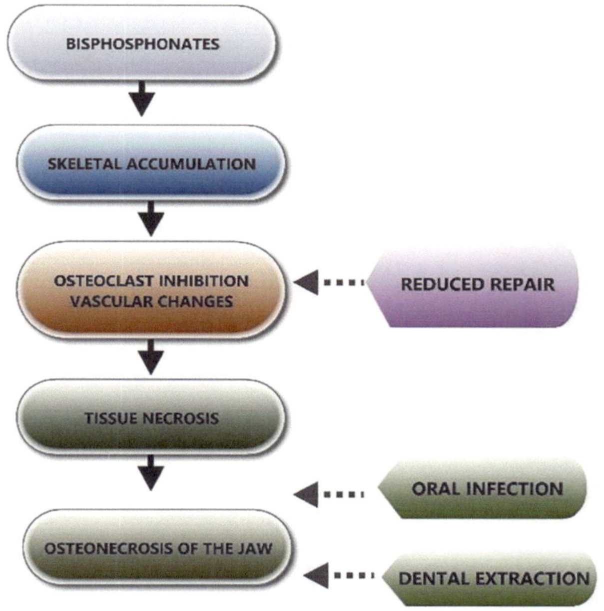

Figure 2.
Schematic diagram showing the possible mechanism of development of BP-associated osteonecrosis. BP, bisphosphonate (adapted and modified from Anil et al. [83]).

jaw [84, 87]. Incidents of osteonecrosis of the jaw have been reported in persons using BPs and undergoing invasive dental treatment procedures, including tooth extraction, dental implant placement, and surgical and nonsurgical periodontal treatment [88, 89]. Although BPs have been reported to cause oral mucosal alterations, the changes occurring in the jaw bone are of greater significance to the dentist [90, 91]. Osteonecrosis of the jaw is less often reported among patients who have received treatment with oral BPs at lower doses, used for osteoporosis, than among patients who have received treatment with higher doses, used for metastatic cancer. Even though the exact incidence of BRONJ is unknown, reports have estimated it to be approximately 1 in 10,000 for intravenous BPs. There is also an incomplete understanding of how BP therapy may affect tissue healing and the success rate of dental implantation [75, 80]. Advanced cases of BRONJ can lead to pathological fractures, especially in edentulous patients with long-standing oral implants [92].

6. Bisphosphonate-related osteonecrosis of the jaw

BPs alter the bone tissue metabolism by inhibiting bone resorption and reducing bone turnover. At the cellular level, BPs affect the recruitment of osteoclasts, their viability, the bioavailability of their progenitors, and their effect on bone. From a molecular point BPs have been proposed to modulate the function of osteoclasts by reacting with a surface receptor or with an intracellular enzyme [93]. BRONJ is defined as an area of exposed bone in the maxillofacial region that does not heal within 8 weeks in a patient who is receiving treatment with a BP. BRONJ develops secondary to the mechanisms of action of BPs in anti-osteoclastic and antiangiogenic

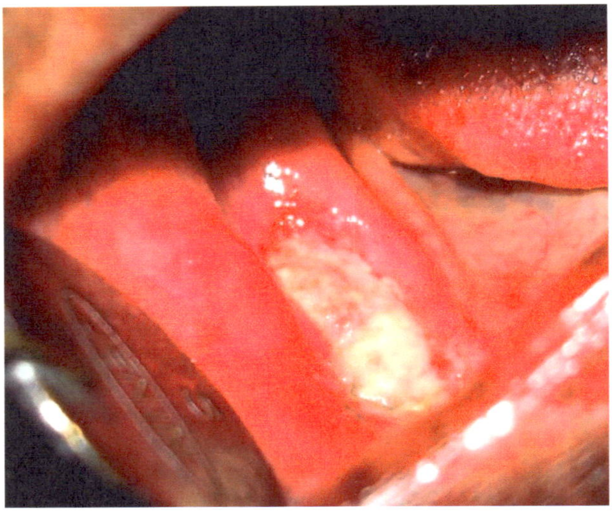

Figure 3.
BRONJ in a 63-year-old woman subsequent to extraction of mandibular molar. The patient was on intravenous zoledronate for 1 year (adapted and modified from Anil et al. [83]).

activities, which alter bone metabolism, inhibit bone resorption and reduce bone turnover. Additional signs and symptoms may include pain, swelling, paresthesia, suppuration, soft tissue ulceration, intra- or extraoral sinus tract formation, tooth loosening, and radiographic variability. These symptoms most commonly occur at sites of previous tooth extractions or other dental surgical interventions but may occur spontaneously. The exact role of BPs remains to be determined, and alterations in bone homeostasis coupled with odontogenic or surgical insult, or both, may be key to the development of osteonecrosis of the jaw [88, 93]. Cases of BRONJ are more common when frequent doses of intravenous BPs are used in treating malignancy than when oral BP regimens are used in treating osteoporosis [94].

The diagnosis of BRONJ is primarily based on the patient's history and the findings of a clinical examination. Most of the time, these patients have necrotic bone exposure ranging from a few millimeters to larger areas and can be asymptomatic for weeks, months, or years (**Figure 3**). The incidence of BRONJ is higher in the mandible than in the maxilla and in areas of thin mucosa overlying bony prominences, such as tori and the mylohyoid ridge. The management of BRONJ mainly comprises pain control measures, antibiotic therapy, mouth rinsing, BP discontinuation, hyperbaric chamber therapy, laser therapy, and surgical debridement [95, 96]. Assessments of markers of bone resorption, such as the serum C-terminal telopeptide of type I collagen; CTx or ITCP) test, can be used to assess the risk of developing BRONJ. Patients with a CTx level lower than 150 pg./mL should consider discontinuation of BP therapy for a period of 4–6 months.

7. Conclusion

Osteoporosis is a common skeletal disorder characterized by reduced bone mass and altered bone architecture, leading to an increase in bone fragility and the risk of fracture. This condition is associated with a decrease in bone quality and quantity, which might affect dental implant osseointegration. The placement of dental implants in patients with osteoporosis is still debated because of the quality of the bone, which is a key factor that determines the success of dental implantation. Although osteoporosis is not considered a risk factor for dental implant failure, the initial implant stability can be influenced by both the local and skeletal bone density, and the healing time is prolonged in osteoporotic patients. While the risk of osteonecrosis of the jaw in patients on BPs is low, patients should be informed of this risk and sign a consent form including this specific point. Based on the available literature, it can be concluded that implants placed in patients with systemic osteoporosis did not present higher failure rates than those placed in patients without osteoporosis.

Conflict of interest

The authors declare no conflict of interest.

Author details

Sara Gibreel[1], Hasaan Gassim Mohamed[2], Amartya Raj Suraj[1] and Sukumaran Anil[1,3]*

1 Department of Dentistry, Oral Health Institute, Hamad Medical Corporation, Doha, Qatar

2 Dentistry Department, Primary Health Care Corporation, Doha, Qatar

3 College of Dental Medicine, Qatar University, Doha, Qatar

*Address all correspondence to: anil@graduate.hku.hk

References

[1] Johnell O, Kanis JA: An estimate of the worldwide prevalence and disability associated with osteoporotic fractures. Osteoporos Int 2006, 17(12):1726-1733.

[2] Gadeleta SJ, Boskey AL, Paschalis E, Carlson C, Menschik F, Baldini T, Peterson M, Rimnac CM: A physical, chemical, and mechanical study of lumbar vertebrae from normal, ovariectomized, and nandrolone decanoate-treated cynomolgus monkeys (Macaca fascicularis). Bone 2000, 27(4):541-550.

[3] Feng X, McDonald JM: Disorders of bone remodeling. Annu Rev Pathol 2011, 6:121-145.

[4] Li Y, He S, Hua Y, Hu J: Effect of osteoporosis on fixation of osseointegrated implants in rats. J Biomed Mater Res B Appl Biomater 2017, 105(8):2426-2432.

[5] Basudan AM, Shaheen MY, Niazy AA, van den Beucken J, Jansen JA, Alghamdi HS: Histomorphometric Evaluation of Peri-Implant Bone Response to Intravenous Administration of Zoledronate (Zometa(®)) in an Osteoporotic Rat Model. Materials (Basel) 2020, 13(22).

[6] Ozawa S, Ogawa T, Iida K, Sukotjo C, Hasegawa H, Nishimura RD, Nishimura I: Ovariectomy hinders the early stage of bone-implant integration: histomorphometric, biomechanical, and molecular analyses. Bone 2002, 30(1):137-143.

[7] Chen H, Liu N, Xu X, Qu X, Lu E: Smoking, radiotherapy, diabetes and osteoporosis as risk factors for dental implant failure: a meta-analysis. PLoS One 2013, 8(8):e71955.

[8] de Medeiros F, Kudo GAH, Leme BG, Saraiva PP, Verri FR, Honório HM, Pellizzer EP, Santiago Junior JF: Dental implants in patients with osteoporosis: a systematic review with meta-analysis. Int J Oral Maxillofac Surg 2018, 47(4): 480-491.

[9] Darcey J, Horner K, Walsh T, Southern H, Marjanovic EJ, Devlin H: Tooth loss and osteoporosis: to assess the association between osteoporosis status and tooth number. British Dental Journal 2013, 214(4):E10-E10.

[10] Tarantino U, Cerocchi I, Scialdoni A, Saturnino L, Feola M, Celi M, Liuni FM, Iolascon G, Gasbarra E: Bone healing and osteoporosis. Aging Clin Exp Res 2011, 23(2 Suppl):62-64.

[11] Marco F, Milena F, Gianluca G, Vittoria O: Peri-implant osteogenesis in health and osteoporosis. Micron 2005, 36(7-8):630-644.

[12] Du Z, Chen J, Yan F, Xiao Y: Effects of Simvastatin on bone healing around titanium implants in osteoporotic rats. Clinical Oral Implants Research 2009, 20(2):145-150.

[13] Dudeck J, Rehberg S, Bernhardt R, Schneiders W, Zierau O, Inderchand M, Goebbels J, Vollmer G, Fratzl P, Scharnweber D *et al*: Increased bone remodelling around titanium implants coated with chondroitin sulfate in ovariectomized rats. Acta Biomater 2014, 10(6):2855-2865.

[14] Abtahi J, Agholme F, Sandberg O, Aspenberg P: Effect of local vs. systemic bisphosphonate delivery on dental implant fixation in a model of osteonecrosis of the jaw. J Dent Res 2013, 92(3):279-283.

[15] Fujimoto T, Niimi A, Sawai T, Ueda M: Effects of steroid-induced osteoporosis on osseointegration of titanium implants. Int J Oral Maxillofac Implants 1998, 13(2):183-189.

[16] Nasu M, Amano Y, Kurita A, Yosue T: Osseointegration in implant-embedded mandible in rats fed calcium-deficient diet: a radiological study. Oral Dis 1998, 4(2):84-89.

[17] Tuck SP, Francis RM: Osteoporosis. Postgraduate Medical Journal 2002, 78(923):526-532.

[18] Poole K, Compston J: Osteoporosis and its management. British Medical Journal 2006, 333(7581):1251.

[19] Jeffcoat M: The association between osteoporosis and oral bone loss. Journal of periodontology 2005, 76(11-s):2125-2132.

[20] Riggs B, Khosla S, Melton III L: Sex steroids and the construction and conservation of the adult skeleton. Endocrine reviews 2002, 23(3):279.

[21] Vidal O, Lindberg M, Hollberg K, Baylink D, Andersson G, Lubahn D, Mohan S, Gustafsson J, Ohlsson C: Estrogen receptor specificity in the regulation of skeletal growth and maturation in male mice. Proceedings of the National Academy of Sciences of the United States of America 2000, 97(10):5474.

[22] Weitzmann MN, Pacifici R: Estrogen deficiency and bone loss: an inflammatory tale. J Clin Invest 2006, 116(5):1186-1194.

[23] Nakamura T, Imai Y, Matsumoto T, Sato S, Takeuchi K, Igarashi K, Harada Y, Azuma Y, Krust A, Yamamoto Y *et al*: Estrogen prevents bone loss via estrogen receptor alpha and induction of Fas ligand in osteoclasts. Cell 2007, 130(5):811-823.

[24] Khosla S, Oursler MJ, Monroe DG: Estrogen and the skeleton. Trends Endocrinol Metab 2012, 23(11):576-581.

[25] Mödder UI, Clowes JA, Hoey K, Peterson JM, McCready L, Oursler MJ, Riggs BL, Khosla S: Regulation of circulating sclerostin levels by sex steroids in women and in men. J Bone Miner Res 2011, 26(1):27-34.

[26] Prestwood K, Pilbeam C, Burleson J, Woodiel F, Delmas P, Deftos L, Raisz L: The short-term effects of conjugated estrogen on bone turnover in older women. Journal of Clinical Endocrinology & Metabolism 1994, 79(2):366.

[27] Albertsson D, Mellstrom D, Petersson C, Thulesius H, Eggertsen R: Hip and fragility fracture prediction by 4-item clinical risk score and mobile heel BMD: a women cohort study. BMC Musculoskelet Disord 2010, 11:55.

[28] Robbins J, Aragaki AK, Kooperberg C, Watts N, Wactawski-Wende J, Jackson RD, LeBoff MS, Lewis CE, Chen Z, Stefanick ML *et al*: Factors associated with 5-year risk of hip fracture in postmenopausal women. JAMA : the journal of the American Medical Association 2007, 298(20):2389-2398.

[29] Kelepouris N, Harper K, Gannon F, Kaplan F, Haddad J: Severe osteoporosis in men. Annals of internal medicine 1995, 123(6):452.

[30] White SC, Rudolph DJ: Alterations of the trabecular pattern of the jaws in patients with osteoporosis. Oral Surg Oral Med Oral Pathol Oral Radiol Endod 1999, 88(5):628-635.

[31] White SC: Oral radiographic predictors of osteoporosis.

Dentomaxillofac Radiol 2002, 31(2):84-92.

[32] Barbu HM, Comaneanu RM, Andreescu CF, Mijiritsky E, Nita T, Lorean A: Dental Implant Placement in Patients With Osteoporosis. Journal of Craniofacial Surgery 2015, 26(6).

[33] Devlin H, Horner K: Diagnosis of osteoporosis in oral health care. Journal of Oral Rehabilitation 2008, 35(2):152-157.

[34] Qi MC, Zhou XQ, Hu J, Du ZJ, Yang JH, Liu M, Li XM: Oestrogen replacement therapy promotes bone healing around dental implants in osteoporotic rats. Int J Oral Maxillofac Surg 2004, 33(3):279-285.

[35] Hwang D, Wang HL: Medical contraindications to implant therapy: part I: absolute contraindications. Implant Dent 2006, 15(4):353-360.

[36] Op Heij DG, Opdebeeck H, van Steenberghe D, Quirynen M: Age as compromising factor for implant insertion. Periodontol 2000 2003, 33:172-184.

[37] Hwang D, Wang HL: Medical contraindications to implant therapy: Part II: Relative contraindications. Implant Dent 2007, 16(1):13-23.

[38] Alsaadi G, Quirynen M, Komárek A, Van Steenberghe D: Impact of local and systemic factors on the incidence of oral implant failures, up to abutment connection. Journal of clinical periodontology 2007, 34(7):610-617.

[39] Tenenbaum HC, Shelemay A, Girard B, Zohar R, Fritz PC: Bisphosphonates and periodontics: potential applications for regulation of bone mass in the periodontium and other therapeutic/diagnostic uses. J Periodontol 2002, 73(7):813-822.

[40] Friberg B, Ekestubbe A, Mellström D, Sennerby L: Brånemark implants and osteoporosis: a clinical exploratory study. Clin Implant Dent Relat Res 2001, 3(1):50-56.

[41] Shibli JA, Aguiar KC, Melo L, d'Avila S, Zenóbio EG, Faveri M, Iezzi G, Piattelli A: Histological comparison between implants retrieved from patients with and without osteoporosis. Int J Oral Maxillofac Surg 2008, 37(4):321-327.

[42] Liu Y, Hu J, Liu B, Jiang X, Li Y: The effect of osteoprotegerin on implant osseointegration in ovariectomized rats. Arch Med Sci 2017, 13(2):489-495.

[43] Shibli JA, Aguiar KC, Melo L, Ferrari DS, D'Avila S, Iezzi G, Piattelli A: Histologic analysis of human peri-implant bone in type 1 osteoporosis. J Oral Implantol 2008, 34(1):12-16.

[44] Wagner F, Schuder K, Hof M, Heuberer S, Seemann R, Dvorak G: Does osteoporosis influence the marginal peri-implant bone level in female patients? A cross-sectional study in a matched collective. Clin Implant Dent Relat Res 2017, 19(4):616-623.

[45] Becker W, Hujoel PP, Becker BE, Willingham H: Osteoporosis and implant failure: an exploratory case-control study. J Periodontol 2000, 71(4):625-631.

[46] von Wowern N, Gotfredsen K: Implant-supported overdentures, a prevention of bone loss in edentulous mandibles? A 5-year follow-up study. Clin Oral Implants Res 2001, 12(1):19-25.

[47] Amorim MA, Takayama L, Jorgetti V, Pereira RM: Comparative study of axial and femoral bone mineral density and parameters of mandibular bone quality in patients receiving dental implants. Osteoporos Int 2007, 18(5):703-709.

[48] Alsaadi G, Quirynen M, Komarek A, van Steenberghe D: Impact of local and systemic factors on the incidence of late oral implant loss. Clin Oral Implants Res 2008, 19(7):670-676.

[49] Alsaadi G, Quirynen M, Michiles K, Teughels W, Komárek A, van Steenberghe D: Impact of local and systemic factors on the incidence of failures up to abutment connection with modified surface oral implants. Journal of clinical periodontology 2008, 35(1):51-57.

[50] Holahan CM, Koka S, Kennel KA, Weaver AL, Assad DA, Regennitter FJ, Kademani D: Effect of osteoporotic status on the survival of titanium dental implants. Int J Oral Maxillofac Implants 2008, 23(5):905-910.

[51] Dvorak G, Arnhart C, Heuberer S, Huber CD, Watzek G, Gruber R: Peri-implantitis and late implant failures in postmenopausal women: a cross-sectional study. Journal of clinical periodontology 2011, 38(10):950-955.

[52] de Souza JG, Neto AR, Filho GS, Dalago HR, de Souza Júnior JM, Bianchini MA: Impact of local and systemic factors on additional peri-implant bone loss. Quintessence Int 2013, 44(5):415-424.

[53] Famili P, Zavoral JM: Low Skeletal Bone Mineral Density Does Not Affect Dental Implants. J Oral Implantol 2015, 41(5):550-553.

[54] Siebert T, Jurkovic R, Statelova D, Strecha J: Immediate Implant Placement in a Patient With Osteoporosis Undergoing Bisphosphonate Therapy: 1-Year Preliminary Prospective Study. J Oral Implantol 2015, 41 Spec No:360-365.

[55] Temmerman A, Rasmusson L, Kübler A, Thor A, Quirynen M: An open, prospective, non-randomized, controlled, multicentre study to evaluate the clinical outcome of implant treatment in women over 60 years of age with osteoporosis/osteopenia: 1-year results. Clin Oral Implants Res 2017, 28(1):95-102.

[56] de Souza Faloni AP, Schoenmaker T, Azari A, Katchburian E, Cerri PS, de Vries TJ, Everts V: Jaw and long bone marrows have a different osteoclastogenic potential. Calcif Tissue Int 2011, 88(1):63-74.

[57] Bonewald LF: The amazing osteocyte. J Bone Miner Res 2011, 26(2):229-238.

[58] Gowen LC, Petersen DN, Mansolf AL, Qi H, Stock JL, Tkalcevic GT, Simmons HA, Crawford DT, Chidsey-Frink KL, Ke HZ *et al*: Targeted disruption of the osteoblast/osteocyte factor 45 gene (OF45) results in increased bone formation and bone mass. J Biol Chem 2003, 278(3):1998-2007.

[59] Alghamdi HS, van den Beucken JJ, Jansen JA: Osteoporotic rat models for evaluation of osseointegration of bone implants. Tissue Eng Part C Methods 2014, 20(6):493-505.

[60] Korn P, Kramer I, Schlottig F, Tödtman N, Eckelt U, Bürki A, Ferguson SJ, Kautz A, Schnabelrauch M, Range U *et al*: Systemic sclerostin antibody treatment increases osseointegration and biomechanical competence of zoledronic-acid-coated dental implants in a rat osteoporosis model. Eur Cell Mater 2019, 37: 333-346.

[61] Duarte PM, César Neto JB, Gonçalves PF, Sallum EA, Nociti j F: Estrogen deficiency affects bone healing around titanium implants: a histometric

study in rats. Implant Dent 2003, 12(4):340-346.

[62] Giro G, Gonçalves D, Sakakura CE, Pereira RM, Marcantonio Júnior E, Orrico SR: Influence of estrogen deficiency and its treatment with alendronate and estrogen on bone density around osseointegrated implants: radiographic study in female rats. Oral Surg Oral Med Oral Pathol Oral Radiol Endod 2008, 105(2): 162-167.

[63] de Melo L, Piattelli A, Lezzi G, d'Avila S, Zenóbio EG, Shibli JA: Human histologic evaluation of a six-year-old threaded implant retrieved from a subject with osteoporosis. J Contemp Dent Pract 2008, 9(3):99-105.

[64] Shibli JA, Grande PA, d'Avila S, Iezzi G, Piattelli A: Evaluation of human bone around a dental implant retrieved from a subject with osteoporosis. Gen Dent 2008, 56(1):64-67.

[65] Madrid C, Sanz M: What impact do systemically administrated bisphosphonates have on oral implant therapy? A systematic review. Clin Oral Implants Res 2009, 20 Suppl 4:87-95.

[66] Peter B, Gauthier O, Laib S, Bujoli B, Guicheux J, Janvier P, van Lenthe GH, Muller R, Zambelli PY, Bouler JM *et al*: Local delivery of bisphosphonate from coated orthopedic implants increases implants mechanical stability in osteoporotic rats. Journal of biomedical materials research Part A 2006, 76(1):133-143.

[67] Greenspan S, Harris S, Bone H, Miller P, Orwoll E, Watts N, Rosen C: Bisphosphonates: safety and efficacy in the treatment and prevention of osteoporosis. American Family Physician 2000, 61(9):2731-2736.

[68] Fleisch HA: Bisphosphonates: preclinical aspects and use in osteoporosis. Ann Med 1997, 29(1):55-62.

[69] Russell RG, Rogers MJ, Frith JC, Luckman SP, Coxon FP, Benford HL, Croucher PI, Shipman C, Fleisch HA: The pharmacology of bisphosphonates and new insights into their mechanisms of action. J Bone Miner Res 1999, 14:53-65.

[70] Sparidans RW, Twiss IM, Talbot S: Bisphosphonates in bone diseases. Pharm World Sci 1998, 20(5):206-213.

[71] Drake MT, Clarke BL, Khosla S: Bisphosphonates: mechanism of action and role in clinical practice. Mayo Clinic proceedings 2008, 83(9): 1032-1045.

[72] Coleman R: Risks and benefits of bisphosphonates. Br J Cancer 2008, 98(11):1736-1740.

[73] Greenspan S, Harris S, Bone H, Miller P, Orwoll E, Watts N, Rosen C: Bisphosphonates: safety and efficacy in the treatment and prevention of osteoporosis. Am Fam Physician 2000, 61(9):2731-2736.

[74] Goss A, Bartold M, Sambrook P, Hawker P: The nature and frequency of bisphosphonate-associated osteonecrosis of the jaws in dental implant patients: a South Australian case series. J Oral Maxillofac Surg 2010, 68(2):337-343.

[75] Javed F, Almas K: Osseointegration of dental implants in patients undergoing bisphosphonate treatment: a literature review. J Periodontol 2010, 81(4):479-484.

[76] Stadelmann V, Gauthier O, Terrier A, Bouler J, Pioletti D, Nantes F: Implants delivering bisphosphonate locally increase periprosthetic bone density in

an osteoporotic sheep model. A pilot study. Eur Cell Mater 2008, 16:10-16.

[77] YIldIz A, Esen E, Kürkçü M, Damlar I, DaglIoglu K, Akova T: Effect of zoledronic acid on osseointegration of titanium implants: an experimental study in an ovariectomized rabbit model. J Oral Maxillofac Surg 2010, 68(3):515-523.

[78] Shabestari GO, Shayesteh YS, Khojasteh A, Alikhasi M, Moslemi N, Aminian A, Masaeli R, Eslami B, Treister NS: Implant placement in patients with oral bisphosphonate therapy: a case series. Clin Implant Dent Relat Res 2010, 12(3):175-180.

[79] Starck W, Epker B: Failure of osseointegrated dental implants after diphosphonate therapy for osteoporosis: a case report. Int J Oral Maxillofac Implants 1995, 10(1):74-78.

[80] Kasai T, Pogrel MA, Hossaini M: The prognosis for dental implants placed in patients taking oral bisphosphonates. J Calif Dent Assoc 2009, 37(1):39-42.

[81] Shirota T, Nakamura A, Matsui Y, Hatori M, Nakamura M, Shintani S: Bisphosphonate-related osteonecrosis of the jaw around dental implants in the maxilla: report of a case. Clin Oral Implants Res 2009, 20(12):1402-1408.

[82] Serra M, Llorca C, Donat F: Oral implants in patients receiving bisphosphonates: a review and update. Med Oral Patol Oral Cir Bucal 2008, 13:E755-E760.

[83] Anil S, Preethanath RS, AlMoharib HS, Kamath KP, Anand PS: Impact of osteoporosis and its treatment on oral health. Am J Med Sci 2013, 346(5):396-401.

[84] Bagan J, Scully C, Sabater V, Jimenez Y: Osteonecrosis of the jaws in patients treated with intravenous bisphosphonates (BRONJ): A concise update. Oral Oncol 2009, 45(7):551-554.

[85] Kawahara M, Kuroshima S, Sawase T: Clinical considerations for medication-related osteonecrosis of the jaw: a comprehensive literature review. Int J Implant Dent 2021, 7(1):47.

[86] Rupel K, Ottaviani G, Gobbo M, Contardo L, Tirelli G, Vescovi P, Di Lenarda R, Biasotto M: A systematic review of therapeutical approaches in bisphosphonates-related osteonecrosis of the jaw (BRONJ). Oral Oncol 2014, 50(11):1049-1057.

[87] Hoff AO, Toth BB, Altundag K, Johnson MM, Warneke CL, Hu M, Nooka A, Sayegh G, Guarneri V, Desrouleaux K *et al*: Frequency and risk factors associated with osteonecrosis of the jaw in cancer patients treated with intravenous bisphosphonates. J Bone Miner Res 2008, 23(6):826-836.

[88] Marx RE: Pamidronate (Aredia) and zoledronate (Zometa) induced avascular necrosis of the jaws: a growing epidemic. J Oral Maxillofac Surg 2003, 61(9):1115-1117.

[89] Ficarra G, Beninati F, Rubino I, Vannucchi A, Longo G, Tonelli P, Pini Prato G: Osteonecrosis of the jaws in periodontal patients with a history of bisphosphonates treatment. Journal of clinical periodontology 2005, 32(11):1123-1128.

[90] Gonzalez-Moles MA, Bagan-Sebastian JV: Alendronate-related oral mucosa ulcerations. J Oral Pathol Med 2000, 29(10):514-518.

[91] Demerjian N, Bolla G, Spreux A: Severe oral ulcerations induced by

alendronate. Clin Rheumatol 1999, 18(4):349-350.

[92] Pogrel M: Bisphosphonates and bone necrosis. J Oral Maxillofac Surg 2004, 62(3):391-392.

[93] Ruggiero SL, Mehrotra B, Rosenberg TJ, Engroff SL: Osteonecrosis of the jaws associated with the use of bisphosphonates: a review of 63 cases. J Oral Maxillofac Surg 2004, 62(5):527-534.

[94] Bamias A, Kastritis E, Bamia C, Moulopoulos LA, Melakopoulos I, Bozas G, Koutsoukou V, Gika D, Anagnostopoulos A, Papadimitriou C *et al*: Osteonecrosis of the jaw in cancer after treatment with bisphosphonates: incidence and risk factors. J Clin Oncol 2005, 23(34):8580-8587.

[95] Vescovi P, Merigo E, Manfredi M, Meleti M, Fornaini C, Bonanini M, Rocca JP, Nammour S: Nd:YAG laser biostimulation in the treatment of bisphosphonate-associated osteonecrosis of the jaw: clinical experience in 28 cases. Photomed Laser Surg 2008, 26(1):37-46.

[96] Magopoulos C, Karakinaris G, Telioudis Z, Vahtsevanos K, Dimitrakopoulos I, Antoniadis K, Delaroudis S: Osteonecrosis of the jaws due to bisphosphonate use. A review of 60 cases and treatment proposals. Am J Otolaryngol 2007, 28(3):158-163.

Chapter 3

Growth Factors and Dental Implantology

Deeksha Gupta

Abstract

Normal healing procedure of bone involves various sequential events to develop bone and bridge the bone -to- bone gap. When this healing occurs with a metal (titanium) fixture on one side, it is called as osseointegration. After extensive studies on this topic, it is found that this procedure occurs in presence of various biologic constituents that are spontaneously released at the site. Thus, to accelerate normal healing after implant placement and make results more predictable, it has been proposed to use these autologous factors in the osteotomy site. Since it is the beginning of a new revolution in dental implantology, right now it is essential to analyze all possible combinations of host conditions, bone quality and quantity and bio factors being used. This can definitely be a boon for the patients with compromised systemic or local conditions.

Keywords: Osseointegration, bone healing, growth factors, platelet rich concentrates, concentrated growth factor

1. Introduction

Repair and regeneration are one of the most complex multi-cellular physiological processes in human body. These are responsible for restitution of normal structure and function in the body. The complex biological course occurs in a cascade of events wherein the release and action of one chemical substance causes the release/inhibition of the other. The substances released in the course of action are chemical mediators causing migration, infiltration, proliferation, and differentiation of the cells to culminate in an inflammatory response, formation of a new tissue and finally wound closure [1]. The entire procedure is a well synchronized one regulated by a signaling network. This network is a self regulatory system controlled by several growth factors, cytokines and chemokines.

Growth factors are substances released by the body at various stages of tissue healing. Healing is a coordinated process that involves harmonized efforts of several cell types including keratinocytes, fibroblasts, endothelial cells, macrophages, and platelets [1]. Cytokines and Chemokines act by activating the migration of [mainly] inflammatory cells to the wound site up regulating their own production.

By definition inflammation is redness, swelling, pain, and/or a feeling of heat in an area of the body. This is a protective reaction of the tissues to injury, disease, or irritation [2]. This reaction is exhibited by every cell of body in an attempt to control/prevent the tissues from further injury. It also initiates recovery of the damaged tissues.

It is initiated in any cell of the body after a tissue injury. This injury can have various end results including death of the tissue to complete restoration of form and function. However, general injuries usually result in an intermediate outcome, i.e., partial tissue regeneration, fibrosis, and/or chronic inflammation [3].

Chronic wounds are defined as; 'defects that have not proceeded through orderly and timely repair to regain structural and functional integrity. Since any lesion has the potential to become chronic, chronic wounds are classified on the basis of their underlying cause'. Apart from compromised nutritional or immunological status and advanced age; vascular insufficiency, diabetes mellitus, and local-pressure effects are the major causes for wounds to become chronic non healing wounds [4].

When bone is subjected to trauma or an adverse stimulus, the resident cells release numerous cytokines, chemokines, and other substances that initiate local vasodilatation and efflux of inflammatory cells from the circulation. This terminates the adverse event and initiates the healing process [3]. Bone healing and bone formation is explained under 3 basic principles of: Osteoinduction, Osteogenesis and Osteoconduction.

Bone matrix stores growth factors that activate and maintain cellular processes during bone formation and healing. These growth factors are potent enough to accelerate bone formation and bone healing when applied locally to both intact and healing bone tissue. Normally, these proteins are produced by osteoblasts and incorporated into the extracellular matrix during bone formation, but many times, small amounts remain trapped into the matrix. Then these bone growth factors exhibit their effects by stimulating neighboring bone cells to proliferate and increase matrix protein synthesis [5–7].

Smoking, diabetes, or radiation therapy in patients with compromised local or systemic vascularity pose clinical challenge to bone grafts and dental implants due to impaired bone healing and an increase in peri implant complication [8, 9]. The success of dental implants essentially depends on adequate bone volume, density, and vascularity [10].

2. Cascade of wound healing

It takes a well managed system to control the secretion and migration of mediators to their correct places. Also a self regulatory feedback system ensures inhibition of right molecules at the right time. As soon as an injury takes place, bleeding is induced, all organisms including humans evoke an immediate, programmed, non-antigen specific immune response to preserve the organism's integrity and re-establish homeostasis [3].

In the **Table 1** [1, 10] we can have a quick brush through the events involved and release of growth factors at specific time to initiate specific actions in a healing cascade in the body.

This outline of the flow or spontaneity of the release of the various growth factors at the wound site illustrate the importance of each factor that is released at a specified time. As completion of one episode initiate second one. Thus the beginning of this process requires an injury of any/all tissues in the body.

As we talk about dental implants, it is implicated that we implant a foreign body, that is inert enough not to cause any antigenic activity, into the bone after creating

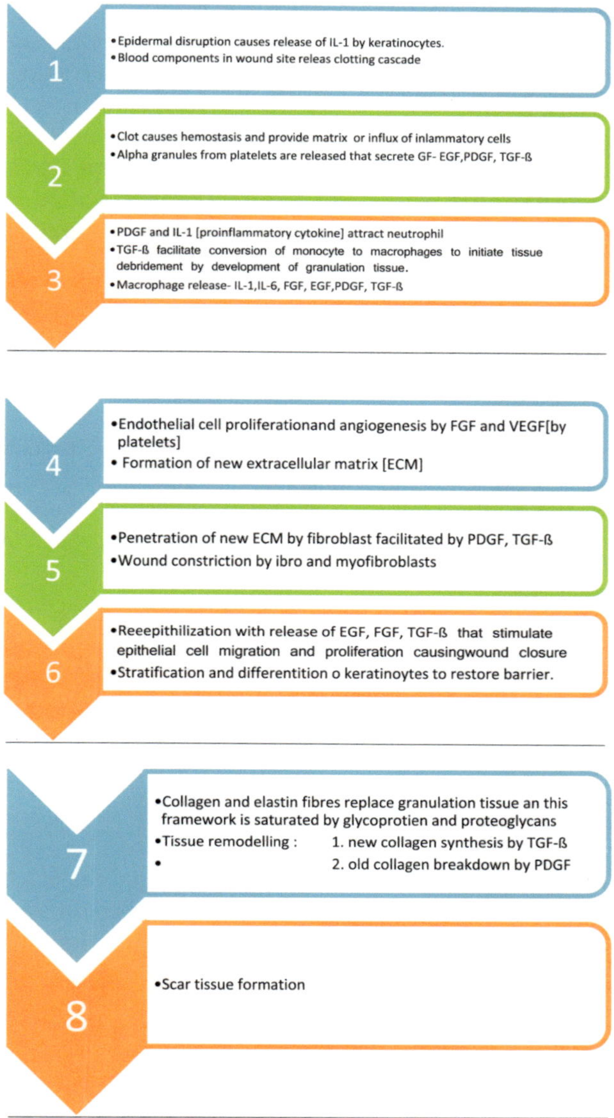

Table 1.
Sequential release of growth factors to initiate and terminate healing.

an osteotomy site. This site preparation is a planned injury into the otherwise intact healthy bone (usually considered apt for implantation in ideal case).

Hence soon after the injury to the bone, starts the cascade of bone healing. We shall understand the physiology of bone healing before the healing around the implants.

3. Bone healing

Bone is a living tissue responsible for the structural support and calcium metabolism in the body [11]. It is constituted by bone cells and bone matrix. Bone cells are of three main types' viz. osteoblasts, osteocytes and osteoclasts. These cells are differentiated by the mesenchymal cells, (during growth, at the time of trauma or general remodeling), to become osteoprogenitor cells and later take up the function of specific bone cells.

Bone matrix is composed of 35% organic and 65% inorganic components. Calcium and phosphate ions mainly constitute the inorganic part. Type I collagen forms the major part (90%) of the bone matrix which is impregnated with minerals and calcium salts. Minerals are in form of hydroxyapatites. Bone matrix also consists of non- collagenous proteins (10%) like osteocalcin, osteonectin, osteopondin etc. which function to regulate mineralization and interaction of collagenous and non-collagenous proteins, mediate cell to matrix binding.

Besides the bone matrix also consists of small amount of potent regulatory proteins that are produced by osteoblasts and incorporated by the extracellular matrix during bone formation. These are called as Growth Factors [5].

These are protein molecules that regulate osteoblast and osteoclast metabolism during bone remodeling and/or initiate and control healing response after bone trauma. They can exhibit their effects in the local environment only. Thus, to facilitate cell proliferation and matrix production at the site, they effect by paracrine or autocrine mechanism.

The extensive number of growth factors being discovered and researched lays consideration on the significance of their existence. When we try to understand bone metabolism it is empirical to read about the hormones that effect changes in bone matrix. It has been researched and found that the growth factors mediate the response of these systemic hormones, locally by augmenting the cell replication and initiating the cell differentiation by binding to membrane bound receptors [5].

3.1 Important growth factors in bone healing

Here is a list of the growth factors (**Table 2**) majorly required at a healing site. Apart from the main ones there are various other factors required by different tissues of the body during healing. We will discuss in detail the factors affecting bone healing.

3.1.1 Transforming growth factor-beta (TGF-ß)

This multifactorial cytokine basically regulates growth and differentiation of the cells. It stimulates the cells of mesenchymal origin and inhibits those of ectodermal origin. Although almost all body cells posses this factor but bone and platelets have approximately 100 times more TGF-ß than others and osteoblasts bear highest number of TGF-ß receptors [12]. TGF- ß 1, TGF- ß 2, and TGF- ß3 are found in mammals, but TGF- ß 1 predominates in cutaneous wound healing.

TGF- ß 1 facilitates the recruitment of additional inflammatory cells and augments macrophage mediated tissue debridement. It deactivates superoxide production from macrophages in vitro protecting the surrounding healthy tissue and prepares the wound for granulation tissue formation. When overexpressed, TGF- ß 1 has been shown to stimulate connective tissue growth factor (CTGF) also shown to play an important role in the development of hypertrophic and keloid scars [1].

TGF- ß 2 is also involved in recruiting inflammatory cells and fibroblasts to the wound site. In vivo experiments show that TGF- ß 2 stimulates the formation of granulation tissue by inducing angiogenesis. 121,122 During matrix formation and

S. no.	Growth factor	Important Subtypes	Secreted by	Functions
1	Transforming growth factor -ß superfamily	• TGF- ß 1 • TGF- ß 2 • TGF- ß 3 • Bone morphogenetic proteins • Activins	Platelets Keratinocytes Macrophages Lymphocytes Fibroblasts Osteoblasts Chondrocytes Osteoclasts	• Granulation tissue formation, • Re-epithelialization, –Matrix formation, remodeling
1a	Bone morphogenetic proteins	12	Osteoblasts Chondrocytes Osteoclasts	• Cartilage growth/repair, • Bone growth/repair
1b	Activins		Fibroblasts Keratinocytes	• Inhibits keratinocyte proliferation, • Induces terminal differentiation of keratinocytes
2	Platelet derived growth factors	• PDGF-AA,1 • PDGF-AB,1 • PDGF- BB,1 • PDGF-CC,1 • PDGF-DD	Platelets Keratinocytes Macrophages Endothelial cells Fibroblasts	• Granulation tissue formation, • Re-epithelialization, –Matrix formation, remodeling, • Bone repair
4	Insulin like growth factors	• IL-1 • IL-6	Neutrophils Monocytes Macrophages Keratinocytes Osteoblasts	• Angiogenesis, • Re-epithelialization, • Bone repair
5	Fibroblast growth factors	7 • aFGF • bFGF	Keratinocytes Mast Cells Fibroblasts Endothelial cells Smooth muscle cells Chondrocytes	• Granulation tissue formation, • Re-epithelialization, –Matrix formation, remodeling
6	VEGF		Platelets Neutrophils Macrophages Endothelial cells Smooth muscle cells Fibroblasts	• Granulation tissue formation, • Cartilage growth/repair, • Bone growth/repair
7	EGF		Platelets Macrophages Fibroblasts	• Re-epithelialization
8	TNF-α		Neutrophils Macrophages	• Inflammation • Re epithelialization

Table 2.
Important bone forming growth factors.

remodeling, TGF- ß 2 increases protein, DNA, and collagen production. By stimulating recruitment of fibroblasts to the wound site, the combined result is increased collagen deposition (particularly type I and III) and scar formation in vivo.

TGF- ß 3 promote wound healing by recruiting inflammatory cells and fibroblasts to the wound site and by facilitating keratinocyte migration. Furthermore, it has been demonstrated that TGF- ß 3 is a potent inhibitor of DNA synthesis in human keratinocytes. TGF- ß 3 inhibits scarring and promotes better collagen organization in vivo [1].

Due to abundance of TGF-ß in body cells, it is necessary to regulate its action in specific sites at the time of need. Hence it is released in a biologically inactive form i.e. latent TGF-ß. Its activation occurs in acidic environment through an enzymatic reaction [13] which probably regulates the exhibition of its effects.

3.1.2 Bone morphogenetic proteins (BMP)

BMP's were first discovered with formation of a completely mineralized woven bone with marrow, ectopically. It was achieved with the experiments done by Marshall Urist [14] using demineralized bone matrix placed in the subcutaneous tissue.

BMPs are currently well known to induce expression of osteoblast markers and stimulate bone formation in vivo [15]. It is believed that BMP are the most potent proteins to stimulate the mesenchymal stem cell differentiation in a chondroblastic and osteoblastic origin. They work by stimulating bone formation from the periphery of the implant, while matrix is laid down towards the center until it is entirely replaced by trabecular bone [16]. Their release is initiated from traumatized bone tissue during early-stage o fracture healing.

Today 12 types of BMP's have been isolated which exert their effects through specific receptor complexes. To utilize the action of these protein, they should be produced in large amounts. Also, a special carrier protein can be used to exhibit their action in low doses [5]. The function of the carrier protein is to immobilize the bone inducing protein at a site for the required time. E.g., Collagen matrix, demineralized bone matrix, synthetic polysaccharide matrices.

A recent prospective, randomized, controlled clinical trial showed the ability of recombinant human BMP-2 (rhBMP-2) applied to a collagen sponge to accelerate fracture and wound healing in patients with open tibia fractures [17].

3.1.3 Platelet derived growth factors (PDGF)

A powerful chemotactic factor, that is responsible for mitogenesis, angiogenesis and chemotaxis of fibroblasts and osteoblasts at the wound site. Glycoprotein by nature it has a crucial role in bone formation which was evident when reduced intramembranous bone was recorded on usage of PDGF inhibitors. Rat calvaria defect studies also demonstrate new bone formation in 2 weeks when PDGF is used with a poly L-lactide membrane.

3.1.4 Insulin growth factors (IGF)

Earlier designated as somatomedin-C and skeletal growth factor, these peptides are found to be synthesized by several tissue of body including bone. The secretion of IGF in bone tissue is controlled by parathyroid hormone and growth hormone. These hormones regulate the longitudnal growth and metabolism of cartilage by stimulating the chondroblastic IGF [18, 19].

The subtype IGF-II is found 10–20 times more than IGF-I in the bone matrix. Both subtypes stimulate osteoblast replication thereby increasing the bone matrix synthesizing cells. This in turn lead to new bone formation. However IGF-I is 4–7 times more potent than IGF-II. Apart from these, IGF also stimulates collagen production and inhibits collagen degradation.

It is observed in animal studies, that a single subcutaneous injection of growth hormone resulted in increase in serum IGF-1 during fracture healing in pig tibias [20]. Mesenchymal stromal cells transfected with IGF-1 and administered to a mouse femur fracture site, increased bone healing [21].

3.1.5 Fibroblast growth factors (FGF)

This polypeptide growth factor exerts proliferative effect on osteoblasts thus contributing in increasing the bone collagen. They are recognized as mitogenic factors for cells of mesenchymal and neuroectodermal origin and also play significant role in angiogenesis during the healing phase. Out of the 7 members of the FGF family, FGF-1 is acidic and FGF-2 is basic. Basic FGF (bFGF) is considered more potent and is believed that it has stimulatory effect on TGF-ß secretion by osteoblasts. Various animal studies have also concurred with this fact.

3.1.6 Vascular endothelial growth factors (VEGF)

VEGF is a powerful angiogenic growth factor that has been studied extensively in the oncologic and wound healing literature [22, 23]. It is released from endothelial cells, platelets, megakaryocytes, lymphocytes, and plasma cells. The major functions it takes care, are angiogenesis, neovascularization, and wound healing [24]. It is also mitogenic to endothelial cells, increases vascular permeability, and increases tissue oxygenation [25]. Individual administration of these growth factors shows the improvement of fracture healing and the potential for use in alveolar bone defects in preparation for implant placement [10].

4. Osseointegration and role of growth factors

"Osseointegration, (as defined by Zarb &Albrektsson) is a time dependent healing process whereby clinically asymptomatic rigid fixation of alloplastic materials is achieved, and maintained, in bone during functional loading" [26].

Clinically it has been demonstrated that the implants were anchored in bone without intervening fibrous tissue. Experimentally this data was researched at the ultrastructural level. Collagen filaments approaching the titanium oxide surface were seen that were separated only by a 20–40 nm thick Proteoglycan layer [27].

Branemark and Albrektsson [28] in their study evaluated the outcome of all implants inserted during 1 year and then followed them up for 5 years. They found an implant success rate of 96.5% in the mandible. This improved success rate compared to the data published by Adell et al. [29] reflects a true improvement in the outcome. This success was attributed to meticulous surgical and prosthodontic techniques.

Direct bone healing occurs in defects, primary fracture healing and in osseointegration. It is activated by any lesion of the pre-existing bone matrix. Once activated; the process continues in a biologically determined program. Thus, osseointegration also is programmed healing of the bone by developing a direct structural and functional connection between ordered, living bone and the surface of a load-bearing implant [30].

Osseointegration is facilitated on a precise fitting (anatomical reduction), primary stability (stable fixation) and adequate loading during the healing period. Osseointegration requires a bioinert or bioactive material and surface configurations that are conducive for bone deposition (osteophilic) [31].

4.1 Stages of osseointegration

On an event of trauma, when the bone matrix is exposed to extra cellular fluid, non-collagenous proteins and growth factors are set free and activate bone repair [32]. These facilitate chemotaxis of osteoprogenitor cells of the bone marrow and from the endocortical and periosteal bone envelopes. They proliferate and differentiate into osteoblast precursors and osteoblasts that begin bone opposition from the defect wall proceeding towards implant surface.

As the process gets initiated, it proceeds into a well-planned cascade in 3 stages:

- Incorporation by woven bone formation;
- Adaptation of bone mass to load (lamellar and parallel-fibered bone deposition);
- Adaptation of bone structure to load (bone remodeling).

4.1.1 Incorporation by woven bone formation

The first bone tissue formed is a primitive type, characterized by randomly oriented collagen fibrils, numerous, irregularly shaped osteocytes developing into an initially low-density bone: the woven bone. Its major role is to provide a scaffold of rods and plates thereby spreading out into the surrounding at a rapid rate. Simultaneous growth of elaborate vascular nets forming primary spongiosa bridging gaps rom bone to implant takes place for next 4–6 weeks.

4.1.2 Adaptation of bone mass to load (lamellar and parallel-fibered bone deposition

From the second month onwards, the microscopic architecture shifts towards either the well-known lamellar bone. Lamellar bone consists of parallel packing of the collagen fibrils with alternating course gives it the highest ultimate strength. Talking about its growth pattern it merely grows by apposition on a preformed solid base unlike the woven bone. This apposition can occur on 3 surfaces that can provide a solid base, viz., woven bone formed in the first period of osseointegration, preexisting or pristine bone surface and the implant surface.

4.1.3 Adaptation of bone structure to load (bone remodeling

Bone remodeling characterizes the last stage of osseointegration beginning around third month. With an initial high activity, it slows down again to later continue for life. In cortical and cancellous bone, remodeling occurs in discrete units, often called a bone multicellular unit, as proposed by Frost [33]. Remodeling starts with osteoclastic resorption, followed by lamellar bone deposition.

However, initially osseointegration was conceived differently. The debate started with Collins (1954) who stated "Although histologically inert, an implanted object never becomes incorporated into the bone". Later in 1970 Southam et al. came up with their ideology that "When any metallic appliance is implanted in bone, a layer of fibrous tissue will always develop around the appliance which subsequently will never be as secure in the bone as it was at the time it was implanted".

It was believed by some authors like Jacobs (1976, 1977), Muster & Champy (1978) that a direct contact between implant and bone is possible only when implant is made up of ceramic. However, many researches done on implant biomaterial advocate use of various materials for osseointegration like stainless steel (Linder & Lundskog 1975), vitaltium (Klawitter & Weinstein 1974, Linder & Lundskog 1975, Weiss 1977), tantalum (Grundschober et al. 1980) and titanium (Branemark et al. 1969, 1977, Linder & Lundskog 1975, Karagianes et al. 1976, Schroeder et al. 1976, Juillerat & Kuffer 1977).

The point to note here is that titanium on contact with atmosphere instantaneously develops an oxide layer of about 100 Å thickness [TiO, Ti02, Ti,03 and Ti,O], thereby preventing a direct contact between bone and metal.

To further dissect the ultrastructure of the tissue adherent to the bone and implant in Osseo integrated implants, T. Albrektsson [34] investigated the interface zone between bone and implant using X-rays, SEM, TEM and histology.

Thirty-eight stable and integrated implants implanted in maxilla, mandible and temporal regions were removed for various reasons from 18 patients. The SEM study showed a dense adherent network of collagen fibers between titanium and bone. The pattern of the anchorage of collagen filaments to titanium appeared to be similar to that of Sharpey's fibers to bone. No wear products of titanium were seen in the bone or soft tissues in spite of implant loading times up to 90 months. The soft tissues were also closely adhered to the titanium implant, thereby forming a biological seal, preventing microorganism infiltration along the implant. This caused no adverse tissue effects. An intact bone-implant interface was analyzed by TEM, revealing a direct bone-to implant interface contact also at the electron microscopic level, thereby suggesting the possibility of a direct chemical bonding between bone and titanium.

4.2 Osseointegration in compromised cases

Any surgery on a human body requires a thorough understanding of the procedure as well as the systemic condition of the patient. Many times, we have encountered patients willing for an implant surgery with a compromised medical history. Researchers have always tried to find answers to.

Documentations of a comparative study by Moy et al. [35] done to evaluate the success and failure rate of dental implants on patients suffering with and without various risk factors, such as smoking, coronary artery disease, asthma, chronic steroid use, chemotherapy, head and neck radiation, diabetes, hypertension, and postmenopausal status suggest absence of any statistically significant difference between the two groups. However, when in the same study specific medical risk were evaluated, patient suffering from diabetes, history of head and neck irradiation and people with tobacco use showed significant increase in implant failure.

4.2.1 Diabetes mellitus

Diabetes mellitus impairs/delays normal healing hence plays a direct role on implant success rate. Thus, it has been mentioned as a relative contraindication to implant placement. Olson et al. [36] found that duration of diabetes and implant length were statistically significant predictors of implant failure. Diabetic patients face problems of delayed wound healing, increase in micro vascular and macro vascular disease, impaired response to infection, and susceptibility to periodontal disease.

In animal models, growth factors with vascular properties have been used by Kawaguchi [37] to evaluate wound healing. He reported that" rhbFGF shows to improve fracture healing in normal rats and rats with diabetes, facilitating the repair process in normal rats and improving the impaired healing ability in rats with diabetes". bFGF also has shown increased angiogenesis, decreased wound complications, and improved bone mineral density in rat healing sternal wounds [38]. It can be comprehended by this that angiogenic and osteoinductive properties of growth factors improve bony and soft-tissue wound healing thus playing an important role in patients with diabetes.

4.2.2 Head and neck radiation

Patients are living a longer and a good quality life after cancer resection surgeries and consequent rehabilitation. Prosthesis plays a major role for these patients in uplifting their confidence of self-image. Dental implants have served to improve the success of these prostheses compromising oral and facial structures.

Radiation has many deleterious effects, the most relevant to bony and soft-tissue healing being hypocellularity, hypovascularity, and hypoxemia. Thus, increasing the failure rate during the osteophyllic or osteoconductive phases of osseointegration.

Before beginning with application on human beings, growth factors loaded on suitable carriers are inserted in animals to delineate their effects in all possible conditions. One such study evaluated the effect of BMP-2 on irradiated and non-irradiated rabbits. The irradiation dose was 20 Gy of 6-MeV electron beams. After irradiation, hydroxyapatite discs coated with rBMP-2 were applied subperiosteally in the snout area. Histological analysis demonstrated that rBMP-2 was equally effective in bone formation in irradiated and non-irradiated tissue [39]. Two other studies also found improved bone regeneration after treatment with BMP-2 or BMP-3 in animal cranial bone defects.

Recent studies reveal a marked reduction in TGF- ß, PDGF, and bFGF expression in cortical and cancellous bones post radiation up to range of 60-70Gy. (T.L. Aghaloo et al., unpublished data). Local TGF- ß administration may overcome radiation-induced impaired wound healing by increasing wound breaking strength, possibly via an increase in the synthesis of type I collagen by fibroblasts.

Another study evaluated the effect of grafting material that was pretreated with bFGF. It was found to cause induction of angiogenesis and osseous healing of irradiated mandibular resection sites. Also active bone formation and re-establishment of mandibular contours occurred in the bFGF-treated rabbits, but control animals experienced sequestration, necrosis, and failure to heal [40].

4.2.3 Smoking

Smoking has shown a large role in peri-implant bone loss. This is attributed to the carbon monoxide; oxidating radicals, nitrosamines, and nicotine that are released during smoking. This nicotine plays havoc in the system of an individual. It causes a systemic increase in epinephrine and norepinephrine thereby decreasing blood flow, increasing platelet aggregation, causing polymorphonuclear lymphocyte dysfunction, and increasing fibrinogen, hemoglobin, and thus blood viscosity.

Nicotine also causes local vasoconstriction from direct absorption into oral mucous membrane. This delays the wound healing. The effect of growth factors VEGF, bFGF, and BMP-2, −4, and − 6 gene expression is significantly inhibited, leading to suppression of bone healing and vascularity [41].

In animal studies, osteoinductive bovine bone protein plus autogenous bone grafting completely overcomes the inhibitory effect of nicotine [42].

5. Platelet concentrate revolution

Various pathological etiologies may result in oral defects or dysfunction thereby affecting the quality of life in patients. The greatest challenge in clinical research is to develop bioactive surgical additives, that can help to increase the speed of healing process or/and regulate inflammation. Solution to this challenge was found to be *tissue engineering.* This had to be aided with some type of '*biofuel*'. Since the triad forming the base of tissue engineering with a reparative objective is formed by the following: matrices or scaffolds, with various presentations (gels, fibrous matrices, and permeable membranes), progenitor cells (undifferentiated stem cells, or cells with preliminary differentiations) and growth factors. Thus, various platelet-derived products or platelet concentrates have been introduced that act as biological mediators aiding the healing response [43].

In dental implantology, the process of osseointegration determines the success of the implanted fixture. The prosthetic loading depends on the stability of the implant attained by osseointegration which is calculated to be complete between 0 and 6 months [44].

To increase bone-implant surface connectivity and accelerate healing few changes in implant surface properties and design can be made that increase primary stability and help the peri-implant tissue remain healthy. Secondly, to accelerate osseointegration, modulation of healing after the placement of the implant can be done. This modulation is achieved by *bioactive molecules* that increase osteoblastic differentiation and accelerate bone healing around the implant [45].

In 1974, platelets regenerative potentiality was introduced, and Ross *et al*, [46] were first to describe a growth factor from platelets. After activation of the platelets which are trapped within fibrin matrix, growth factors were released that could stimulate the mitogenic response in the bone periosteum during normal wound healing for repair of the bone [47].

The platelet-containing preparations derived from human blood contain many growth factors such as bone morphogenetic protein (BMP), platelet-derived growth factor (PDGF), insulin-like growth factor (IGF), vascular endothelial growth factor (VEGF), transforming growth factor-β1 (TGF-β1), and transforming growth factor-β2 (TGF-β2). These are considered to play a crucial role in bone healing [48, 49]. These growth factors, as explained earlier, attract the undifferentiated mesenchymal cells to the wound site, thus facilitating angiogenesis, chemotaxis, and cell proliferation [44].

C.Pirpir [50] et al. concurred with the above information and he concluded from his study that application of Concentrated growth factor enhanced stability of implants and accelerated osseointegration in the early period. His study demonstrated that CGF has positive effects on the ISQ value at the first week and fourth week.

Many other studies have been undertaken by Ji-Min Kim and Dong-Seok Sohn [51], S. Manoj [52], Andrea Forabosco [53] and Sila Cagri Isler [54] to evaluate bone regeneration around immediate post extraction implants, in sinus floor augmentation and cases of peri-implantitis who have given their affirmation towards increased bone healing with application of platelet containing preparations. Since blood has long been recognized as the torch bearer of healing process in the body, it has potential to accelerate wound healing when added to wounded tissues or surgical sites.

5.1 Platelet rich plasma (PRP)

Platelet-rich plasma (PRP), also known as autologous conditioned plasma, first introduced in dentistry by Whitman et al. is a concentrate of platelet-rich plasma protein derived from whole blood, centrifuged to remove red blood cells. This concentrate, full of various essential growth factors is introduced to the surgical site, enriching the natural blood clot. This hastens the wound healing and stimulates bone regeneration [55]. Specific protocols and automated systems for preparing PRP have been developed and commercialized, including Ace, PRGF, PRP-Landesber, Curasan, PCCS, Harvest SmartPReP, Vivostat, Friadent-Schutze, Regen, Fibrinet and Plateltex. Dohan Ehrenfest and colleagues offer an excellent comparison between these traditional systems.

A natural human blood clot consists of 95% red blood cells (RBCs), 5% platelets, less than 1% white blood cells (WBCs), and numerous amounts of fibrin strands. A PRP blood clot, on the other hand, contains 4% RBCs, 95% platelets, and 1% WBCs [56].

The PRP preparation protocol requires collection of blood with an anticoagulant, centrifugation in two steps, and induced polymerization of the platelet concentrate using calcium chloride and bovine thrombin [57]. PRP can be used in conjunction with different grafting materials in bone augmentation procedures. However, the addition of bovine-derived thrombin to handle PRP may increase the risk of life-threatening coagulopathies [58].

5.2 Platelet rich fibrin (PRF)

PRF represents a step ahead in the platelet revolution. Choukroun *et al.*, [59] developed the PRF in 2001 to accumulate platelets and released cytokines in a fibrin clot. Cytokines are immediately used and destroyed in a healing wound. The harmony between cytokines and their supporting fibrin matrix is the magic wand of the or real therapeutic potential of PRF. Also, this technique does not require any gelling agent [60].

Today PRF is increasingly being investigated and used worldwide by clinicians as an adjunctive autologous biomaterial to promote bone and soft tissue healing and regeneration [61]. In surgical procedures, PRF could serve as a resorbable membrane for guided bone regeneration (GBR), preventing the migration of non-desirable cells into bone defect and providing a space that allows the immigration of osteogenic and angiogenic cells and permits the underlying blood clot to mineralize. However, a normal PRF membrane has rapid degradability (1–2 weeks), but if fibers are cross-linked, it could provide resistance against enzymatic degradation and could be more stable during the healing time.

PRF technology has grabbed the attention of clinicians because of its excellent advantages.

a. Derived from patient's own blood so no chance of adverse reaction.

b. Easy to prepare at chairside and easy to use.

c. Financially realistic for patient

d. May be used alone or in combination with bone grafts, promoting hemostasis, bone growth, and maturation.

It is also concluded and concurred by various authors in their studies, that PRF is a good regenerative option with bone grafts in intra bony defects [62], treatment of peri-implantitis [63], reconstruction of large defects after cancer surgery [64]. Other applications include to accelerate healing in maxillary sinus augmentation, socket healing after tooth extraction, filling of the cyst cavity, treatment of furcation defects in periodontology, and soft tissue injuries [65].

They can be used as an adjunct, as a graft stabilizing membrane or used alone in dental (immediate) implant procedures [66]. Collagen Membrane has been used successfully in these regenerative procedures. An additional use or total replacement with platelet concentrates can provide further regenerative advantages due to the presence of biochemical agents of healing.

Simonpieri A. [67] also stated that, PRF membranes protects the surgical site; promotes soft tissue healing; and when its fragments mixes with graft material, it functions as a "biological connector" between the different elements of graft and acts as a matrix which supports neo angiogenesis, capture of stem cells, and migration of osteoprogenitor cells to the center of graft.

5.3 Concentrated growth factor

Concentrated growth factor, (CGF) another milestone towards regenerative dentistry was defined by Sacco in 2006 [68]. CGF also has its own centrifugal technique in a manner similar to that of obtaining PRF. It is seen to form rich layers of growth factors that include TGF-β1, VEGF, PDGF, IGF, EGF, FGF, and BMP which are delivered at the site of application. The positive effects of these blood products have triggered the development of various platelet products in different concentrations.

The concentrated growth factor used the advantage of longer and denser fibrin matrix with higher growth factor content. While CGF has been stated to be an improved formulation of PRF, it has also been proposed that a different term is used for CGF because of the use of a different centrifuge machine (MEDIFUGE, Silfradent srl, S. Sofia, Italy) and centrifugation speed (2400 to 3000 rpm). This produces a three layered structure: red blood cell layer at the bottom, platelet-deprived plasma layer (without cell) at the top, and fibrin gel with concentrated growth factor and platelet aggregation in the middle (**Figure 1**) [50]. Furthermore, CGF has been found to be almost identical to self-clotted advanced-PRF (A-PRF) in respect of mechanical and degradation properties [69].

Many studies have now come up with positive effects from local administration of CGF at the defect site. It is proved to increases bFGF or VEGF release. This increases angiogenesis, as well as enhances neutrophil migration by performing integrin release. It has also been shown that CGF contains such growth factors and CD34-positive cells that also provide angiogenesis, neovascularization, and vascular continuity [68].

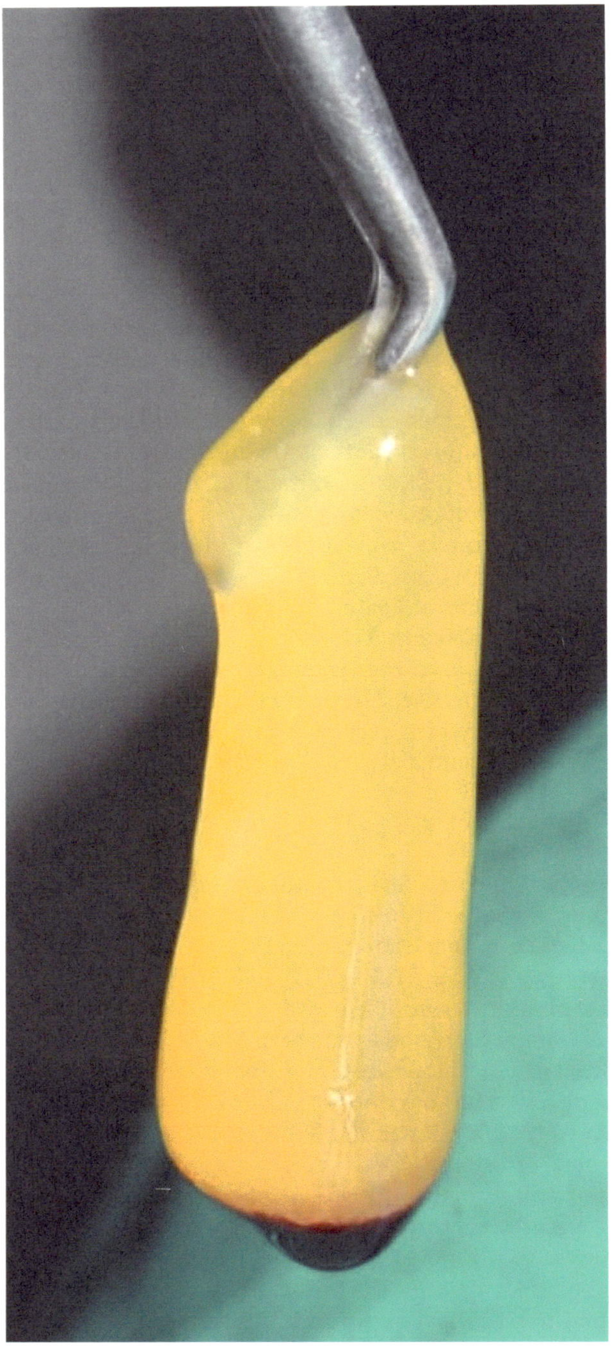

Figure 1.
Freshly prepared concentrated growth factor.

It is also validated that autogenous bone is the gold standard for grafting in the defects, implant sites or sinus lift procedures, but it is always associated with problems of 'second' surgical site and the associated morbidity of the donor tissue. As an alternative, allograft and xenografts are also used, which have the risk of cross-infection [52].

Along with the choice of graft material being a topic of debate, in many procedures like filing the jumping distance, the additional use of a membrane is also a matter of controversy. Various studies have documented some of the complications due to the use of membranes in these sites [70]. The use of CGF has been proposed as a substitute to fill the jumping distance in order to overcome certain disadvantages associated with various graft materials and membranes including increased treatment costs.

One animal study was conducted on CGF, PRF, and PRP placed separately in the defects in the rabbit skull compared with control groups with empty defect or self healing. Histomorphometric analysis revealed statistically significant differences between control and study groups in the growth of new bone formation at 6 and 12 weeks. In the study group, the greatest bone formation was observed in the CGF-treated group but this difference was not statistically significant [71]. In a study by Takeda et al. [72] performed on rats, it was observed that cell proliferation and osteoblastic differentiation in the cell culture from the CGF-treated group was significantly higher than in the other groups.

6. Mode of application

The growth factors are the naturally occurring molecules responsible for completing the healing process. However, there are instances where the systemic, metabolic or local compromise of the patient can lead to inadequacy of these factors, delaying or inhibiting healing.

In solution to these problems, many in vitro and animal studies have been conducted to determine the potency of added growth factors on the healing sites. The most important criteria of clinical use of these molecules must always be biocompatibility, biodegradability, hydrophilicity, and modulation of the osteoinductive response.

The various BMP carriers and delivery systems used in studies include collagen sponge, hyaluronan sponge, polylactic acid, polylactic-polyglycolic acid, fibrin glue, xenograft, and demineralized freeze-dried bone allograft [73, 74].

Orthopedic studies also show the use of polylactide-coated implants as local delivery mechanisms for IGF-1, TGF-b1, and BMP-2. These studies have shown predictable with favorable results on fracture healing. Adding to advantage is absence of systemic side effects and more effective delivery than systemic delivery of growth factors [75].

7. Futuristic approach

Tissue engineering was initiated with the aim of developing genetically engineered autologous cells and tissues without causing donor site morbidity. Although growth factors are naturally occurring molecules, a laboratory made tissue engineered component would definitely aid in faster healing of tissues even in the compromised cases.

Holy et al. suggested a recent biomimetic strategy to engineer bone. This is conducted by involving autologous osteogenic cells that are seeded, in vitro on a biodegradable polymer scaffold that mimics the architecture of trabecular bone to create a scaffold-cell hybrid called a tissue engineering construct [76].

Growth factor delivery mechanism in-vivo, makes use of Gene therapy approaches. This is used with BMPs that elicit osteoinductive and bone healing effects [77, 78].

Given the complex osteogenic cascade of bone regeneration at implant development site, a combination of different BMPs and other angiogenic growth factors shall definitely improve the success rates of dental implants, particularly at compromised host sites.

Advances in growth factor vector design, gene regulation, and tissue targeting are in their infancy which will soon establish themselves or future human clinical trials and eventual use in daily dental and surgical practice.

8. Conclusion

The osseointegrated implant interface remains in a very delicate balance where adverse individual tissue reactions may combine with the foreign body reaction to cause unwanted sequel in form of marginal bone loss or implant failure. There are many other predictable factors leading to implant failure. Thus, to get this spectrum high up on success of dental implants, apart from the factors of implant design, osteotomy site preparation and the available bone, the addition of biomimetic molecules to the host tissues has been abundantly researched however the great heterogeneity of the available studies and the limited number of RCTs do not allow to draw a robust conclusion.

The autologous preparation, dense concentration of growth factors and affirmative (*in vitro, in vivo and animal)* study results has opened avenues of their progressive research in dental implantology. This can be a boon for hosts receiving any kind of surgery, who have an underlying systemic/metabolic compromise. Many human studies and trials are also underway for devising carriers for these bioactive agents (direct vs. indirect), the dosage, the timing of administration, as well as the possibility of combining different agents to promote synergistic effects.

Conflict of interest

None.

Author details

Deeksha Gupta
Department of Prosthodontics, Manubhai Patel Dental College and Hospital, Vadodara, Gujarat, India

*Address all correspondence to: dr.deeksha.sharma@gmail.com

References

[1] Barrientos S, Stojadinovic O, Golinko MS, Brem H, Tomic-Canic M. Growth factors and cytokines in wound healing. Wound Rep Reg. 2008;**16**:585-601

[2] National Cancer Institute's Dictionary of Cancer Terms

[3] Stuart B. Goodman, Jukka Pajarinen, Zhenyu Yao, Tzuhua Lin. Inflammation and bone repair: From particle disease to tissue regeneration. Frontiers in Bioengineering and Biotechnology. 2019; 7:1-11. https://doi.org/10.3389/fbioe.2019.00230

[4] Eming SA, Martin P, Tomic-Canic M. Wound repair and regeneration: Mechanisms, signaling, and translation. Science Translational Medicine. 2014;**6**(265):265sr6

[5] Lind M. Growth factor stimulation of bone healing Effects on osteoblasts, osteomies, and implants fixation [THESIS]. Acta Orthopaedica Scandinavica. 1998;**69**(sup 283):i-37. acta orthop sca (supp23)

[6] CanalisE MCTL, Centrella M. Growth factors and the regulation of bone remodeling. The Journal of Clinical Investigation. 1988;**81**:277-281

[7] Joyce ME, Jingushi S, Bolander ME. Transforming growth factor-8 in the regulation of fracture repair. The Orthopedic Clinics of North America. 1992;**21**:199-209

[8] Moy PK, Aghaloo TL, Medina DM. Implants in Medically Compromised Patients [Abstract]. Boston: Presented at the Academy of Osseointegration; 2003

[9] Werkmeister R, Szulczewski D, Walteros-Benz P, Joos U. Rehabilitation with dental implants of oral cancer patients. Journal of Cranio-Maxillo-Facial Surgery. 1999;**27**:38-41

[10] Aghaloo TL, Anh DL. Growth factors in implant site development. Oral Maxillofacial Surg Clin N Am. 2004;**16**:111-125

[11] Garg AK. Bone physiology for dental implantology. In: Bone: Biology, Harvesting, Grafting for Dental Implants. Rationale and Clinical Applications. Illinois: Quintessence Publishing Co. Inc.; 2004. pp. 3-17. Ch-1

[12] Robey PG, Young MF, Flanders KC, Roche NS, Kondaiah P, Reddi AH, et al. Osteoblasts synthesize and respond to transforming growth factor-type 8 (TGF-8) in vitro. J Cell Bioi. 1987; **105**:457-463

[13] Lawrence DA, Pircher R, Jullien P. Conversion of a high molecular weight latent TGF-8 from chicken embryo fibroblasts into a low molecular weigth active TGF-8 under acidic conditions. Biochemical and Biophysical Research Communications. 1985;**133**:1026-1032

[14] Urist MR, DeLange RJ, Finerman GAM. Bone cell differentiation and growth factors. Science. 1983;**220**:680-686

[15] Coffey RJ Jr, Derynck R, Wilcox JN, Bringman TS, Goustin AS, Moses HL, et al. Production and auto-induction of transforming growth factor-alpha in human keratinocytes. Nature. 1987;**328**:817-820

[16] Nanney LB, McKanna JA, Stoscheck CM, Carpenter G, King LE. Visualization of epidermal growth factor receptors in human epidermis. The

Journal of Investigative Dermatology. 1984;**82**:165-169

[17] Pullar CE, Isseroff RR. The beta 2-adrenergic receptor activates pro-migratory and pro-proliferative pathways in dermal fibroblasts via divergent mechanisms. Journal of Cell Science. 2006;**119**(Pt 3):592-602

[18] Mohan S, Baylink DJ. Bone growth factors. Cl in Orthop. 1991;**263**:30-48

[19] Isgaard J, Nilsson A, Lindahl A, Jansson JO, Isaksson OG. Effects of local administration of GH and IGF-1 on longitudinal bone growth in rats. The American Journal of Physiology. 1986;**250**:E367-E372

[20] Falanga V, Eaglstein WH, Bucalo B, Katz MH, Harris B, Carson P. Topical use of human recombinant epidermal growth factor (h-EGF) in venous ulcers. The Journal of Dermatologic Surgery and Oncology. 1992;**18**:604-606

[21] Corsini E, Primavera A, Marinovich M, Galli CL. Selective induction of cell-associated interleukin-1alpha in murine keratinocytes by chemical allergens. Toxicology. 1998;**129**:193-200

[22] Choi JS, Leong KW, Yoo HS. In vivo wound healing of diabetic ulcers using electrospun nanofibers immobilized with human epidermal growth factor (EGF). Biomaterials. 2008;**29**:587-596

[23] Pittelkow MR, Cook PW, Shipley GD, Derynck R, Coffey RJ Jr. Autonomous growth of human keratinocytes requires epidermal growth factor receptor occupancy. Cell Growth & Differentiation. 1993; **4**:513-521

[24] Rappolee DA, Mark D, Banda MJ, Werb Z. Wound macrophages express TGF-alpha and other growth factors in vivo: analysis by mRNA phenotyping. Science. 1988;**241**:708-712

[25] Hashimoto K. Regulation of keratinocyte function by growth factors. Journal of Dermatological Science. 2000;**24**(Suppl. 1):S46-S50

[26] Parithimarkalaignan S, Padmanabhan TV. Osseointegration: An Update. J Indian Prosthodont Soc. 2013;**13**(1):2-6

[27] Small IA, Misiek DJ. A sixteen-year evaluation of the mandibular staple bone plate. J Oral Maxillofacial Surg. 1986;**44**:60-66

[28] Branemark P-I, Albrektsson T. Endosteal dental implants in the treatment of the edentulous jaw. The Branemark implant. In: Fonseca RJ, Davis WH, editors. Reconstructive preprosthetic oral and maxillofacial surgery. W.B ed. Philadelphia: Saunders Co.; 1986. pp. 210-224

[29] Adell R, Lekholm U, Rockler B, Branemark P-I. A 15-year study of osseointegrated implants in the treatment of the edentulous jaw. International Journal of Oral Surgery. 1981;**10**:387-416

[30] Listgarten MA, Lang NP, Schroeder HE, Schroeder A. Periodontal tissues and their counterpart around endosseous implants. Clinical Oral Implants Research. 1991;**21**:1-19

[31] Schenk RK, Buser D. Osseointegration: A reality. Periodontology. 2000;**17**(1998):22-35

[32] Callaghan JJ. The clinical results and basic science to total hip arthroplasty with porous-coated prostheses. Journal of Bone and Joint Surgery. 1993; **75A**:299-310

[33] Frost HM. Bone Dynamics in Osteoporosis and Osteomalacia. The Henry Ford Hospital Surgical Monographs. Index. Illinois: Springfield, CC Thomas Publisher; 1966

[34] Albrektsson T, Branemark H, Lindstrom J. Osseointegrated titanium implants. Requirements for Ensuring a Long-Lasting, Direct Bone-to-Implant Anchorage in Man. Acta Orthopaedica Scandinavica. 1981;**52**:155-170

[35] Moy PK, Aghaloo TL, Medina DM. Implants in Medically Compromised Patients [abstract]. Boston: Presented at the Academy of Osseointegration; 2003

[36] Olson JW, Shernoff AF, Tarlow JL, Colwell JA, Scheetz JP, Bingham SF. Dental endosseous implant assessments in a type 2 diabetic population: A prospective study. The International Journal of Oral & Maxillofacial Implants. 2000;**15**:811-818

[37] Kawaguchi H, Kurokawa T, Hanada K, Hiyama Y, Tamura M, Ogata E, et al. Stimulation of fracture repair by rhbFGF in normal and streptozotocin-diabetic rats. Endocrinology. 1994;**135**:774-778

[38] Iwakura A, Tabata Y, Tamura N, Doi K, Nishimura K, Nakamura T, et al. Gelatin sheet incorporating bFGF enhances healing of devascularized sternum in diabetic rats. Circulation. 2001;**104**(12 Suppl. 1):1325-1329

[39] Howard BK, Brown KR, Leach JL, Chang CH, Rosenthal DI. Osteoinduction using BMP in irradiated tissue. Archives of Otolaryngology – Head & Neck Surgery. 1998;**124**:985-988

[40] Eppley BL, Connolly DT, Winkelmann T, Sadove AM, Heuvelman D, Feder J. Free bone graft reconstruction of irradiated facial tissue: experimental effects of bFGF stimulation. Plastic and Reconstructive Surgery. 1991;**88**(1):1-11

[41] Thesis SM, Boden SD, Hair G, Titus L, Morone MA, Ugbo J. The effect of nicotine on gene expression during spine fusion. Spine. 2000;**25**(20): 2588-2594

[42] Silcox DH, Boden SD, Schimandle JH, Johnson P, Whitesides TE, Hutton WC. Reversing the inhibitory effect of nicotine on spinal fusion using an osteoinductive protein extract. Spine. 1998;**23**(3):291-296

[43] Khiste SV, Tari RN. Platelet-rich fibrin as a biofuel for tissue regeneration. International Scholarly Research Notices. 2013;**2013**(627367). 6 pages. DOI: 10.5402/2013/627367

[44] Raghavendra S, Wood MC, Taylor TD. Early wound healing around endosseous implants: A review of the literature. The International Journal of Oral & Maxillofacial Implants. 2005;**20**(3):425-431

[45] Oncu E, Bayram B, Kantarci A, Gulsever S, Alaaddinoglu EE. Positive effect of platelet rich fibrin on osseointegration. Medicina Oral, Patología Oral y Cirugía Bucal. 2016; **21**(5):e601-e607

[46] Ross R, Glomset J, Kariya B, Harker L. A platelet-dependent serum factor that stimulates the proliferation of arterial smooth muscle cells *in vitro*. Proceedings of the National Academy of Sciences of the United States of America. 1974;**71**:1207-1210

[47] Gassling V, Douglas T, Warnke PH, Açil Y, Wiltfang J, Becker ST. Platelet-rich fibrin membranes as scaffolds for periosteal tissue engineering. Clinical Oral Implants Research. 2010;**21**(5): 543-549

[48] Anitua E, Andia I, Ardanza B, Nurden P, Nurden AT. Autologous platelets as a source of proteins for healing and tissue regeneration. Thrombosis and Haemostasis. 2004; **91**(1):4-15

[49] Anitua E, Orive G, Pla R, Roman P, Serrano V, Andia I. The effects of PRGF on bone regeneration and on titanium implant osseointegration in goats: a histologic and histomorphometric study. Journal of Biomedical Materials Research. Part A. 2009;**91**(1):158-165

[50] Pirpir C, Yilmaz O, Candirli C, Balaban E. Evaluation of effectiveness of concentrated growth factor on osseointegration. International Journal of Implant Dentistry. 2017;**3**:7

[51] Kim J-M, Sohn D-S, Bae M-S, Moon J-W, Lee J-H, In-Sook Park D. Flapless transcrestal sinus augmentation using hydrodynamic piezoelectric internal sinus elevation with autologous concentrated growth factors alone. Implant Dentistry. 2014;**23**:168-174

[52] Manoj S, Punit J, Chethan H, Nivya J. A study to assess the bone formed around immediate postextraction implants grafted with Concentrated Growth Factor in the mandibular posterior region. JO. 2018;**10**(4):121-129

[53] Forabosco A, Gheno E, Spinato S, Garuti G, Forabosco E, Consolo U. Concentrated growth factors in maxillary sinus floor augmentation: A preliminary clinical comparative evaluation. International Journal of Growth Factors and Stem Cells in Dentistry. 2018;**1**(1):2-7

[54] Isler SC, Soysal F, Ceyhanlı T, Bakırarar B, Unsal B. Regenerative surgical treatment of peri-implantitis using either a collagen membrane or concentrated growth factor: A 12-month randomized clinical trial. Clinical Implant Dentistry and Related Research. 2018;**20**(5):1-10. DOI: 10.1111/cid.12661

[55] Soffer E, Ouhayoun JP, Anagnostou F. Fibrin sealants and platelet preparations in bone and periodontal healing. Oral Surgery, Oral Medicine, Oral Pathology, Oral Radiology, and Endodontics. 2003;**95**:521-528

[56] Nevins M, Giannobile WV, McGuire MK, Kao RT, Mellonig JT, Hinrichs JE, et al. Platelet-derived growth factor stimulates bone fill and rate of attachment level gain: Results of a large multicenter randomized controlled trial. J Periodontal. 2005;**76**:2205-2215

[57] Marx RE, Carlson ER, Eichstaedt RM, Schimmele SR, Strauss JE, Georgeff KR. Platelet-rich plasma: Growth factor enhancement for bone grafts. Oral Surgery, Oral Medicine, Oral Pathology, Oral Radiology, and Endodontics. 1998; **85**:638-646

[58] Gupta V, Bains VK, Singh GP, Mathur A, Bains R. Regenerative potential of platelet rich fibrin in dentistry: Literature review. Asian J Oral Health Allied Sci. 2011;**1**(1):22-28

[59] Choukroun J, Adda F, Schoeffler C, Vervelle A. Une opportunité en paro-implantologie: Le PRF. Implantodontie. 2001;**42**:55-62

[60] Naik B, Karunakar P, Jayadev M, Marshal VR. Role of Platelet rich fibrin in wound healing: A critical review. Journal of Conservative Dentistry. 2013;**16**(4):284-293

[61] Borie E, Oliví DG, Orsi IA, Garlet K, Weber B, Beltrán V, et al. Platelet-rich fibrin application in dentistry: A literature review. International Journal of Clinical and Experimental Medicine. 2015;**8**(5):7922-7929

[62] Chang YC, Zhao JH. Effects of platelet-rich fibrin on human periodontal ligament fibroblasts and application for periodontal infrabony defects. Australian Dental Journal. 2011;**56**:365-371

[63] Shah R, Shah H, Shetty O, Mistry G. A novel approach to treat peri implantitis with the help of PRF. The Pan African Medical Journal. 2017;**27**:256

[64] Reyes M, Montero S, Cifuentes J, Zarzar E. Extraction technique and surgical use of the plasma rich in growth factors (P. R.G.F.): Update. Revista Dental de Chile. 2002;**93**:25-28

[65] Prakash S, Thakur A. Platelet concentrates: Past, present and future. J Maxillofac Oral Surg. 2011;**10**(1): 45-49

[66] Simonpieri A, Del Corso M, Vervelle A, Jimbo R, Inchingolo F, Sammartino G, et al. Current knowledge and perspectives for the use of platelet-rich plasma (PRP) and platelet-rich fibrin (PRF) in oral and maxillofacial surgery part 2: Bone graft, implant and reconstructive surgery. Current Pharmaceutical Biotechnology. 2012;**13**: 1231-1256

[67] Simonpieri A, Del Corso M, Sammartino G, Dohan Ehrenfest DM. The relevance of Choukroun's platelet-rich fibrin and metronidazole during complex maxillary rehabilitations using bone allograft. Part II: Implant surgery, prosthodontics, and survival. Implant Dentistry. 2009;**18**:220-229

[68] Rodella LF, Favero G, Boninsegna R, Buffoli B, Labanca M, Scari G, et al. Growth factors, CD34 positive cells, and fibrin network analysis in concentrated growth factors fraction. Microscopy Research and Technique. 2011;**74**(8): 772-777

[69] Masuki H, Okudera T, Watanebe T, et al. Growth factor and pro-inflammatory cytokine contents in platelet-rich plasma (PRP), plasma rich in growth factors (PRGF), advanced platelet-rich fibrin (A-PRF), and concentrated growth factors (CGF). Int J Implant Dent. 2016;**2**:19

[70] Becker W, Dahlin C, Becker BE, et al. The use of e-PTFE barrier membranes bone promotion around titanium implant placed in extraction socket: A perspective multi-centre study. The International Journal of Oral & Maxillofacial Implants. 1994;**9**:31-40

[71] Kim TH, Kim SH, Sandor GK, Kim YD. Comparison of platelet-rich plasma (PRP), platelet-rich fibrin (PRF), and concentrated growth factor (CGF) in rabbit-skull defect healing. Archives of Oral Biology. 2014;**59**(5): 550-558

[72] Takeda Y, Katsutoshi K, Matsuzaka K, Inoue T. The effect of concentrated growth factor on Rat bone marrow cells in vitro and on calvarial bone healing in vivo. The International Journal of Oral & Maxillofacial Implants. 2015;**30**(5):1187-1196

[73] Choi SH, Kim CK, Cho KS, Huh JS, Sorensen RG Wozney JM, et al. Effect of rhBMP-2/absorbable collagen sponge on healing in 3-wall intrabony defects in dogs. Journal of Periodontology 2002;**73**(1):63 –72.

[74] Howell TH, Fiorellini JP, Paquette DW, Offenbacher S, Giannobile WV, Lynch SE. A phase I/II clinical trial to evaluate a combination of rhPDGF-BB and rhIGF-1 in patients with periodontal disease. Journal of Periodontology. 1997;**68**(12):1186-1193

[75] Schmidmaier G, Wildemann B, Heeger J, Gabelein T, Flyvbjerg A,

Bail HJ, et al. Improvement of fracture healing by systemic administration of growth hormone and local application of IGF-1 and TGF-b1. Bone. 2002; **31**(1):165-172

[76] Holy CE, Fialkov JA, Davies JE, Shoichet MS. Use of a biomimetic strategy to engineer bone. Journal of Biomedical Materials Research. 2003;**65A**(4):447-453

[77] Baltzer AW, Lattermann C, Whalen JD, Wooley P, Weiss K, Grimm M, et al. Genetic enhancement of fracture repair: healing of an experimental segmental defect by adenoviral transfer of the BMP-2 gene. Gene Therapy. 2000;**7**(9):734-739

[78] Alden TD, Varady P, Kallmes DF, Jane JA, Helm GA. Bone morphogenetic protein gene therapy. Spine. 2002; **27**(16S):S87-S93

Chapter 4

Implant Stability Quotient (ISQ): A Reliable Guide for Implant Treatment

Gaurav Gupta

Abstract

Implant stability is a prerequisite for successful dental implants and osseointegration. To determine the status of implant stability, continuous monitoring in an objective and qualitative manner is important. To measure implant stability two different stages are there: Primary and secondary. Primary implant stability at placement is a mechanical phenomenon that is related to the local bone quality and quantity, the type of implant and placement technique used. Primary stability is checked from mechanical engagement with cortical bone. Secondary stability is developed from regeneration and remodeling of the bone and tissue around the implant after insertion and affected by the primary stability, bone formation and remodeling. Implant stability is essential for the time of functional loading. Classical benchmark methods to measure implant stability were radiographs or microscopic analysis, removal torque, push-through and pull-through but due to lack of feasibility, time consumption and ethical reasons other methods have been propounded over period of time like measurement of implant torque, model analysis and most important ISQ which has the ability to monitor osseointegration and the life expectancy of an implant. ISQ is a valuable diagnostic and clinical tool that has far-reaching consequences on implant dentistry and this article throws light on advanced and reliable methods of assessing ISQ.

Keywords: implant stability, implant stability quotient (ISQ), osseointegration, osstell instrument, primary stability, resonance frequency analysis

1. Introduction

Implant treatment has become the first choice of treatment for replacement of missing teeth and oral rehabilitation over last few years. Osseointegration is the most important requirement for long term success of dental implant procedure. Many techniques have been experimented to reduce the failure rate of dental implants in long term. So far, insertion torque value and implant stability quotient (ISQ) obtained by the Osstell instrument are common clinical methods to assess the initial stability of an implant for a predictable loading procedure. The ISQ-values are used as an indicator for mechanical implant stability, and are believed to have predictive power for clinical outcome. Nowadays in clinical practice ISQ readings are used as gauging factor to decide the time interval for practical implant loading and to decide the prognosis of implant procedure [1]. Quantitative measurement of implant stability is of high clinical significance so various principles have been used to estimate this parameter accurately like, the periotest assay and resonance frequency analysis (RFA). A device called Osstell was formulated which works on the principle of RFA. The instrument measures the resonance frequency through the transducer attached to a implant fixture and display the result ISQ value on a scale of 1 to 100. It is an objective method of measuring implant stability. Higher ISQ value denotes higher primary stability. Usually ISQ value of 55–80 is considered optimal for implant success. In our clinical practice we have observed higher ISQ values in mandible cases than maxilla. The ISQ scale has a non-linear correlation to micro mobility [2]. Finite element analysis also has been recently used to analyze the mechanical and vibration behavior of the three dimensionally designed structure [3–6].

In our cases we found out that if ISQ value is on higher side of the scale initially, a small dip in values normally compensated with time and should be considered as a normal event which does necessitate alteration of routine treatment plan [2]. All implants with ISQ values higher than 54 considered for immediate loading.

But on the contrary, if values fall drastically then it should be taken as warning sign for unsuccessful implant in future and appropriate actions should be considered in terms of more follow-up schedule and to take additional precautionary measurements to wait before loading, to check for signs of infection and mechanical trauma. Lower values are expected to increase after the healing period in some cases.

2. Discussion

2.1 Principle: resonance frequency analysis

This diagnostic method computes implant stability and bone density by vibrational and structural analysis in noninvasive manner [7]. Two devices have been developed commercially to measure implant stability, one is electrical and other is based on magnetic principle. First method uses direct wire connection between transducer and resonance frequency analyzer. The second method based upon measurement of magnetic frequencies between transducer and resonance frequency analyzer by a wireless probe (**Figures 1** and **2**). Both methods are competent for measuring similar changes; however the magnetic device results in higher ISQ value when measuring the stability of non submerged dental implant (**Figures 3–6**) [8].

These methods can reveal considerable increase or decrease in implant stability which could not be appraised clinically. Various factors can affect the readings like effective implant length (length of the exposed threads and abutment height), implant shape and diameter and bone quality and quantity [9].

Measuring implant stability by implant oscillation frequency of bone can be assessed by RFA. Meredith et al. 1998 described the noninvasive method of assessing implant stability by OSSTELL devices. In 1999, OSSTELL devices was designed by the Integration Diagnostics Ltd., Sweden. Over last few years, various types of Osstell devices have developed to extemporize the implant stability measurements, namely, OSSTELL™, OSSTELL Mentor, and OSSTELL ISQ.

In 2009 the last and latest generation of this device was developed, OSSTELL ISQ, which includes a new control unit with a probe connected to it by means of a cable. These devices are gaining popularity due to reliability and ease of assessing implant

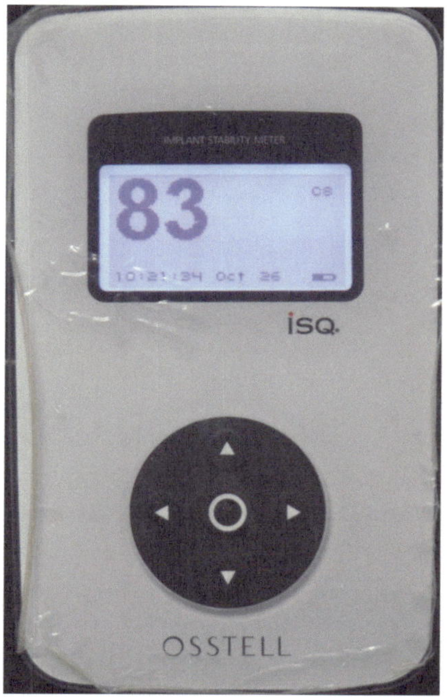

Figure 1.
Osstell devices: Electrical and magnetic RFA based devices.

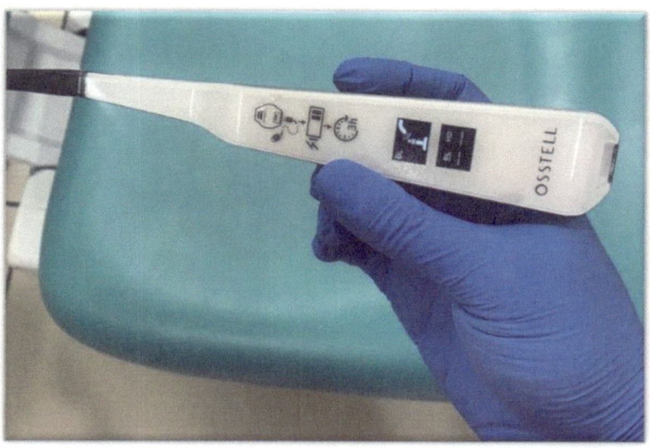

Figure 2.
Osstell Beacon cordless device: Electrical and magnetic RFA based devices.

stability. These measurements are independent of intra and inter observer variability and reproduce accurate results.

Nedir et al. [2] estimated the implant primary stability as an indicator of osseointegration. As per his study, ISQ value of more than 49 will osseointegrate over period of three months and those with values higher than 54 can be loaded immediately.

Primary stability of implants which was assessed through RFA using OSSTELL Mentor devices was underestimated to analyze the comparability and reproducibility [10]. Clinical trials concluded the almost perfect replicability and high reliability of ISQ

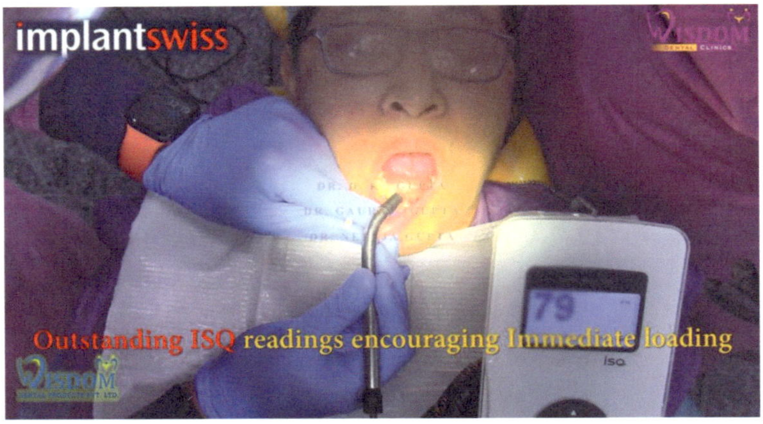

Figure 3.
Outstanding ISQ readings by Osstell device encouraging for immediate loading in lower front region.

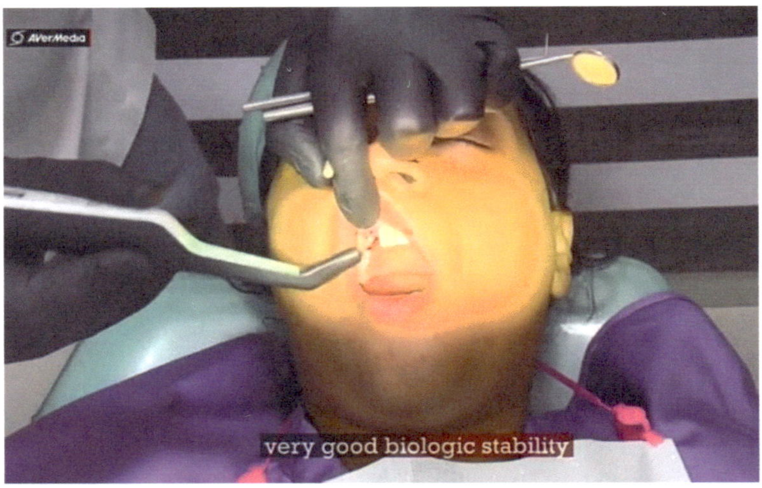

Figure 4.
Measurement of ISQ by advanced RFA bases magnetic Osstell device immediately after implant placement.

measurements with Osstell devices [11]. ISQ measurement by OSSTELL Mentor device during immediate and delayed loading implant cases concluded that it offers an objective method to determine the implant stability and for immediate loading [12].

Comparison of OSSTELL Mentor and OSSTELL ISQ in measuring implant stability was evaluated and the mean values of ISQ for OSSTELL ISQ and OSSTELL Mentor were 72.87 and 72.04 respectively, suggesting perfect compliance, consistency and recreatability between these devices [13].

There are various factors which affect the ISQ readings like anatomical direction of measurement in patient's mouth, gender of the patient, intraoral location of the implant [14], sex of the patient, immediate versus delayed implantation, diameter and length of implant, designing of implant, insertion torque [15, 16], bone type at the site of implant, contact surface area of implant. Various research studies indicated the possible interplay of insertiuon torque and ISQ values. Insertion torque was

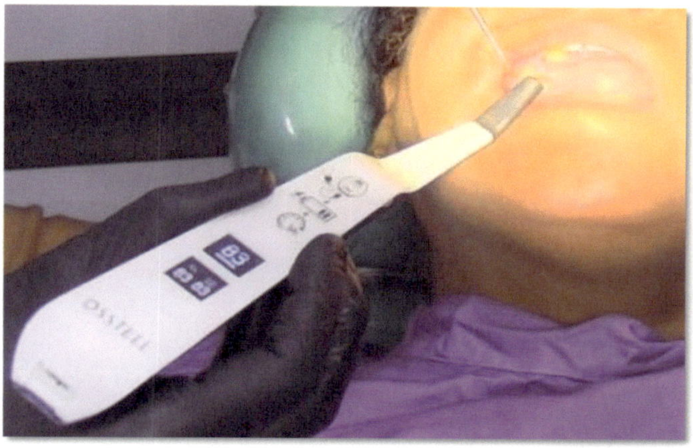

Figure 5.
Measurement of ISQ by Osstell device 3 months after implant placement depicting good biologic stability.

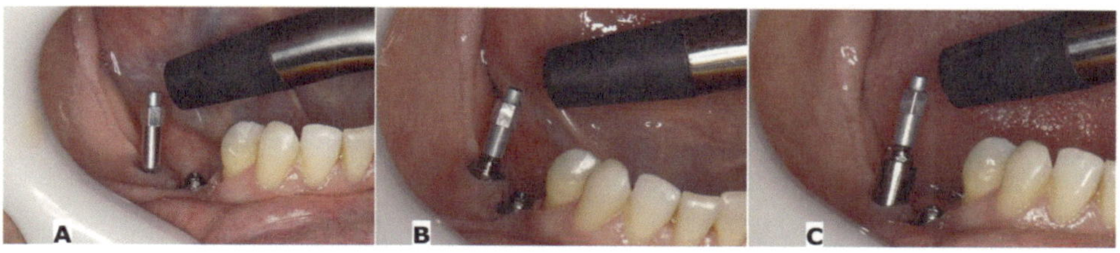

Figure 6.
Implant stability on the abutment and platform level Resonance Frequency Analysis by Osstell (a) Implant platform (b) 1 mm microvunit (c) 5 mm microvunit.

introduced to assess the primary stability of the implant and accordingly plant the surgical procedure on solid backgrounds. Good cortical bone thickness results in increased ISQ values due to better osseointegration, whereas less trhickness results in reduced stability and lesser ISQ. In last few decades immediate implant protocol has become more popular due to less clinical treatment time. If the favorable preclinical condition exist, immediate implant results in almost similar ISQ values when compared to delayed implant procedures. After 3 months when loading begins in delayed implant cases, secondary stability equalize to the level of ISQ values of similar magnitude as those achieved in primary stability phases.

In our practice we compared the ISQ values of successful implants at the time of loading and post operatively with the ISQ values of implant failure cases, which manifested significant difference in values. However, ISQ distributions at implant insertion denoted overlapping which indicated that there was no correlation among the data that could be used to predict successful osseointegration. The predictiveness of ISQ values were enigmatic [17].

3. Conclusion

Though the connection between bone density/quality and resonance frequency analysis is still enigmatic but our clinical practice suggested a significant interrelation between RFA measurement by Osstell device and implant success. Further studies are needed to evaluate a correlation of RFA with bone quality analysis and implant stability, which can ascertain success, failure or long-term prognosis of an implant.

Author details

Gaurav Gupta[1,2,3,4]

1 Sawai Man Singh Medical College and Hospital, Jaipur, India

2 Preventive and Pediatric Dentistry, India

3 California, USA

4 Implantology (AOI & ISOI), India

*Address all correspondence to: dr.gauravgupta99@gmail.com

References

[1] Dottore AM, Kawakami PY, Bechara K. Stability of implants placed in augmented posterior mandible after alveolar osteotomy using resorbable nonceramic hydroxyapatite or intraoral autogenous bone: 12-month follow-up. Clinical Implant Dentistry and Related Research. 2014;**16**(3):330-336

[2] Nedir R, Bischof M, Szmukler-Moncler S, Bernard JP, Samson J. Predicting osseointegration by means of implant primary stability. Clinical Oral Implants Research. 2004;**15**:520-528

[3] Deng B, Tan KB, Liu GR, Lu Y. Influence of osseointegration degree and pattern on resonance frequency in the assessment of dental implant stability using finite element analysis. The International Journal of Oral & Maxillofacial Implants. 2008;**23**:1082-1088

[4] Chun HJ, Cheong SY, Han JH, Heo SJ, Chung JP, Rhyu IC, et al. Evaluation of design parameters of osseointegrated dental implants using finite element analysis. Journal of Oral Rehabilitation. 2002;**29**:565-574

[5] Lang LA, Kang B, Wang RF, Lang BR. Finite element analysis to determine implant preload. The Journal of Prosthetic Dentistry. 2003;**90**: 539-546

[6] Huang HM, Lee SY, Yeh CY, Lin CT. Resonance frequency assessment of dental implant stability with various bone qualities: A numerical approach. Clinical Oral Implants Research. 2002;**13**:65-74

[7] Valderrama P, Oates TW, Jones AA, Simpson J, Schoolfield JD, Cochran DL. Evaluation of two different resonance frequency devices to detect implant stability: A clinical trial. Journal of Periodontology. 2007;**78**:262-272. Back to cited text no. 14

[8] Lages FS, Willya Douglas-de-Oliveira D, Ibelli GS, Assaf F, Queiroz TP, et al. Relationship between implant stability on the abutment and platform level by means of resonance frequency analysis: A cross-sectional study. PLOS ONE. 2017;**12**(7):e0181873. DOI: 10.1371/journal.pone.0181873

[9] Meredith N, Alleyne D, Cawley P. Quantitative determination of the stability of the implant-tissue interface using resonance frequency analysis. Clinical Oral Implants Research. 1996;**7**:261-267. Back to cited text no.

[10] Snijders RS, van Wijk AJ, Lindeboom JA. A comparative study of the Osstell™ versus the Osstell Mentor™ to evaluate implant stability in human cadaver mandibles. Journal of Oral Rehabilitation. 2013;**40**:774-779

[11] Herrero-Climent M, Santos-García R, Jaramillo-SantosR,Romero-RuizMM,Fernández-Palacin A, Lázaro-Calvo P, et al. Assessment of Osstell ISQ's reliability for implant stability measurement: A cross-sectional clinical study. Medicina Oral, Patología Oral y Cirugía Bucal. 2013;**18**:e877-e882

[12] González-Jaranay M, Moreu-Burgos G, Gómez-Moreno G, Rubio-Roldán J, Machuca-Portillo G, Perrotti V, et al. Changes in resonance frequency analysis assessed by Osstell mentor during osseointegration: Comparison between immediately loaded implants and control implants without load. Journal of Osseointegration. 2014;**6**:51-55

[13] Jaramillo R, Santos R, Lázaro P, Romero M, Rios-Santos JV, Bullón P, et al. Comparative analysis of 2 resonance frequency measurement devices: Osstell mentor and osstell ISQ. Implant Dentistry. 2014;**23**:351-356

[14] Guler AU, Sumer M, Duran I, Sandikci EO, Telcioglu NT. Resonance frequency analysis of 208 Straumann dental implants during the healing period. The Journal of Oral Implantology. 2013;**39**(2):161-167

[15] Brizuela-Velasco A, Alvarez-Arenal A, Gil-Mur FJ. Relationship between insertion torque and resonance frequency measurements, performed by resonance frequency analysis, in micromobility of dental implants: an in vitro study. Implant Dentistry. 2015;**24**(5):607-611

[16] Gehrke SA, Neto UTD, Del Fabbro M. Does implant design affect implant primary stability? A resonance frequency analysis-based randomized split-mouth clinical trial. The Journal of Oral Implantology. 2015;**41**(6):E281-E286

[17] Krafft T, Graef F, Karl M. Osstell resonance frequency measurement values as a prognostic factor in implant dentistry. The Journal of Oral Implantology. 2015;**41**:e133-e137

Chapter 5

RFA and Its Use in Implant Dentistry

Charles D. Schlesinger

Abstract

For over two decades the use of resonance frequency analysis or RFA has been used as a tool to determine the stiffness of implants in bone. Through the years the technology has become better, smaller and more accurate. Today, the use of RFA has been proven to be far superior to other clinical techniques to determine implant stability and is used not only to increase the level of success for implantologists around the world, but also to further the study of implant technology development.

Keywords: Implants, Stability, RFA, Treatment decisions

1. Introduction

Over the last two and half decades, the use of RFA instrumentation has gone from being an experimental gadget to an everyday and necessary instrument in determining implant stability and the overall health of the peri-implant/implant interface. This chapter will delve into the technology and its use in the modern day practice as well as ongoing research.

Clinicians generally agree that it is important to verify the status of implant–bone interface before attachment of prosthetic abutment, after completion and insertion of the definitive prosthesis [1].

Modern implantology has progressed to a point where our treatments are predictable, our outcomes better and our healing times shorter. Much of this is a direct result of better micro and macro implant characteristics. The modern implant with its osteo-promotive surface, better thread geometry and internal prosthetic connection allows clinicians to treat patients that historically would have had a guarded-prognoses at best.

Resonance Frequency Analysis, other was known as RFA is a technology that has become the standard by which an implantologist can measure the degree of integration not only prior to restoring an implant, but it can also be used to determine the progression of integration during the healing phase.

Prior to the development of these instruments and use of RFA for the determination of implant stability, the measurement of implant stability was rudimentary at best. It relied on blunt tapping, reverse torque, Seating torque, a Periotest device or time. Each of these methods have their limitations and ultimately are not reliable predictors of implant stability.

Before we delve into the specifics or RFA, lets first look at the other methods of determining implant stability.

IntechOpen

2. Blunt tapping

The use of a blunt instrument such as a mirror handle has been used to determine, in a very crude fashion, the stability of an implant. The metallic mirror handle is tapped against an implant, a cover screw, a healing abutment or a definitive abutment. The clinician then listens to the sound that occurs and relates that to the stability of the implant in the peri-implant bone. As you can imagine, there is a lot of room for interpretation and experience is the key to predictability in this method.

3. Torque at implant placement

Studies and anecdotal evidence have shown that 30 N/cm is the value considered to be sufficient for primary stability. Below this level, an implant has always been considered highly susceptible to failure by lack of stability. There are two types of torque that we see when placing an implant — insertion torque and seating torque. When immediately loading dental implants, it is the final insertion torque that is the key to successful treatment. In order to follow an immediate load protocol, a minimum seating torque value of 45 N/cm-50 N/cm is necessary [2].

Webster's Dictionary defines *torque* as a force to rotate an object about an axis. By Newton's Third law of Motion, we can confidently deduce that the torque value a practitioner gets when placing an implant is equal to the resistance to the original rotational force. Basically, you can turn the implant, which is a screw, until it either cannot move axially in a downward direction anymore or the bone around the implant exceeds its deformational limit and can no longer resist the axial rotation (stripping). This deformational limit will vary from a high value in D1 cortical bone to a lower value in D4 medullary bone.

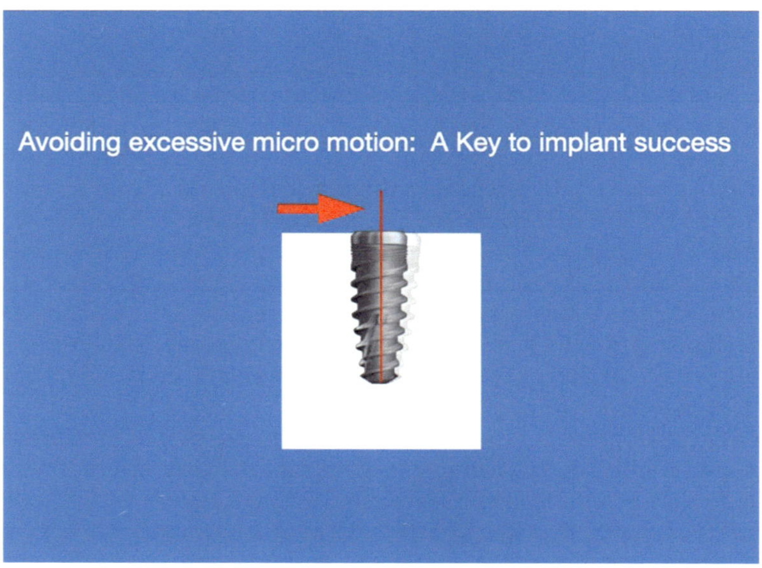

Figure 1.
100–150 microns of lateral movement will result in soft tissue encapsulation.

The limitation of just looking at torque is that it does not take into account the stability of the implant in lateral directions (**Figure 1**). It is this lateral stability, or resistance to sliding motion between the implant and the osteotomy, that is crucial to success. Therefore, it is possible to have a low torque value with high lateral stability or the opposite situation where you have high rotational stability (torque) and low lateral stability (ISQ) [3].

4. Reverse torque

This type of evaluation of implant stability carries with it a potentially high possibility of a negative outcome. This test uses a torque wrench set at 20-30 N/cm and the implant is then subjected to a rotational force in the counter-clockwise direction. Though, in most integrated situations this should not be an issue, it is possible to break integration in softer bone types such as D4 bone or if done too early in the healing process in other bone types.

5. Periotest

The Periotest device was originally designed to measure the mobility of teeth by using a pneumatic plunger that would read the deflection of the tooth in the natural peridontium. In 1990, Olive et al. used it to test the stability of dental implants [4]. The values reported by the device range from −8 to +50. **Figure 2** shows the values for interpreting implant stability, and **Figure 3** shows the values associate with natural teeth.

Unfortunately, because the Periotest value is strongly related to the excitation direction and position, the reading from the method does not always correspond precisely to a biomechanical parameter [5]. Another possible cause for a false reading is that the clinicians hand, or ability to not move that hand becomes part of the equation. If some of the percussive force is either resisted too much or absorbed too much, the readings will not be true.

Periotest Value Range	Interpretation
-8 to 0	Good osseointegration; the implant is well integrated and pressure can be applied to it
+1 to +9	A clinical examination is required: the application of pressure on the implant is generally not (yet) possible
+10 to +50	Osseointegration is insufficient and no pressure may be allowed to act on the implant

Figure 2.
Periotest value range.

Clinical degree of loosening	Periotest value
0	-08 to +09
I	+10 to +19
II	+20 to +29
III	+30 to +50

Figure 3.
Periodontal mobility classification vs. Periotest values.

6. Time

Historically the integration of implants was based on the data collected on natural bone healing and the integration times of the early non-coated implants developed by Branemark. A healing phase of 4–6 months was not uncommon and in many practices all implants were placed in this specified healing time frame.

The issue with this is that every individual is unique. Though the majority of individuals fall into the averages for the time required for integration, the advent of new technology and the differences in individual biology can greatly alter the time to restoration.

7. Bone healing

Osseointegration follows a common, biologically determined program that is subdivided into 3 stages:

- Incorporation by woven bone formation;
- Adaptation of bone mass to load (lamellar and parallel-fibered bone deposition)
- Adaptation of bone structure to load (bone remodeling).

Osseointegration is also a measure of implant stability, which can occur at 2 different stages: primary and secondary. Primary stability of an implant mainly comes from mechanical engagement with compact bone. Secondary stability, on other hand, offer biological stability through bone regeneration and remodeling. The former is a requirement for secondary stability. The latter, however, dictates the time of functional loading [6].

In order to understand RFA and what it is measuring, one must understand implant stability and the factors that influence it. At the time of implant placement, 100% of the stability comes from the relationship between the geometry of the implant and the peri-implant bone. The implants macro geometry; such as thread patter and size, shape of the body of the implant (tapered or parallel walled) and the roughness of the surface coating, or micro-geometry all effect the mechanical locking ability in bone. On the other side of this equation there is the bone itself. The initial stability, or mechanical retention is directly affected by the quality of the bone that the implant is inserted into, with bone types ranging from D1 to D4.

D1 bone has very little medullary bone and therefore mainly consists of cortical bone which is very dense and highly mineralized. As we move down the progression scale towards poorer bone quality, we see an increase in medullary or cancellous bone, with its large non-mineralized spaces between the trabeculae. On the opposite side of the spectrum there is D4 bone which has a very thin mineralized cortical shell that surrounds spongy bone with very little mineralized content and a higher percentage of collagen.

As expected, mechanical stability is usually very high in D1 bone and for the most part very poor in D4 bone with ISQ values supporting this [7].

Biologic stability is attributed to the surface interaction and maturation of bone surrounding the dental implant. The bone, as it is moving through its three stages of change has a direct effect on the stability of the implant. Even after high initial mechanical stability, there is usually a drop off in overall stability during the 3–6 week time period post-placement. This is due to the natural remodeling that occurs as the healing process progresses. There is resorption of bone by osteoclastic activity followed by the deposition of osteoblasts on the surface of the implant. At this point the un-organized

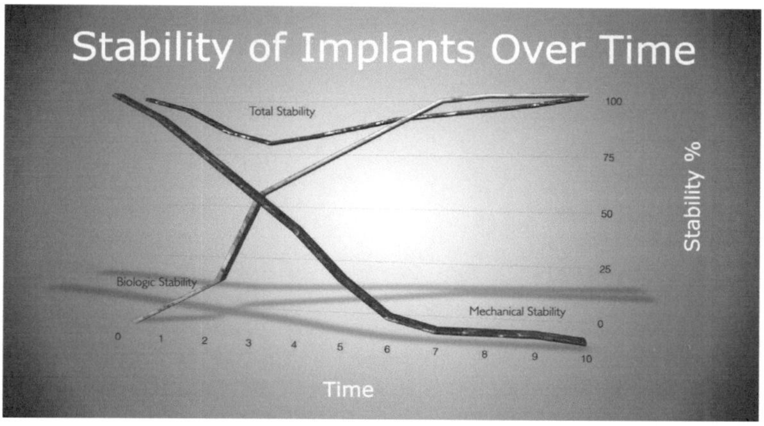

Figure 4.
Comparison of mechanical vs. biologic stability.

woven bone starts to become organized and the formation of lamellar bone occurs. It is at this point that we see an increase in implant stability afforded by the progression of osseointegration. The next step in the process is maturation and then it is followed by the adaptation of the peri-implant bone to the forces of mastication and load. This cross-over can be seen in the diagram above (**Figure 4**).

8. RFA

Resonance Frequency Analysis for implant stability was first proposed by Merideth in his 1996 [8]. The first resonance frequency device was developed by Osstell and the device consisted of an L-shaped receiver that mounted on the implant and a transducer that pulsed it with a magnetic frequency.

Resonance Frequency Analysis (RFA) is the measurement of the frequency with which a device vibrates (**Figure 5**). RFA measurements reflect the micro-mobility of dental implants, which in turn is determined by the bone density at the implant site [9].

A transducer connected to the implant is excited by means of an electric or magnetic impulse (depending on the type of transducer used). Thus, the implant is subjected to slight lateral force that causes lateral displacement due to elastic deformation of the bone. The frequency of the registered oscillation depends on the stiffness of bone-implant attachment: the stiffer the system is, the higher the transducer's oscillation frequency will be. While most tests render subjective results, RFA allows objective, noninvasive assessment of implant stability [10].

Why is the measurement of lateral stability important? If an implant repeatedly moves laterally in the range of 100–150 microns, the body will not form bone at the implant-bone interface, instead, soft tissue will form and the resulting encapsulation of the implant in soft tissue will result in a failure.

ISQ is short for *Implant Stability Quotient.* The ISQ-scale runs from 1 to 100 and corresponds to the resonance frequency in a close to linear way. The scale was determined in 2003, and ISQ 1 correspond approximately to 1,000 Hz and ISQ 100 correspond approximately to 10,000 Hz. The early scientific studies were used to determine how the ISQ scale should relate to Hz and numerous clinical studies after that have put the ISQ-scale in a clinical context, relating to treatment and loading protocols.

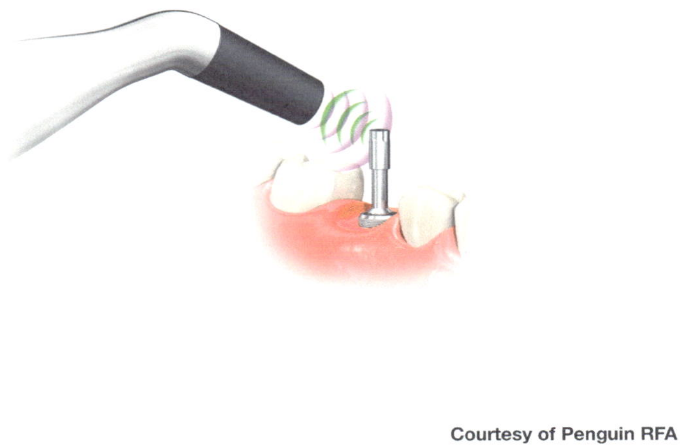

Figure 5.
How RFA works.

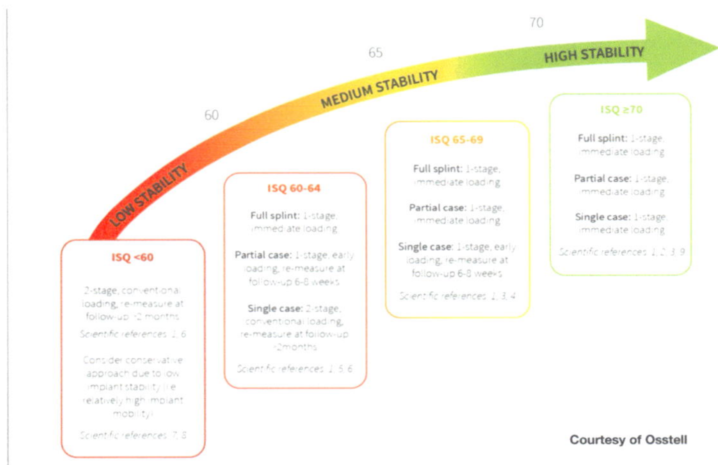

Figure 6.
The ISQ scale provided by Osstell.

The developed ISQ scales which are used today give the practitioner a way to quantitatively assess an implants stability. Developed over time by comparing clinical outcomes to ISQ values, thousands of scientific articles have been written that back up the validity of this type of testing device.

The following chart shows the various landmark values for ISQ and what they mean clinically (**Figure 6**). These values are pivotal to successful treatment and not only help direct the initial treatment with regard to deciding on a one stage vs. two stage surgery, but also the progression of healing and the correct time period in which to restore.

9. RFA devices

The two major players in the arena of RFA are Osstell and Penguin. They both work in similar fashion, but the systems differ a bit in their armamentarium.

10. Osstell

Starting in 2001, the first commercially available RFA device was released for clinical use. Over the years the Osstell family of devices has evolved to become more accurate and ultimately smaller (**Figure 7**). The features available to the clinician are broad with the large library of clinically backed literature available at www.osstell.com, and clinical tracking ability through www.osstellconnect.com.

The newest Osstell device is the Beacon which is smaller than previous iterations and lights up with either red, yellow or green to correspond to the values on the ISQ scale (**Figure 8**).

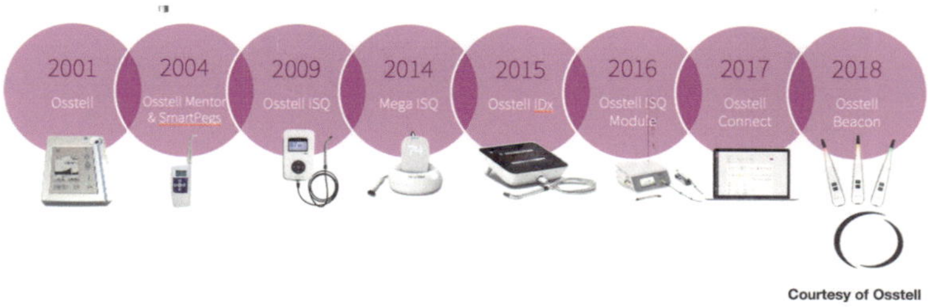

Figure 7.
The evolution of the Osstell device.

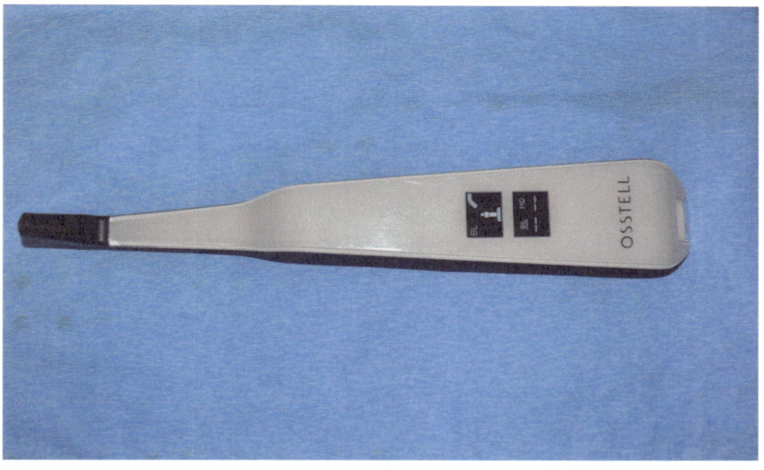

Figure 8.
The Osstell Beacon.

11. Penguin RFA

Emerging onto the scene in 2015, The Penguin RFA device uses similar technology as the Osstell and when it was introduced, was the first device to decrease the overall size of an RFA device to the size of a portable curing light (**Figure 9**).

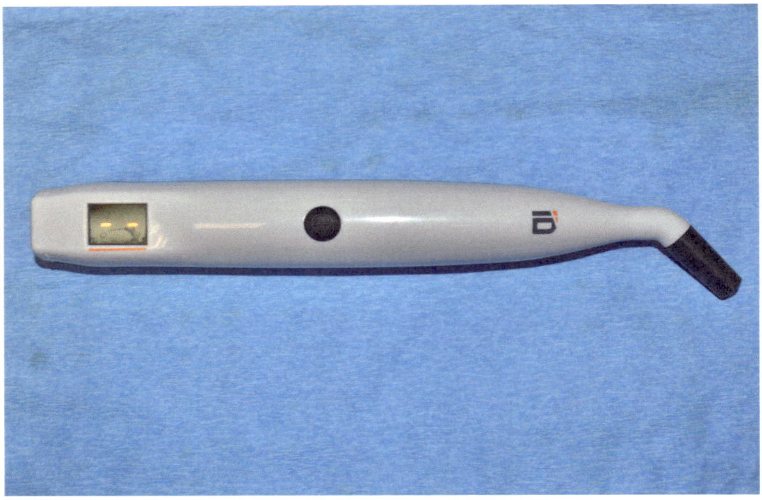

Figure 9.
The penguin RFA device.

12. Comparing the two devices

Both devices utilize a peg that is screwed into the abutment connection of the implant. These pegs are not only platform diameter specific, but also implant/abutment interface type specific. Therefore, you must have different pegs for different implants.

The Osstell unit utilizes single use Smartpegs which are made of aluminum (**Figure 10**). The use of aluminum was chosen in order to prevent accidental

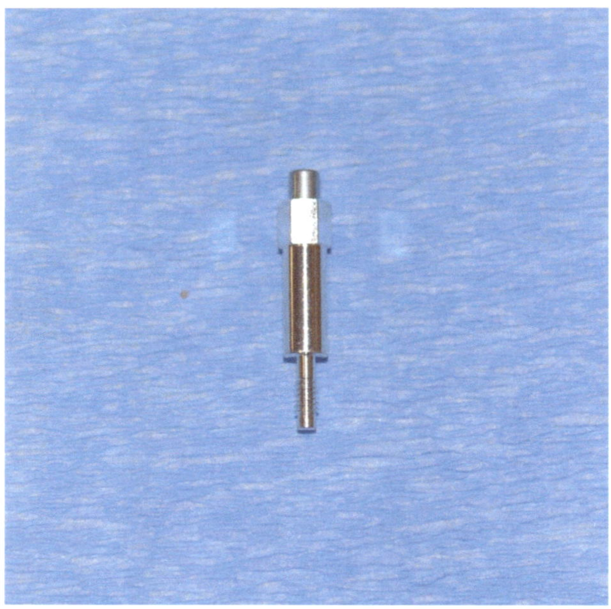

Figure 10.
Osstell Smartpeg.

cross-threading of the peg from damaging the threads inside the implant. On the other hand, the penguin RFA unit uses Multipegs made of titanium (**Figure 11**). These pegs are multi-use and can be sterilized and re-used approximately 20 times before replacing. The reason they must be replaced is that after repeated thermal cycling in an autoclave, the ductility of the titanium peg can change and I have seen the small magnet become corroded, both of which can result in inaccurate readings.

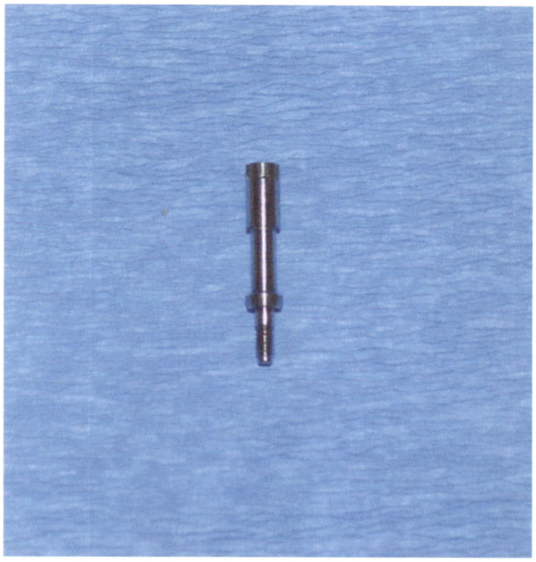

Figure 11.
Penguin multipeg.

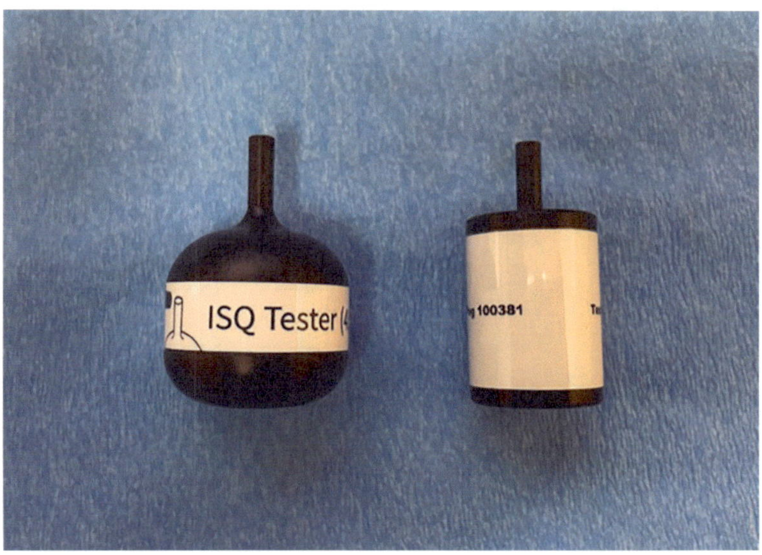

Figure 12.
Penguin (L) and Osstell (R) calibration pegs.

Both the Osstell and Penguin RFA units have calibration pegs (**Figure 12**) which are available. The Osstell peg is set to give an ISQ of 55 and the Penguin will give a reading of 45-55. Since the Osstell pegs are single use and calibrated at the factory, further calibration of the unit is not necessary according to the manufacturer. The Penguin on the other hand, with its multi-use pegs may benefit from the ability to check calibration as they are being re-used.

13. Discussion

The success of dental implants is affected by various factors according to the oral and general health of the patient, and it has been reported that the ISQ values vary in a range between 58 and 84, with a mean of 68 after 8–12 months [11].

When trying to provide not only predictability, but also expedient treatment, the use of an RFA device is invaluable. These devices provide a much better indicator of the level of osseointegration than all the other methods available. They are easy to use and only take a few moments to get ISQ values. Measurements are taken in the BL direction and in the MD direction while directing the transducer at an angle of 45 degrees to the peg (**Figure 13**).

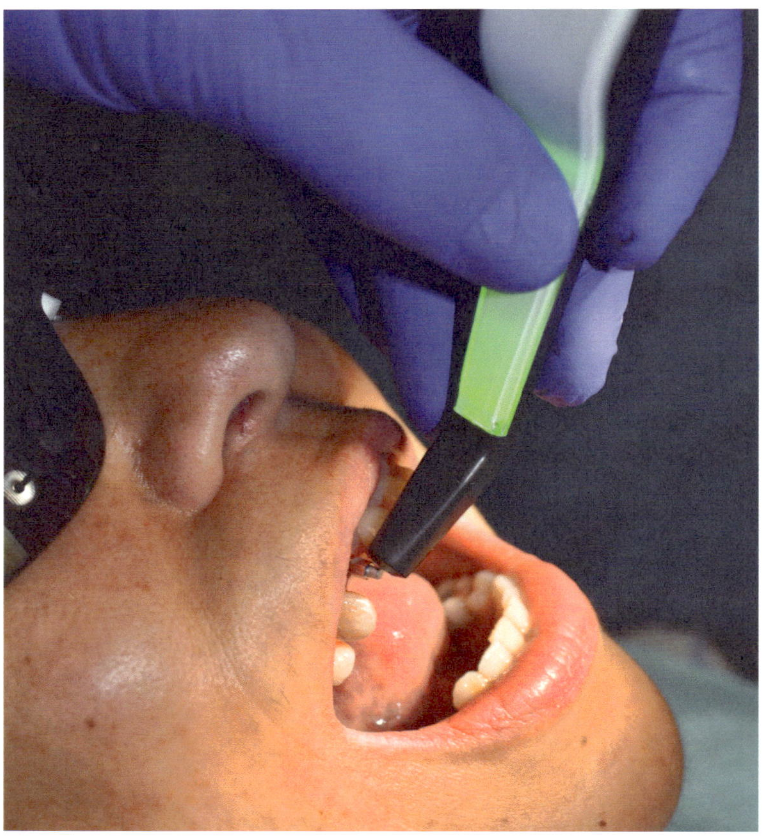

Figure 13.
Angle to test stability showing "green" ISQ value.

Intra-operatively it is a simple procedure and provides the data you need to make intelligent clinical decisions (**Figure 14**). At placement an ISQ value of 55 is equivalent to the use of torque value where a measurement of 30 would indicate sufficient primary stability in order to safely place a healing abutment for a 1 stage or early loading protocol. Any lower ISQ would indicate to the clinician that a two-stage protocol by burying the implant would be prudent. If a stability of 70 or above then immediately loading a single implant could be done safely.

In my clinical protocol, I take measurements at placement and then again at 8 weeks. At that time, I can make a determination of where the implant is in the healing spectrum. If the ISQ number has reached a minimum of 70, then I will proceed to the restorative phase with confidence. If it is somewhere between my initial measurement and 70, then I will wait another month and re-check.

Clinically this is not only tracked in my digital notes, but also on the Osstellconnect site (**Figure 15**). Conversely, if the ISQ number has dropped significantly below my initial reading at placement, it indicates a failing or failed implant and the decision to remove it is discussed with the patient. Even though this is an event that no one wants,

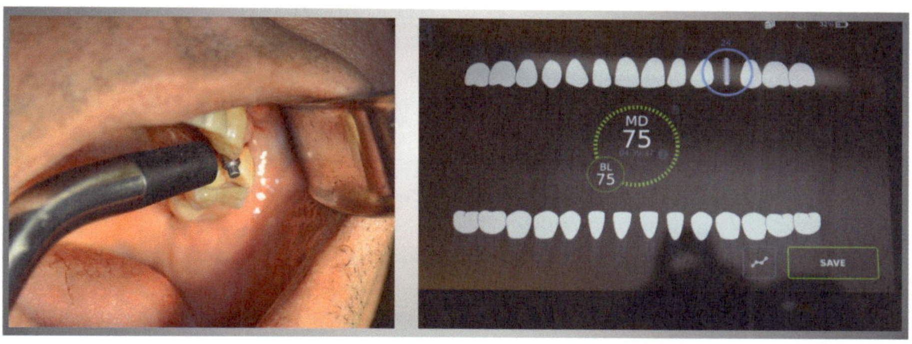

Figure 14.
Osstell IDX being used clinically.

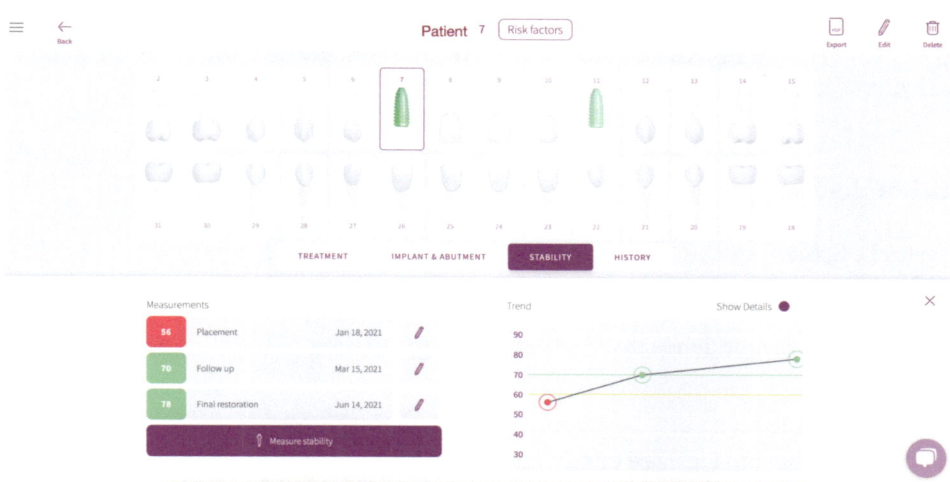

Figure 15.
Screenshot of clinical interface on Osstell connect.

at least it is identified early enough that a new implant can be placed and the patient only loses two months in the overall treatment time.

When compared with the use of RFA, Osstell™ system proved to be more reliable compared to Periotest® system in measuring dental implant stability in hard and in soft interfaces [12]. In 2020 when comparing the Osstell to the Penguin, Bural et al. saw no statistical difference in their readings [13].

Today, RFA is being used in clinical research to quantify differences in implant designs and surface technology. It was used to determine the difference in stability and bone loss associated with implants with differing crestal macro structures and thread designs [14].

Also, RFA was able to show that rehabilitations with splinted crowns combining 4- and 10-mm implants demonstrated a favorable 1-year performance in a shortened maxillary dental arch [15].

These instruments are allowing clinical researchers to dissect the parameters and minutia that contribute to overall implant success. For example, the use of RFA has shown that there is no differences in stability of implant or failure rate between men and women [16].

Yet, in Peter Andersson's 2019 publication, he did find that women had lower ISQ values than men, which he and his colleagues attributed to the incidence of osteoporosis in female patients. These diametrically opposed outcomes will spur further studies into the differences in success between the sexes and what critical factors may be responsible.

He Also found that there was a significantly higher risk for failure for implants with an ISQ value below 70 and 75 than for implants with higher stability at placement. Moreover, the risk for failure increased further if the ISQ value was still below 70 and 75 after 3–4 months of healing [17].

As you can imagine, research like this, is and will allow, us to treat more patients effectively and predictably.

The use of RFA is helping to develop better techniques for regeneration and help quantify the role that biologics like platelet-rich fibrin may have in enhancing healing and contributing to better implant stability [18].

Todays world of implantology if filled with wonderful technology to help practitioners and patients alike. CBCT technology, digital CAD/CAM and 3D printing all are used to provide the very best in patient care. RFA allows for a better understanding of primary stability, the healing process of osseointegration and takes the guesswork out of know when to restore.

Author details

Charles D. Schlesinger
FICOI, Albuquerque, New Mexico, USA

*Address all correspondence to: cdschlesinger@gmail.com

References

[1] Walker L., Morris H.F., Ochi S. Periotest values of dental implants in the first 2 years after second-stage surgery: DICRG interim report no. 8. Dental implant clinical research group. *Implant Dent.* 1997;6:207-212.

[2] Schlesinger CD. Immediately loading dental implants: doing it right for long term success. *Dent Today.* 2016; 35(5):84-89.

[3] Schlesinger C. Torque Vs RFA in Implant Placement. Implant Practice US August/September 2016.

[4] Olive J., Aparicio C. Periotest method as a measure of osseointegrated oral implant stability. *Int. J. Oral Maxillofac. Implants.* 1990;5:390-400.

[5] Caulier H., Naert I., Kalk W., Jansen J.A. The relationship of some histologic parameters, radiographic evaluations, and Periotest measurements of oral implants: an experimental animal study. *Int. J. Oral Maxillofac. Implants.* 1997;12:380-386.

[6] Parithimarkalaignan S, Padmanabhan T. Osseointegration: An Update, J Indian Prosthodont Soc. 2013 Mar;13(1):2-6.

[7] Yoon H, Yeo S. Effect of bone quality and implant surgical technique on implant stability quotient (ISQ) value J Adv Prosthodont. 2011 Mar;3(1):10-15.

[8] Merideth N, Alleyne D, Cawley P. Quantitative determination of the stability of the implant-tissue interface using resonance frequency analysis. Clin Oral Implants Res 1996 Sep;7(3):261-7.

[9] Pagliani L, Sennerby L, Petersson A, Verrocchi D, Volpe S & Andersson P The relationship between resonance frequency analysis (RFA) and lateral displacement of dental implants: an in vitro study *Journal of Oral Rehabilitation 2012*

[10] Degidi M, Daprile G, Piattelli A. Determination of primary stability: a comparison of the surgeon's perception and objective measurements. *Int J Oral Maxillofac Implants.* 2010;25:558-61.

[11] Bafijari D, Bendedetti A, Stamatoski A, et al. Influence of Resonance Frequency Analysis (RFA) Measurements for Successful Osseointegration of Dental Implants During the Healing Period and Its Impact on Implant Assessed by Osstell Mentor Device. Open Access Maced J Med Sci. 2019 Dec 15;7(23):4110-4115.

[12] Al-Jetaily S, Al-dosari A. Assessment of Osstell™ and Periotest® systems in measuring dental implant stability (in vitro study). Saudi Dent J. 2011 Jan;23(1):17-21.

[13] Bural C, Dayan C, Geckili O. Initial Stability Measurements of Implants Using a New Magnetic Resonance Frequency Analyzer With Titanium Transducers: An Ex Vivo Study. J Oral Implantol 2020 Feb 1;46(1):35-40.

[14] Ranabhatt R, Singh K, Siddarth R, Tripathi S, Arya D. A randomized clinical study to compare implant stability and bone loss using early loading protocol in two implant systems with different design. J Indian Prosthodont Soc. Jan-Mar 2021;21(1):74-80.

[15] Gaspersic R, Dard M, Linder S, Oblak C. One-Year Results Assessing the Performance of Prosthetic Rehabilitations in the Posterior Maxilla

Supported by 4-mm Extrashort Implants Splinted to 10-mm Implants: A Prospective Case Series. J Oral Maxillofac Implants. Mar-Apr 2021;36(2):371-378.

[16] Ganguly R, Measurement of dental implant stability by resonance frequency analysis: a study. IJOMS Supplement 1 , 95-96, March 01, 2017.

[17] Andersson P, Pagliani L, et al. Factors Influencing Resonance Frequency Analysis (RFA) Measurements and 5-Year Survival of Neoss Dental Implants. International Journal of Dentistry. Research Article | Open Access Volume 2019 |Article ID 3209872

[18] Soni R, Priya A, Agrawal R, Bhatnagar A, Kumar L. Evaluation of efficacy of platelet-rich fibrin membrane and bone graft in coverage of immediate dental implant in esthetic zone: An *in vivo* study. Natl J Maxillofac Surg. Jan-Jun 2020;11(1):67-75.

Section 2

Current Trends and Biomaterials in Clinical Relevance

Chapter 6

Incorporation of Novel Elements in Bioactive Glass Compositions to Enhance Implant Performance

Joy-anne N. Oliver, Olanrewaju Akande and Melanie Ecker

Abstract

Increasing popularities of bioactive-glasses and their potential medical applications have led to countless studies into improving their material characteristics and overall performance. Some scientists hope to create new bioactive-glass compositions, while others seek to merely modify existing ones such as the novel 45S5 bioactive-glass composition; created by Dr. Larry Hench. These modifications aim to address potential complications that may arise at a site following implantation such as bacterial infections. In other cases, the incorporation of a selected element or compound may aim to improve the implant functioning by increasing cell proliferation. Although possibilities are plentiful, researchers avoid compromising the typical bioactive glass characteristics when doping with elements such as silver, or gold to achieve additional properties. This chapter elaborates on the incorporation of popular elements by doping bioactive-glass compositions to introduce desired properties based on the implant application.

Keywords: doping, bioactive glass, hydroxyapatite, angiogenesis, osteogenesis, osteoconductive, biocompatibility, cell proliferation

1. Introduction

A bioactive material is one that is able to elicit a specific biological response at the interface of a material that results in bond formation between the body tissues and the material that they surround [1]. Common bioactive materials include bioactive glasses, and from that derived bioactive glass-ceramics and bioactive ceramics.

Bioactive glass was first introduced in the late 1960's by Dr. Larry Hench after an enlightening conversation with an army officer while attending a scientific conference. During their discussion, they connected on the common tragic injuries that the soldiers were experiencing during the Vietnam War that was occurring at that time. These types of injuries involved those to the limbs, and during that time, the treatment quite often involved amputation due to the absence of a material capable of effectively supporting the hands or the feet. Over the next few years, Hench and his students developed a soda-calcia-phosphate-silicate based glass composition, which was proven to stimulate bone [2]. The result of this development in 1969 was the well-known and copyrighted 45S5 Bioglass. This discovery was the beginning of a new generation of materials, acting as temporary substrates for supporting damaged tissues [3], and since then launched products formed from variations of bioactive glasses and glass-cermaics such as calcium phosphates and synthetic hydroxyapatite [4–7].

The main purpose of such substrates was to create implants that react to the body's process unlike the implants that were in use at that time which were inert or unreactive. His continued study focused on revealing the mechanism on why his novel glass composition, 45S5, was able to interact with the body as a result of by-products from the dissolution of the glass components in the body [8, 9].

When a glass is designed to function as a potential implant and possess bioactive features, its behavior is monitored as certain criteria must be achieved before confirming bioactivity. This can be done by determining its surface type. There are five surface type characteristics of silica-based glasses. Type I surfaces undergo only a thin surface layer hydration when exposed to the bodily aqueous environment. In a case like that, the bulk composition is similar to that of the surface composition. Type II surfaces consists of a silica-rich protective film that occurs as a result of selective alkali ion removal. Type III surfaces are known for their ability to form dual surface layers, known to contribute to durability in both acidic and alkali solutions. Type III surface interactions are characteristic of an ideal bioactive glass. Type IV surfaces have the ability to form a silica-rich layer, however, the silica concentration is not high enough to protect the glass from further attack by network dissolution. Therefore, they are known to have poor durability. Glasses that undergo congruent dissolution with equivalent loss of alkali and silica exhibit that of a Type V glass surface [10].

2. What constitutes an effective bioactive glass?

The original purpose for creating a bioactive glass was to form a chemical bond with bone, and this was achieved by Dr. Larry Hench as stated prior. It is important to understand the mechanism of how this interaction became possible. According to Hench, further thermodynamic studies allowed us to understand that there is a formation of an organic structure being derived from an inorganic one. He was able to determine that the stability of Bioglass® came as a direct result of the formation of a Type III surface [10]. This usually occurs as the result of the presence of phosphorus pentoxide P_2O_5 in its composition or in some cases, aluminum(III) oxide Al_2O_3, forming an additional surface layer of either alumina-silicate or calcium-phosphate species on the surface of the silica-rich layer. This comes as a result of dealkalization, surface structural modifications or precipitation from solution [9, 10]. Glasses like these tend to be very durable in both acidic and alkaline solutions, which contribute to the formation of a hydroxyapatite layer capable of creating a bond with tissue.

Hench, his students, and his second wife, June Wilson, a clinical biologist, also noted that this mechanism contributed to 45S5 creating strong bonds to living tissue because of the expression of bone-growth genes [2, 11] in the body that was stimulated by the chemical byproducts of the glass components in the body due to Type III surface interaction [10].

2.1 Mechanism of bioactive glass as an implant and hydroxyapatite (HA) formation

The chemical mechanism that occurs once a bioactive glass is successfully introduced into the body as an implant involves a series of ion transfer reactions, as shown

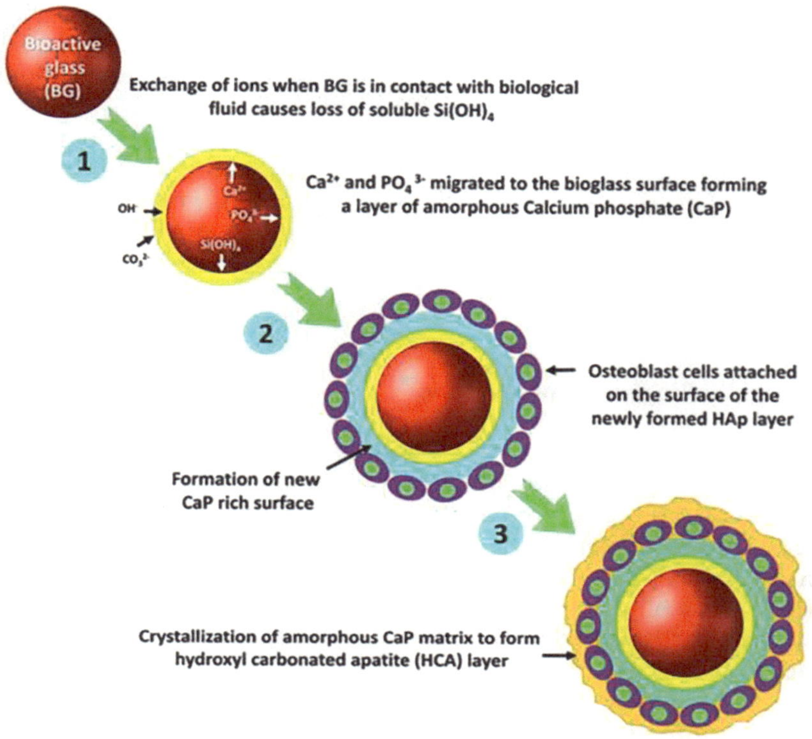

Figure 1.
Illustration of series of ion exchanges involved in the formation of HA [12].

in **Figure 1**, that result in the formation of hydroxyapatite (HA). The HA formation is required for the conformation of bioactivity. When a bioactive glass comes into contact with the bodily environment, a series of reactions occur to confirm bioactivity according to **Figure 1** in a 5-stage process:

1. Cation exchange involving the monovalent and bivalent cations present in the glass with the H^+ from the solution, leading to the formation of Si-OH (silanol) bonds on the glass surface and an increase in pH.

2. The pH continues to increase while Si-O-Si bonds are attacked by hydroxyl ions, causing soluble silica $Si(OH)_4$ to be lost in solution and increases the silanol concentration at the glass surface exposed to the fluid.

3. Condensation and polymerization of silanol groups occur, resulting in the formation of a silica-rich amorphous layer (silica gel).

4. Calcium and phosphate ions diffuse through the silica gel, forming and amorphous $CaO\text{-}P_2O_5$ rich film on the silica gel layer film which later crystalizes.

5. The crystallization of the $CaO\text{-}P_2O_5$ amorphous layer leads to the formation of HA.

Following the confirmation of bioactivity in stage 5, adsorption and desorption of growth factors, produced by the surrounding cells, are enhanced by the HA layers. Thereafter, macrophages prepare the implant site for tissue repair by the elimination of dead cells, followed by the attachment of osteoblast stem cells. The following stage involves the differentiation and proliferation of the osteoblast stem cells toward the mature osteoblast phenotype. This typically occurs within hours to weeks depending on the class of the bioactive material. Thereafter, generation of an extracellular matrix occurs as growth factors stimulate cell division and mitosis and the proteins required for the matrix development. The extracellular matrix becomes mineralized followed by the encasement of mature osteocytes in a collagen-HCA matrix, resulting in bone growth [13].

2.2 The original Bioglass® composition

The novel glass composition Bioglass 45S5 was of the Na_2O-CaO-SiO_2-P_2O_5 glass system and was known to possess a high calcium concentration with its composition close to a eutectic in the Na_2O-CaO-SiO_2 phase diagram [4, 5, 14]. Hench's novel discovery included this glass system in the following mol% concentration: 46.1%SiO_2, 24.4%Na_2O, 26.9%CaO, 2.6%P_2O_5. This glass composition was trademarked Bioglass® and since then has only been used in Ref. to the 45S5 composition and not for any other general bioactive glasses [14]. Its ability to create a bond to bone so strong that it could only be removed once the bone was broken.

2.3 Characterization and measurement of bioactivity

Figure 2 illustrates a ternary plot in increments of 10 wt% of the three base compounds with the addition on P_2O_5 for the formation of the novel Bioglass® composition, and for the design of other potential bioactive glasses and glass ceramics based on

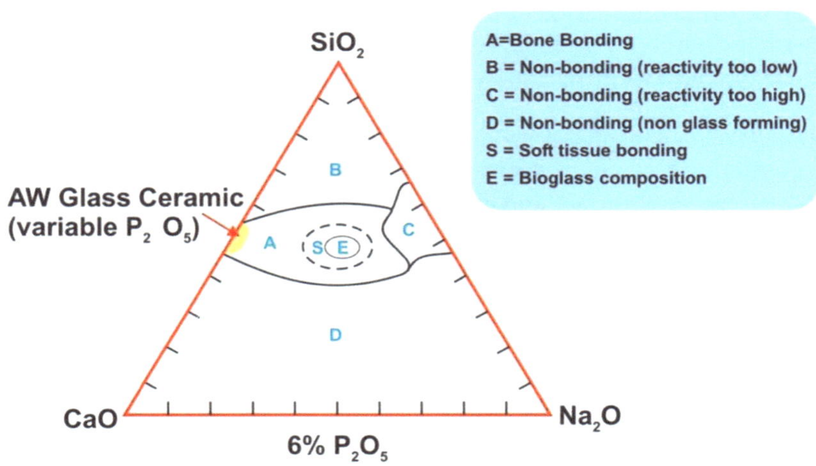

Figure 2.
Compositional dependence (wt%) of bone bonding and soft tissue bonding of bioactive glass and glass-ceramics. The compositions within region a have a constant 6%P_2O_5 apart from AW glass ceramic which consists of concentration of P_2O_5 greater than 6%. Regions S and E both have the ability to interact with and bond to soft tissue and within region E specifically lies the novel bioglass® composition reprinted with permission from [15].

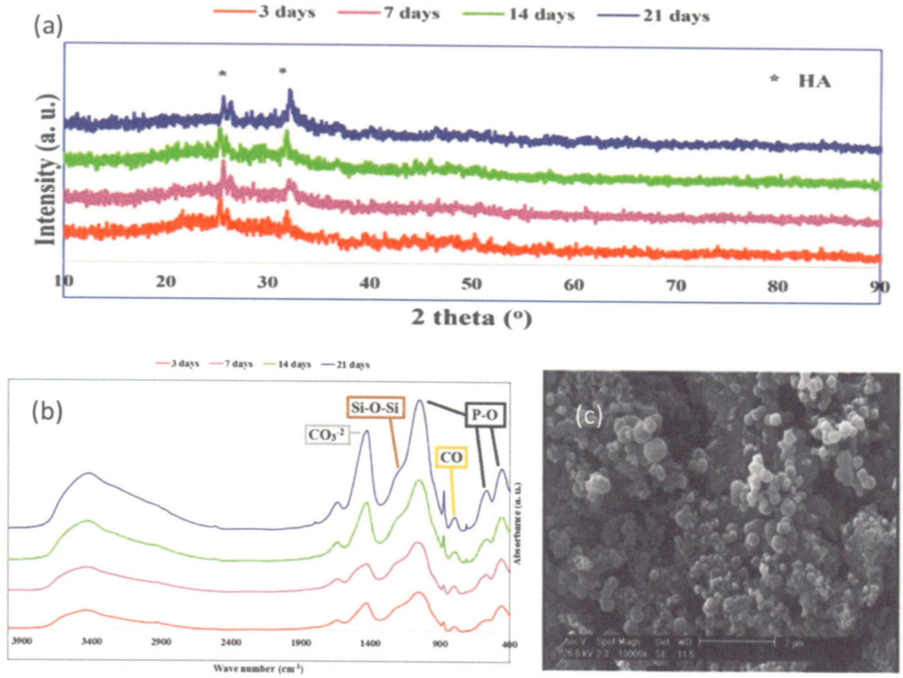

Figure 3.
(a) XRD analysis and identification of HA formation through starred peaks after glass composition S4-Z1 is immersed in SBF solution for 3,7, 14 and 21 days respectively. (b) FTIR analysis of S4-Z1 after immersion in SBF for 3. 7, 14, and 21 days respectively. (c) HA formation identified via SEM analysis after immersion in SBF solution for 21 days. Reprinted with permission [19].

the wt% of each component. Within it identifies regions of bonding type as it relates to the ability to bond to hard or soft tissue. This is a good tool to predict the bioactive behavior of glass compositions within the SiO_2-Na_2O-CaO series and other potential series depending on the compounds involved in the desired composition.

The index of bioactivity, I_B, is used to indicate the measurement of the bioactivity of any material. Introduced by Hench, $I_B = 100/t_{0.5bb}$, where $t_{0.5bb}$ is the time for more than 50% of the implant interface to be bonded to bone [16]. Bioactivity increases as the I_B increases.

Since 1994, bioactive materials were classified into Class A and Class B types. Class A bioactive materials were determined to be osteoproductive materials which elicit both intracellular and extracellular responses at its interface. Therefore, Class A bioactive glasses have the ability to bond with both bone and soft tissue. Class B materials are known as osterconductive materials which elicit only an extracellular response at its interface. Therefore, osteoconductive implants provide a biocompatible interface along which bone migrates. Bioglass® is both osteoproductive and osteoconductive and has an I_B of 10 [17]. Region D in **Figure 2** has an I_B of 0 while there is an I_B of 2 at region A, and it increases as the composition becomes more central on the ternary plot [18].

Experimental processes known to test for bioactivity include *in vivo* or *in vitro* studies. However, many scientists have performed *in vitro* studies such as Simulated Body Fluid (SBF) testing followed by Fourier Transform infrared spectroscopy (FTIR), Scanning electron microscopy (SEM), and X-ray diffraction (XRD). FTIR analysis is performed to detect the presence of HA formation by identifying and evaluating bond bending and stretching inherent to particular functional groups. XRD analysis is possible through the evaluation of phase analysis and identification of peaks absorbed at certain wavelengths, while SEM analysis is used to evaluate the morphology and microstructure of the HA formation. These are indicated in the following **Figure 3** for the analysis of a bioactive glass composition S4-Z1 after submersion in SBF solution at room temperature for 3, 7, 14, and 21 days respectively.

3. Development throughout the years

As Hench's introduction of the novel 45S5 Bioglass® to the medical and engineering era became popular, it birthed future opportunities and advancements for bioactive glasses as researchers sought to make targeted improvements with it to further their knowledge about their applications. Additionally, toxicity of the glasses and environmental factors such as temperature, pressure, and pH must be considered when designing a particular bioactive glass for medical applications. Throughout the years, bioactive glasses have been used in the following areas: dental fillings and treatment, scaffold production, incorporation into other materials such as polymers and for hard and soft bone tissue engineering [20]. Further exploration and experimentation with bioactive glass compositions, led to the formation of many different compositions intended for specific purposes which were achieved by incorporating other compounds to customize them based of the desired characteristics. A few base compositions that have been created overtime is listed in the following **Table 1**.

Most of the bioactive glass compositions in **Table 1** consists of the following four compounds: SiO_2, Na_2O, CaO, and P_2O_5. The original 45S5 composition served to identify which combinations of compounds produced a glass with ideal bioactive properties. While the S53P4 composition comprised of a slight variation of Hench's original 45S5 composition, the 13-93 and 13-93B1 compositions include compounds not found in Hench's original composition. Although these deviations from the 45S5 composition reduces their bioactive potential, other benefits are gained. For example, S53P4 bioactive glass is more stable than the 45S5 composition and borate-based bioactive glasses stimulate faster hydroxyapatite (HA) formation rates. Magnesium ions have been shown to increase bioactive glass antibacterial properties and synergize well with host Mg ions in the body during the bone formation process. Furthermore, the "addition of borate ions into the glass matrix has been proven to increase apatite

	Composition (wt%)									
Name	**SiO_2**	**Na_2O**	**CaO**	**P_2O_5**	**K_2O**	**MgO**	**B_2O_3**	**ZnO**	**CuO**	**Source**
45S5	45.0	24.5	24.5	6.0	•	•	•	•	•	[20]
S53P4	53.0	23.0	20.0	4.0	•	•	•	•	•	[20]
13-93	53.0	6.0	20.0	4.0	12.0	5.0	•	•	•	[20]
13-93B1	34.4	5.8	19.5	3.8	11.7	4.9	19.9	•	•	[20]
13-93B3	•	6.0	20.0	4.0	12.0	5.0	53.0	•	•	[22]
GL1605	•	6.4	20.0	4.0	12.0	5.0	51.6	1.0	0.4	[22]

Table 1.
Composition of various silicate-based bioactive glasses [20].

formation rates" on bioactive glass surfaces. This in turn opens the potential for a faster bone remodeling process [21].

The continuous evolution of bioactive glasses is also revealed through their clinical applications. Silica-base bioactive glasses such as the nominal 45S5 and the S53P4 composition were the original accepted standard in the implantation industry. Their rapid surface reaction time and comparatively low softening temperatures allow for optimal conditions for bone remodeling. Recently, though, borate-based bioactive glasses have gained a foothold in the tissue engineering market. Having been approved in 2016 and 2018 respectively, the 13-93B3 and GL1605 compositions represent the newer borate bioactive glass compositions. Borate glasses on average have been shown to release Na and Ca ions at a faster rate than their silica-based counterparts [22]. They are also responsible for slower regional pH increases than silica glasses due to reduced concentrations of alkali ions and the presence of boron. Whether these features are improvements to silica-based glasses or not is up to researchers and their intended applications, but nevertheless, borate glasses have contributed to the expansion of the bioactive glass market.

3.1 Limitations of bioactive glasses

Like all materials, researchers are continuously testing and expanding the limitations of the base bioactive compositions. For example, some base compositions are more appropriate for environments under constant load while others for those of brief, high load amplitudes. Another factor to consider is the alkalinization of regions introduced to bioactive glasses. While this may not be significant at lower concentrations, it hinders the extent that base bioactive glass compositions can be incorporated into the body since large pH changes can be detrimental to human health. Researchers in response have to determine viable methods of retaining the beneficial effects bioactive glasses present while lessening their control over regional pH. Likewise, the intrinsic brittle nature of bioactive glasses has prompted researchers to consider alternative methods of incorporating them into the body that maintain their biological benefits while increasing their strain to failure nature [23–25]. Rather than diverting valuable resources toward synthesizing different base bioactive glass compositions for singular uses, researchers are now looking to expand base properties through a variety of methods. The goal is to synthesize inorganic bioactive glasses that feature similar properties to materials found within the human body (**Table 2**).

Material	Compressive Modulus (GPa)	Bending Strength (MPa)	Compressive Strength (MPa)	Fracture Toughness (MPa m$^{1/2}$)	Vickers Hardness (MPa)	Structure	Source
HA	35–120	60–120	100–150	0.8–1.2	90–140	Ceramic	[20]
Bioglass® 45S5	60	40	•	0.6	•	Glass	[20]
Bioglass 52S4.6	60	40	•	•	•	Glass	[20]
Trabecular Bone	0.05–0.6	10–20	1.5–7.5	0.1–0.8	40–60	•	[20]
Cortical Bone	7–30	50–150	100–135	2–12	60–75	•	[20]

Table 2.
Mechanical properties of various bioactive glasses, ceramics, and human bones [20].

3.2 Doping-glass performance and manipulation

Customization and improvement of bioactive glasses can be achieved through doping. Doping involves the introduction of impurities or other elements into a base composition that would result in the enhancement in properties (mechanical, biological, structural, thermal, electrical, optical) of the particular product. Wetzel *et al* indicated a limitation of Bioglass® where it easily crystalized during high temperature processing. They deduced that the addition of Mg or Zn on the form of MgO or ZnO even at low concentrations improved the thermal behavior of Bioglass® [24]. Although doping is relatively simple to accomplish, the doping technique implemented can affect the extent of doping taking place. Likewise, there are various parameters one must consider when doping a material or bioglass in this instance. As previously stated, a doping technique must be selected under the assumption that some techniques are more applicable under certain conditions than others. For example, the standard melting technique is relatively straightforward, but the P_2O_5 within the bioactive glass has a much lower melting temperature than the other components [24–26]. A higher temperature processing can lead to the evaporation of a portion of the substance composition, therefore decreasing the overall bioactive potential of the glass along with other properties. Moreover, concentration of dopant material should be determined.

The CaO present in the Bioglass® composition increases its durability. Studies have shown that "when 10 mol% of CaO was substituted with 10 mol% SiO_2 to form 20%Na_2O-10%CaO-70%SiO_2", it exhibited a slower Na^+ dissolution, and a more stabilized SiO_2-rich surface film when compared to the binary 20%Na_2O-80%SiO_2. This is due to the presence of CaO acts as a modifier that increases the coupling reactions between Si-O-Si and NS bonds, stabilizing the SiO_2 rich film by filling the micro voids that form as a result of the Na dissolution, satisfies the bond in this film and prevents any further loss of Na ions [10]. The presence of P_2O_5 allows for the formation of a secondary calcium phosphate film that develops on the side that is in contact with the organic fluid environment.

In some bioactive glass and dopant compositions, low dopant concentrations may not produce the desired properties while high concentrations can. On the other hand, high dopant concentrations may have disadvantages associated with them such as cytotoxic and carcinogenic effects while low concentrations minimize them and provide protection from these drawbacks. Additionally, the application that a bioactive glass will be used for must also be taken into account when doping.

Other functional variables such as load, fatigue, temperature, and the substances that a bioactive glass will experience in its application are essential in the selection of a desired bioactive glass composition. While a doped bioactive glass may function well under minimal stress at room temperature, its properties may not be ideal in its environment of use. Therefore, it is important to consider the dopant material, concentration, and its application to ensure the promotion of ideal properties and the minimization of those that are not wanted.

Transition metals currently make up a large proportion of suitable dopants due to the medical benefits they provide. Elements like iron (Fe), copper (Cu), magnesium (Mg), and zinc (Zn) that already play vital roles within the human body are the focus of these studies [21, 26–30]. Similar interest has also been directed toward the rare earth elements. Various elements like Gadolinium (Gd), Erbium (Er), and Holmium (Ho) that are extensively used in a wide range of medical treatments are attractive avenues for researchers to explore [31–33]. While these make up most target dopant

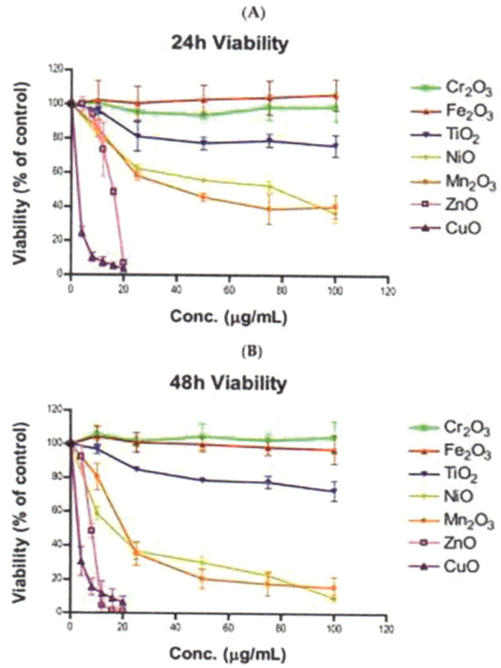

Figure 4.
Cell viability of various transition metal oxides on A549 cells. **Figure 1A** *and* **B** *Model the importance of researchers understanding the biological effects dopant compounds have on the human body. Cell viabilities below 70% are considered to be cytotoxic. While Cr_2O_3 and Fe_2O_3 caused little to no change in cellular viability, the same cannot be said for the oxides of Cu, Zn, Mn, and Ni. However, these ions are also key contributors to various vital functions in the human body [28].*

materials, much work is needed to understand the effects that doping a bioactive glass with one of these compounds will have and their extent. **Figure 4** reveals the cytotoxic effects that various transition element doping oxides have on cell lines. While some compounds may increase desired bioactive glass components, their biocompatibility should also be assessed before wide-spread usage.

3.2.1 Boron oxide (B_2O_5)

It has been experimentally revealed that borate glass systems exhibit greater hydroxyapatite (HA) formation and dissolution rates than their silicate-based relatives (ex: 45S5, 13-19, S53P4). Furthermore, borate glasses have been used for healing applications by medical professionals due to the borate ions possessing inherent antibacterial capabilities. When bioactive glasses are doped with borate ions, there was a "gradual increase in surface apatite formation rates" with increased concentration. [34] Additionally, the antibacterial properties of borate doped glass composition increased with greater doping concentrations. This trend is repeated microstructurally as the glass transition temperature, T_g, decreases with increasing borate concentrations. Moreover, the glass stability factor and crystallization peak temperature, T_p, gradually increased with increasing borate concentrations before decreasing once a concentration threshold is surpassed. This pattern is mirrored in cell proliferation studies and antibacterial tests concerning borate-doped bioactive glasses. Therefore, it is important for researchers to weigh the importance of enhanced HA formation against decreased glass stability, cell proliferation, and antibacterial properties at greater borate concentrations. As with all materials, the conditions these bioactive glasses will be performing in will determine the importance researchers place on these material properties.

3.2.2 Copper (Cu)

Cu is another metallic ion that researchers have incorporated into bioactive glass matrices and scaffolds to increase biological performance. Researchers are drawn to it because of its positive effects on endothelial cells and blood vessel maturation. Cu is also an essential ion in the human body and plays a pivotal role in angiogenesis, so doping bioactive glasses with it serves to enhance these benefits [28, 29]. This is upheld in Cu-doped calcium phosphates and bioactive glass scaffolds that reveal enhanced angiogenesis and stimulated osteogenesis in Cu-doped bioactive glass scaffolds. The Cu^{2+} ion also possesses natural antibacterial properties and works in conjunction with the Ca^{2+} ions in BGs to increase this property. Cu-doped bioactive glasses and scaffolds have also been shown to increase the differentiation levels of mesenchymal stem cells (MSCs) and act as catalyzing agents in endothelial cell proliferation. On the other hand, bioactive glasses and scaffolds doped with Cu are less suitable at elevated temperatures than their non-doped base compositions. This is due to Cu weakening the BG matrix when it is doped which leads to a decreased glass transition temperature, T_g. While this may not change the benefits doping bioactive glasses with Cu provides, it does limit the applications of Cu-doped bioactive glasses and scaffolds.

3.2.3 Gold (Au)

Bioactive glasses doped with gold nanoparticles (AuNPs) have also garnered interest among researchers. This is because AuNPs possess a wide range of biomedical applications like therapy, hygiene, diagnostics, and prevention. It is important to note that AuNPs with small diameters (1–2 nm) are toxic in the human body because they cause damage to cell structures when absorbed [35]. However, particle diameters from 3 to 100 nm appear to not have any toxic effect on cellular structures. Not only does doping with AuNPs increase a BG's biocompatibility, but they also increase the rate of the calcium phosphate layer on the surface, bettering its osteoconductive properties. Greater amplitudes in zeta potentials are also positively correlated with increasing dopant concentrations of AuNPs. In other words, increasing the dopant concentration of AuNP corresponds to greater long-term stability for the bioactive glasses. Interestingly, researchers have also discovered that AuNPs have the possibility of being released into nearby organs from the bioactive glasses they were doped with. This has led some to pursue methods of treatment delivery to specific regions of the body.

3.2.4 Iron (Fe)

Iron was one of the initial elements that were incorporated into bioactive glasses to increase their bioactivity and antibacterial properties [28]. Fe ions have been revealed to enhance the bone metabolism process which is why they were considered as potential doping candidates into bioactive glasses. Fe-doped bioactive glasses have characteristically lower crystallization temperatures than their non-doped counterparts and also have greater storage modulus values [27]. This is turn correlates to larger elastic modulus values for Fe-doped bioactive glasses, making them more suitable for implantation applications into the human body [25]. Likewise, scaffolds created from Fe-doped bioactive glasses have much greater degrees of formability than their base compositions. On the other hand, cytotoxic risks must be considered when doping with high concentrations of Fe which can have detrimental effects within patients and their environment. Interestingly, the magnetic properties present in Fe^{2+} ions are transferred into the base composition they are doped into. Researchers hope to take advantage of this magnetic behavior by expanding upon existing targeted therapeutic treatments.

3.2.5 Magnesium (Mg)

Magnesium is an important trace element in the human body, which is what makes it an excellent candidate for doping into bioactive glasses. The integral role Mg plays in bone development and maintenance drew researchers to include it among the first wave of transition metals to be considered as a suitable doping agent. Bioactive glasses doped with Mg have shown increased rates of HA formation on their surfaces and enhanced bioactive and antibacterial capabilities in comparison to their base concentrations [21]. Additionally, these bioactive glasses have exhibited superior long-term osteoconductive and biocompatibility properties. This is important because researchers are continuously seeking methods to increase biomedical implant lifespans since the percentage of individuals outliving their implants is increasing. Furthermore, Mg-doped bioactive glasses have promising applications in skeletal tissue regeneration due to their lower ionic release rates which do not affect the cellular environment to the extent of those with elevated rates.

3.2.6 Rare earth elements (REE)

Many REE ions have practical medical applications including but not limited to imaging techniques, cancer treatments, and pain relief [32]. Therefore, it is not surprising that some of these elements are viable options for therapeutic bioactive glasses. REE have been shown to promote bone repair and increase osteogenesis rates [31]. This is due to their ability to mimic calcium's role in the bone repair process and open the door to bone density disorder treatments. There are concerns about their cytotoxicity to both patients and the environment (**Table 3**), but that is for researchers to determine what level of risk is acceptable while achieving sought-after results [33]. Furthermore, the sustainability of REE's use as a whole is in question since demand for these naturally occurring elements will soon outweigh their supply. Solutions ranging from increased research into REE recycling and replacement are viable options to consider. However, one may also decide that the resources spent in developing a solution can be otherwise diverted to additional research into other dopant materials.

3.2.7 Silicon nitride (Si_3N_4)

Greater quantities of bone tissue around bioactive glasses have been observed with Si_3N_4-doped BGs [23]. This compound's high strength, fracture toughness, low friction wear, and biocompatibility make it an ideal doping substance for bioactive glasses designed for load-bearing purposes. It is also important to note that Si_3N_4 is an osteoconductive biomaterial with the potential to catalyze osteogenesis. In other words, this compound increases the rate of bone formation by reducing the time it takes bone-forming cells to reach their target regions. Like other viable dopants,

Compound	3 T3 NRU cytotoxicity test		Test *T. tubifex*			Source
	IC_{50} (μg/ mL)	Calculated LD_{50} (mg/ kg b.w.)	EC_{50} (g/ L)	EC_{50} (mol/ L)	$IgEC_{50}$ (mol/ L)	[33]
Erbium (III) chloride hexahydrate	613.1	1135.2	31.6	0.0827	- 1.08	[33]
Lanthanum (III) chloride heptahydrate	379.4	962.6	28.2	0.076	- 1.12	[33]
Praseodymium (III) chloride hydrate	532.4	1085.1	18.7	0.0755	- 1.12	[33]
Europium (III) chloride hexahydrate	530.3	1078.4	26.9	0.0734	- 1.13	[33]
Gadolinium (III) chloride hexahydrate	571.2	1120.7	27.4	0.0736	- 1.13	[33]
Ytterbium (III) chloride hexahydrate	423.1	1001.3	31.0	0.0801	- 1.10	[33]
Samarium (III) chloride hexahydrate	575.6	1124.0	25.1	0.0689	- 1.16	[33]
Thulium (III) chloride anhydrous	440.7	1015.0	22.7	0.0825	- 1.08	[33]
Dysprosium (III) chloride hexahydrate	931.8	1264.0	31.5	0.0836	- 1.08	[33]
Terbium (III) chloride hexahydrate	397.4	979.2	31.6	0.0846	- 1.07	[33]
Holmium (III) chloride hexahydrate	963.6	1205.3	27.1	0.0714	- 1.15	[33]
Lutetium (III) chloride hexahydrate	580.2	1066.5	34.3	0.088	- 1.06	[33]
Yttrium (III) chloride hexahydrate	377.0	959.6	31.0	0.0801	- 1.10	[33]
Neodymium (III) chloride hexahydrate	418.5	966.2	25.8	0.072	- 1.14	[33]
Cerium (III) chloride heptahydrate	501.9	1067.1	31.7	0.0852	- 1.07	[33]
Barium Chloride	661.5	1184.0	15.6	0.075	- 1.12	[33]
Cadmium chloride	0.252	62.7	16.5	0.09	- 1.05	[33]

Table 3.
Cytotoxicity and Ecotoxicity of rare earth compounds [33].

Si_3N_4 promotes MSC differentiation into osteoblasts and improves their adhesion to organic material. This in turn leads to an increased production of collagen and mineralization, enhancing the bone formation process. The increased bone formation also corresponds with an increase in environment pH. This is due to the Na^+ and Ca^{2+} ions being released during bone formation that create hydroxides which contribute to an increase in regional pH. This phenomenon is shared among most bioactive glass compositions, and there are a multitude of methods to negate potential detrimental effects to patients.

3.2.8 Silver (Ag)

Silver was one of the first transition metals that researchers attempted to dope bioactive glasses with. This is due to its inherent antibacterial capability that covers a wide array of diseases. Medical professionals have enjoyed its benefits in surgical applications and researchers sought to expand upon their success. It has been observed that Ag-doped bioactive glasses have greater bioactive and antibacterial capabilities than their non-doped bioactive glass counterparts [28]. Furthermore, Ag particles are able to diffuse uniformly throughout the bioactive glasses in which they are doped. The feature of not forming a separate Ag layer at the glass surface is important because some unintended and potentially dangerous cellular responses can occur [36]. Likewise, the antibacterial and bioactive benefits Ag particles present are countered by their possible cytotoxic effects in the human body at high concentrations. Therefore, researchers' margin of error and the specific application of these bioactive glasses play key roles in determining the extent they are doped with Ag particles.

3.2.9 Zinc (Zn) and strontium (Sr)

Zinc and Strontium have been doped separately and together into bioactive glass compositions to optimize their properties. Zn is responsible for promoting bone formation while Sr. has been found to limit bone resorption and promote bone remodeling [30]. Bioactive glasses, MSC proliferation and differentiation processes are also increased by the doping of Zn and Sr. When Zn is doped into the glass matrix, it is distributed uniformly, and the surface matrix experiences an accelerated growth of its apatite layer. This in turn corresponds to an overall increase in bioactivity. It is important to note that doping the bioactive glass with too much Zn will increase the potential of cytotoxic effects and a create a lower degradation profile. Additionally, solely doping a bioactive glass with Sr. has been found to limit the formation of the apatite layer on the glass surface. Furthermore, the Sr-glass network is looser than the base glass and Zn-glass networks due to Sr's ionic radius being larger than those of Ca, the element being substituted with the dopant material, and Zn. Although extensive research has been done regarding these differences in glass networks, there do not seem to be any significant effects in BG properties when low doping concentrations are used. Likewise, it has been experimentally determined that small molar concentrations of Zn (~2%) and Sr. (~5%) produce optimum cell proliferation and differentiation properties, minimizing negative effects associated with elevated doping concentrations. Co-doping the bioactive glass composition with both Zn and Sr. results in a combination of the two dopant effects. The (Zn + Sr)-glass network promotes cell proliferation and differentiation while also limiting the formation of the glass's surface apatite formation and bone resorption. These represent a few of the various elements and their effects that are considered throughout the glass doping process.

4. Conclusion

Over the past few decades, since the discovery of Bioglass® in 1969, hundreds of other bioactive glass compositions have been derived or attempted, all with the hopes of either improving properties of existing applications such as metal implants, or to personalize a specific composition for a unique application. For instance, using a bioactive glass composition to coat a particular metal alloy for implantation. Over the years, researchers have introduced elements in the form of compounds into base compositions with the aim of achieving distinct properties such as increased bioactivity, anti-bacterial behavior, bone proliferation, etc. Therefore, they have since seen promising outcome when incorporating elements such as magnesium, copper, zinc, boron, and strontium, just to name a few. The evolution of bioactive glasses has already shown promising progress and is expected to be become a staple prat in medical devices and applications within the near future. However, this journey has yet to continue. It is important to evaluate the biological response to the newly developed bioactive glass compositions to fully understand their risks and benefits. We are curious to see where this field is leading us in the next years.

Acknowledgements

A special thanks is directed toward Dr. Vijay Vaidyanathan, Founding Chair of the Biomedical Engineering department at the University of North Texas in Denton, TX, through which all of this is possible.

Conflict of interest

The authors declare no conflict of interest.

Author details

Joy-anne N. Oliver*, Olanrewaju Akande and Melanie Ecker
Biomedical Engineering Department, Materials Science and Engineering, University of North Texas, Denton, TX, USA

*Address all correspondence to: joy-anneoliver@my.unt.edu

References

[1] Hench LL, Kokubo T. Properties of bioactive glasses and glass-ceramics. In: Handbook of Biomaterial Properties [Internet]. Springer US; 1998 [cited 2021 Jun 10]. p. 355-63. Available from: https://link.springer.com/chapter/10.1007/978-1-4615-5801-9_22

[2] Simmons JH, JNCS. The Professional Life of Larry L. Hench – a true renaissance scientist/engineer. J Non Cryst Solids. 2016 Mar 15;436:58-61.

[3] Karlsson KH, Hupa L. Thirty-five years of guided tissue engineering. J Non Cryst Solids. 2008 Jan 15;354(2-9): 717-21.

[4] Jones JR. Reprint of: Review of bioactive glass: From Hench to hybrids. Vol. 23, Acta Biomaterialia. Elsevier Ltd; 2015. p. S53-82.

[5] Hench LL. The story of Bioglass®. In: Journal of Materials Science: Materials in Medicine. 2006. p. 967-78.

[6] Kokubo T. Bioactive glass ceramics: properties and applications. Biomaterials. 1991 Mar 1;12(2):155-63.

[7] Hench LL, Splinter RJ, Allen WC, Greenlee TK. Bonding mechanisms at the interface of ceramic prosthetic materials. J Biomed Mater Res [Internet]. 1971 Nov 1 [cited 2021 Jun 10];5(6):117-41. Available from: https://onlinelibrary.wiley.com/doi/full/10.1002/jbm.820050611

[8] Wilson J, Pigott GH, Schoen FJ, Hench LL. Toxicology and bio-compatibility of bioglasses. J Biomed Mater Res [Internet]. 1981 Nov 1 [cited 2021 May 23];15(6):805-17. Available from: https://onlinelibrary.wiley.com/doi/full/10.1002/jbm.820150605

[9] Clark AE, Hench LL, Paschall HA. The influence of surface chemistry on implant interface histology: A theoretical basis for implant materials selection. J Biomed Mater Res [Internet]. 1976 Mar 1 [cited 2021 May 23];10(2):161-74. Available from: https://onlinelibrary.wiley.com/doi/full/10.1002/jbm.820100202

[10] Hench LL. Physical chemistry of glass surfaces. J Non Cryst Solids. 1977 Sep 8;25(1-3):343-69.

[11] Hench LL, Wilson J. Surface-active biomaterials. Vol. 226, Science. 1984. p. 630-6.

[12] Oliver J anne N, Su Y, Lu X, Kuo PH, Du J, Zhu D. Bioactive glass coatings on metallic implants for biomedical applications. Vol. 4, Bioactive Materials. KeAi Communications Co.; 2019. p. 261-70.

[13] Hench LL, Best SM. Ceramics, Glasses, and Glass-Ceramics: Basic Principles. In: Biomaterials Science: An Introduction to Materials: Third Edition. Elsevier Inc.; 2013. p. 128-51.

[14] Jones JR. Review of bioactive glass: From Hench to hybrids. Vol. 9, Acta Biomaterialia. 2013. p. 4457-86.

[15] Baino F. Bioactive glasses – When glass science and technology meet regenerative medicine. Vol. 44, Ceramics International. Elsevier Ltd; 2018. p. 14953-66.

[16] Koga N, Strnad Z, Šesták J, Strnad J. Journal of Thermal A nalysis and Calorimetry, V ol. Vol. 71. 2003.

[17] Cao W, Hench LL. Bioactive materials. Ceram Int. 1996 Jan 1;22(6): 493-507.

[18] Hench LL. Bioglass: 10 milestones from concept to commerce. J Non Cryst Solids. 2016 Jan 15;432:2-8.

[19] Goudarzi Z, Parvin N, Sharifianjazi F. Formation of hydroxyapatite on surface of SiO2–P2O5–CaO–SrO–ZnO bioactive glass synthesized through sol-gel route. Ceram Int. 2019 Oct 15;45(15):19323-30.

[20] Verrier S, Blaker JJ, Maquet V, Hench LL, Boccaccini AR. PDLLA/Bioglass® composites for soft-tissue and hard-tissue engineering: An in vitro cell biology assessment. Biomaterials. 2004 Jul 1;25(15):3013-21.

[21] Wetzel R, Bartzok O, Hupa L, Brauer DS. Low Mg or Zn substitution for improved thermal properties of Bioglass 45S5. Mater Lett. 2019 Dec 1;256:126599.

[22] Jung S, Day T, Boone T, Buziak B, Omar A. Anti-biofilm activity of two novel, borate based, bioactive glass wound dressings. Biomed Glas [Internet]. 2019 Jan 1 [cited 2021 May 25];5(1):67-75. Available from: https://doi.org/10.1515/bglass-2019-0006

[23] Marin E, Adachi T, Boschetto F, Zanocco M, Rondinella A, Zhu W, et al. Biological response of human osteosarcoma cells to Si3N4-doped Bioglasses. Mater Des. 2018 Dec 5;159:79-89.

[24] Fu Q, Rahaman MN, Sonny Bal B, Brown RF, Day DE. Mechanical and in vitro performance of 13-93 bioactive glass scaffolds prepared by a polymer foam replication technique. Acta Biomater [Internet]. 2008;4:1854-64. Available from: www.sciencedirect.com

[25] Saxena V, Kumar V, Singh A, Singh VK. Effect of reinforcing S53P4 bioactive glass on physio-mechanical and biological properties of Ti-8Nb-2Fe alloy. 2019; Available from: https://doi.org/10.1016/j.ceramint.2019.07.184

[26] Balamurugan A, Balossier G, Kannan S, Michel J, Rebelo AHS, Ferreira JMF. Development and in vitro characterization of sol-gel derived CaO-P 2 O 5-SiO 2-ZnO bioglass. Available from: www.actamat-journals.com

[27] Chiu K-Y, Chen K-K, Wang Y-H, Lin F-H, Huang J-Y. Formability of Fe-doped bioglass scaffold via selective laser sintering. 2020; Available from: https://doi.org/10.1016/j.ceramint.2020.03.216

[28] Gupta N, Santhiya D, Murugavel S, Kumar A, Aditya A, Ganguli M, et al. Effects of transition metal ion dopants (Ag, Cu and Fe) on the structural, mechanical and antibacterial properties of bioactive glass. 2017; Available from: https://doi.org/10.1016/j.colsurfa.2017.11.023

[29] Hoppe A, Meszaros R, Stähli C, Romeis S, Schmidt J, Peukert W, et al. In vitro reactivity of Cu doped 45S5 Bioglassâ derived scaffolds for bone tissue engineering. [cited 2021 Apr 21]; Available from: www.rsc.org/MaterialsB

[30] Wu X, Meng G, Wang S, Wu F, Huang W, Gu Z. Zn and Sr incorporated 64S bioglasses: Material characterization, in-vitro bioactivity and mesenchymal stem cell responses. Mater Sci Eng C. 2015 Jul 1;52:242-50.

[31] Zhu D-Y, lu B, Yin J, Ke Q-F, Xu he, Zhang chang-Q, et al. gadolinium-doped bioglass scaffolds promote osteogenic differentiation of hjBMsc via the akt/gsK3β pathway and facilitate bone repair in vivo. Int J Nanomedicine [Internet]. 2019 [cited 2021 Apr 21];14:1085-100. Available from: http://dx.doi.org/10.2147/IJN.s193576

[32] Giese E. Rare Earth Elements: therapeutic and diagnostic applications in modern medicine. Clin Med Reports. 2018;2(1).

[33] Rucki M, Kejlova K, Vlkova A, Jirova D, Dvorakova M, Svobodova L, et al. Evaluation of toxicity profiles of rare earth elements salts (lanthanides) *. 2020; Available from: https://doi.org/10.1016/j.jre.2020.02.011

[34] Prasad S. S, Datta S, Adarsh T, Diwan P, Annapurna K, Kundu B, et al. Effect of boron oxide addition on structural, thermal, in vitro bioactivity and antibacterial properties of bioactive glasses in the base S53P4 composition. J Non Cryst Solids [Internet]. 2018; 498(May):204-15. Available from: https://doi.org/10.1016/j.jnoncrysol.2018.06.027

[35] Magyari K, Nagy-Simon T, Vulpoi A, Popescu RA, Licarete E, Stefan R, et al. Novel bioactive glass-AuNP composites for biomedical applications. 2017 [cited 2021 May 19]; Available from: http://dx.doi.org/10.1016/j.msec.2017.03.138

[36] Kozon D, Zheng K, Boccardi E, Liu Y, Liverani L, Boccaccini AR. Synthesis of monodispersed Ag-doped bioactive glass nanoparticles via surface modification. Materials (Basel) [Internet]. 2016 [cited 2021 May 20];9(4). Available from: /pmc/articles/PMC5502798/

Chapter 7

Novel Dental Implants with Herbal Composites: A Review

Gopathy Sridevi and Seshadri Srividya

Abstract

Missing a permanent tooth is a miserable condition faced by a common man. A tooth decay, periodontitis, mechanical trauma, or any systemic complications lead to such a complication. These bone defects when left untreated lead to severe resorption of the alveolar bone. A proper dental filling with an appropriate bone substitute material could prevent such resorption and paves a way for subsequent implant placement. Dental implants are considered as the prime option by dentists to replace a single tooth or prevent bone resorption. A variety of bone substitutes are available differ in origin, consistency, particle size, porosity, and resorption characteristics. Herbal composites in dentistry fabricated using biphospho-calcium phosphate, casein, chitosan, and certain herbal extracts of *Cassia occidentalis*, *Terminalia arjuna* bark, *Myristica fragans* also were reported to possess a higher ossification property, osteogenic property and were able to repair bone defects. C. occidentalis was reported to stimulate mineralization of the bone and osteoblastic differentiation through the activation of the PI3K-Akt/MAPKs pathway in MC3T3-E1 cells of mice. This implant proved better osteoconductivity and bioactivity compared to pure HAP and other BCP ratios. Terminalia Arjuna was also worked in the incorporation in the graft to enhance the osteogenic property of the implant and gave good results. Another implant bone graft was synthesized containing BCP, biocompatible casein, and the extracts of *Myristica fragans* and subjected to *in vitro* investigations and the results revealed the deposition of apatite on the graft after immersing in SBF and also the ALP activity was high when treated with MG-63 cells, NIH-3 T3, and Saos 2 cell lines. This study indicates that the inclusion of plant extract enhances the osteogenic property of the graft. Thus, these novel dental implants incorporated with herbal composites evaluated by researchers revealed an enhanced bone healing, accelerates osseointegration, inhibits osteopenia, and inhibits inflammation. This application of herbal composite inclusion in dentistry and its applications has a greater potential to improve the success rate of dental implants and allows the implications of biotechnology in implant dentistry.

Keywords: bone defect, dental filling, implant, hydroxyapatite, osseointegration, herb, osteoconducting

1. Introduction

Human teeth are the hardest substance in the human body that enhances the beauty of a person. It is a highly important structure that helps in food chewing to mechanically break down the food by cutting and crushing them in preparation for swallowing and digesting. It also aids in speech and its articulation of words. Human teeth consist of 20 primary (deciduous, "baby" or "milk") teeth in children and 32 permanent teeth in adults. Teeth are classified as incisors, canines, premolars, and molars. Incisors are primarily used for cutting the food into pieces, canines are used for tearing the tissues of the food, and molars help to grind the food into smaller substances [1].

Teeth are also important for cosmetic purposes as well. Many dental treatments are not purposefully dealt with filling and taking out a tooth, but indeed nowadays people turn out to esthetic dentistry to improve, straighten, lighten, reshape, and repair teeth as well. The field of esthetic dentistry includes the establishment of veneers, crown bridges, implants, tooth-colored filling, and teeth whitening procedures.

1.1 Tooth loss

Tooth exfoliation starts from childhood. A young boy or girl loses the baby teeth, and it gets exfoliated in response to permanent teeth that start developing beneath them. This loss of primary teeth begins around the age of six and continues till 12 years of age. The primary teeth that are vulnerable are the upper and lower lateral incisors that shed at 7–8 years and upper canines are that shed around 10–12 years of age. Only the upper and lower first molars shed at 9–11 years of age and upper and lower second molars shed at 10–12 years of age [2].

1.2 Pathological tooth loss

Tooth loss is a condition that advances with the increase of age. This occurs as a result of mechanical disturbances and abnormal forces that act during the chewing process of hard substances, traumatic injury, etc. Also, a few conditions such as untreated dental caries (tooth decay) and severe periodontal (gum) disease might lead to loss of permanent teeth. Tooth decay is the primary cause of tooth loss. It is caused by the increased plaque retention on the teeth followed by bacterial invasion of the plaque. This ultimately results in dental caries and the formation of cavities. Untreated tooth cavities for a chronic period of time lead to the breakdown of the tooth. This bacterial invasion and retention of plaque deposits also affects the gums and bones attached to the tooth and loses its ability to hold the tooth. Periodontal structures are tissues that support teeth and their attachment to the bone. Diseases of the gums and bones are caused by bacterial invasion of teeth and retention of plaque. It results in diseases of the gums leading to periodontitis and detachment of supporting structures of the teeth and eventually causes tooth loss. So, the ultimate care of oral hygiene is the only preventive measure to prevent tooth loss. Good oral hygiene is the process of maintaining proper brushing of teeth two times a day with fluoridated toothpaste and frequent flossing. Regular dental check-ups every 6 months can be availed to ensure good teeth and prevent tooth loss [3].

1.3 Mechanical trauma and tooth loss

There are a few conditions like bruxism otherwise called teeth grinding that occurs during sleep. This condition is very common in people who tend to be awake by profession at night. This tooth grinding increases the wear and tear action on the tooth and causes mechanical injury. The risk of tooth fractures is common in sportspeople, especially in football and goalie. Research reports claim that smoking is another important cause of tooth loss. Reports from countries, such as the United States, Germany, and

Japan, show a strong relationship between cigarette smoking and tooth loss. The habit of smoking weakens the body's immune response to infection and causes immunosuppression. This makes it harder to guard against a gum infection and takes a longer time to heal. Reports reveal that systemic diseases also relate to tooth loss. Conditions, such as cardiovascular diseases, diabetes mellitus, cancer, and osteoporosis, also lead to permanent tooth loss due to their secondary complications. Therefore, tooth loss is not restricted to poor oral hygiene but poor maintenance of overall health [4–6].

1.4 Treatment options for missing tooth

Missing a permanent tooth is a miserable condition. Years after years the treatment options for missing teeth are dental implants, fixed dental bridges, removable partial dentures. Dental implants are considered as the prime option by dentists to replace a single tooth. This procedure involves the surgical mounting of a titanium metal post or frame on the upper or lower jaw along with mounting the replaced missing tooth. This dental implant acts as a permanent base for the replaced tooth. This procedure is highly advantageous because the replaced dental implant resembles a natural tooth and can last for decades. It also acts independently and does not disturb the adjacent normal tooth. The next treatment option is a fixed dental bridge. This procedure provides bridging between the gaps caused by the lost tooth and involves the employment of a dental prosthesis or an artificial tooth. This dental prosthesis would be attached to adjacent teeth and bonded in place with dental cement. A removable partial denture consists of replacement teeth that are attached to a natural-looking pink base. The natural teeth also act to stabilize and hold the removable plastic base in its position place. This pink base is designed in a way that matches the color of the gums and the color of the normal teeth [7].

2. Dental implants

A dental implant is a material placed in or on the oral tissues that help to support the oral prosthesis. An ideal implant material should possess the following characteristics. It should be biocompatible and possess adequate strength, rigidity, good corrosive, and be capable of wear and fracture resistance. The principles of designing a dental implant should be much compatible with the physical properties of the material. Materials that are used for fabricating a dental implant can be considered according to the chemical composition of the implant and their biological responses. Many reports claim that these dental implants may be made from metals, ceramics, or polymers [8].

2.1 Titanium and its alloys

According to the American Society for testing and materials, there are six distinct types of titanium that are widely available as implant biomaterials. They are grade I, II, III, IV Cp Ti, various combinations of titanium, aluminum like alpha-beta alloy containing 6% Al and 4% V, alpha-beta titanium alloy containing 6% aluminum and 7% niobium, alpha-beta titanium alloy with non-ferrous metal. The physical and mechanical properties, such as tensile strength and osseointegration, elastic modulus, non-toxic nature, are quite different for the different alloys. The most important property related to the oxygen residuals in the metals and the other two titanium is considered as very low interstitial alloys. Among all the available alloys, the commercially prepared pure titanium alloys are generally considered as pure and mentioned in Grade I, Grade II, Grade III, and Grade IV titanium and has wide applications in implant manufacturing. Some trace elements, such as carbon, oxygen, nitrogen, and iron, are also considered in this process. Although titanium possesses many strengthening characteristics, literature reports reveal that it evokes a stronger reaction in the host causing hypersensitivity reactions, failed implants with increased concentration of titanium in peri-implanted tissues, regional nodes, and pulmonary tissues based on animal models, allergy to titanium in the form of urticaria, pruritus of the mucosa or skin, atopic dermatitis, poor fracture healing, necrosis and immunosuppression and weakening of orthopedically implanted titanium [9].

2.2 Ceramics

Ceramics has been widely used as a dental implant coating and it was the first introduced material in the field of implant dentistry. Hydroxyapatite is one of the most known biocompatible materials commonly used as a coating for metal implants. These hydroxyapatite coatings create a good interfacial strength between bone and implant. It provides greater implant stability and improves bone healing that lies adjacent to implants. The use of hydroxyapatite improves the capacity of osseointegration and increases the rate of rehabilitation of patients. This method of implanting decreases the time from implant insertion to final reconstruction of the implant [10]. There are various methods to coat hydroxyapatite on implants, they include sol–gel coating, electrophoretic deposition, plasma spraying, sputter-deposition, and biomimetic precipitation. Ceramic materials that are used for dental implanting and coatings. The materials used are hydroxylapatite (HA), tricalcium phosphate, fluorapatite (FA), tetracalcium phosphate, calcium pyrophosphate, brushite, bioglasses, aluminum oxide, zirconium oxide, etc. (**Figure 1**).

2.3 Metals as dental implants

In the field of dental implanting, metals are widely selected based on factors that involve properties belong to its biomechanical characteristics, machining characteristics, and surface finishing characteristics as well. In the present day, metals, such as

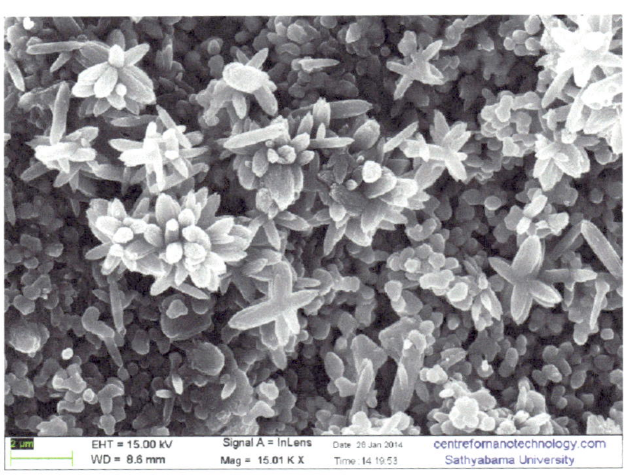

Figure 1.
SEM-image of hydroxyapatite.

Co-Cr, stainless steel, and gold are quite outdated in the dental implant industry and the currently available dental metals are alloys of titanium and zirconium as well. Certain components of dental implants such as the abutment screws and some attachments of the implants are also made of alloys of gold, stainless steel, and Co-Cr. Titanium is mostly considered as an effective material by most of the dentists for its wide intraosseous applications. It has enormous and typical properties, such as lesser readily affected or corroded by the environment, high resistance to chemical dosing, and capability to repair on its own. The resistance to being deformed elastically—modulus of elasticity was very compatible with that of bone and titanium oxide [11, 12]. Although titanium is a typical material suitable for dental implanting, it faces a lot of shortfalls. These drawbacks and detrimental properties of titanium ultimately resulted in prompting the scientists to look and research the new implant from other biomaterials [13].

The next innovation to overcome the said shortfalls led to the development of ceramic implants [14]. And as a result of this zirconia is used as another material for dental inserts. This in turn contrasted with metallic components zirconia demonstrated the least particle discharge and they are thought to be dormant in the body [15]. Zirconia acts as a tooth-like shading and possesses great mechanical properties and has great biocompatibility. In such a way, it is by all accounts an appropriate dental material [16]. The utilization of zirconia implants keeps a strategic distance from the inconvenience and acquiesces to the demand of numerous patients without metal inserts. The material additionally gives high quality, crack sturdiness, and biocompatibility [17]. There are various materials used for fabricating endosseous dental implants like titanium, titanium alloy, stainless steel, alumina, carbon, bioglass, polyurethane, etc. [18–20].

A novel implant, the ceria-stabilized zirconia-alumina-aluminate composite was developed and was established for its significant effect that it is not prone to aging. This implant represents a probable alternative to the yttrium-stabilized zirconia that is used for ceramic oral implants. This implant was evaluated for its long-term stability due to its make with Ce-TZP-comp and it proved a significant lowest fracture load after combined loading/aging [21].

2.4 Polymers

A variety of polymers have been utilized as dental implant materials [22]. A portion of the polymer materials is polymethylmethacrylate, polytetrafluoroethylene, polyethylene, polyurethane, and polysulfone, etc. When polymer acts as a coating layer, inferior mechanical properties, lack of adhesion to living tissues, and adverse immunologic reactions are eliminated [23–26]. In the present day, polymeric materials are constrained to assemble the shock retaining segments joined into the superstructures bolstered by inserts [26]. A wide variety of biomaterials have found profound applications in the form of inserts. This type of insert in implantology requires a suitable biomaterial of choice. The presently available biomaterials, such as bioceramics and other composite biomaterials, are under higher consideration and the precise examination of such biomaterial definitely have a promising future in the field of dental applications.

3. Herbal composites in dentistry

Herbal medicine is an indigenous system of traditional Hindu medicine and is native to the Indian subcontinent. Contemporary practices derived from ayurvedic traditions are also a type of alternative medicine. Ayurveda recommends some daily use therapeutic procedures for the prevention of and maintenance of oral health. It involves Dant Dhavani (brushing), Jivha Lekhana (tongue scrapping), and Gandoosha (gargling) or even oil pulling and tissue regeneration therapies. Various herbs are widely used in dentistry and they are aloe vera [27], cloves [28], eucalyptus [29], peppermint [30], and turmeric [31].

3.1 Icariin

Icariin, one of the traditional Chinese herbal medicines, possesses significant evidence that it strengthens bones, enhances healing of bone, inhibits osteopenic effect, and inhibits inflammation. This idea made scientists incorporate icariin for better osseointegration of dental implants and shorten the rehabilitation time of patients and the results revealed that. Evaluation of the hypothesis: Limited success has been achieved to help implant surgery in icariin significantly improved the success rate of the dental implant [32].

3.2 Ascorbic acid

Another randomized trial of preparing a biocomposite osteogenic nanofiber was developed with the incorporation of polycaprolactone, hydroxyapatite, dexamethasone, gelatin, beta-glycerophosphate, and ascorbic acid along with titanium implants was developed so that it mimics the bone extracellular matrix and eventually induced osteogenesis in the peri-implant niche and also regenerates the osseous tissue. This implant was worked on rabbit models and the results revealed that a coating of osteogenic nanofibrous tissues significantly increased the magnitude of osteogenesis around the zone of peri-implant tissue and also favored the dynamics of osseointegration [33].

3.3 Cassia Occidentalis

Cassia occidentalis Linn belongs to the family Caesalpiniaceae and is commonly called Kasondi in Hindi. It is mostly grown in the southern parts of India and the plant products have been used for various ailments and have a rich medicinal value [34]. C. occidentalis (CO) contains significant bioactive compounds, such as terpenoids, anthraquinones, and carotenoids. The plant products were reported to stimulate mineralization of the bone and osteoblastic differentiation through the activation of the PI3K-Akt/MAPKs pathway in MC3T3-E1 cells of mice [35].

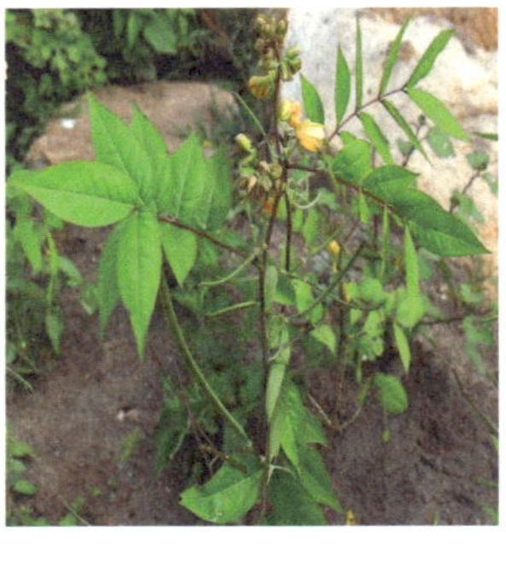

3.4 Cassia Occidentalis

3.4.1 Herbal composite using orange and potato peel, papaya leaf, calendula flower extract

Another novel dental implant synthesized a nanohydroxyapatite using different methods by utilizing the biomolecules from waste products, such as an egg-shell. In this study, an institutional controlled synthesis of nano-sized HAP was performed, which can be employed in the future for another material synthesis thereby an improved bone bonding was obtained by this novel material [36]. A novel implant synthesized with nano HAP rods was performed by an *in situ* method using poly (vinyl alcohol) (PVA). These PVA nano-sized crystals of HAP obtained were further subjected to *in vitro* analysis using simulated body fluid. The nano-sized crystal of HAP composite improved its hardness when treated with PVA and it overcomes the brittleness of pure HAP [37].

3.4.2 Porous scaffolds

A prepared porous scaffold using nano HAP and nylon 6,6 using a salt-leaching technique was a newly handled technique. Here HAP was dispersed on the pore walls of the scaffold bonds well with nylon 6,6 and it increased the stiffness of the scaffold. This porous scaffold acts to be effective as a three-dimensional substrate for bone tissue engineering [38]. Another method developed on dental implanting includes the synthesis of biphospho-calcium phosphate (BCP) for calcium-deficient apatites, such as enamel, dentin, and bone mineral by a process of sintering. The prepared BCP had controlled bioactivity when the HAP/βTCP ratio was controlled. This form of BCP can be used as carriers for growth factors, drug delivery systems, and in tissue engineering [39].

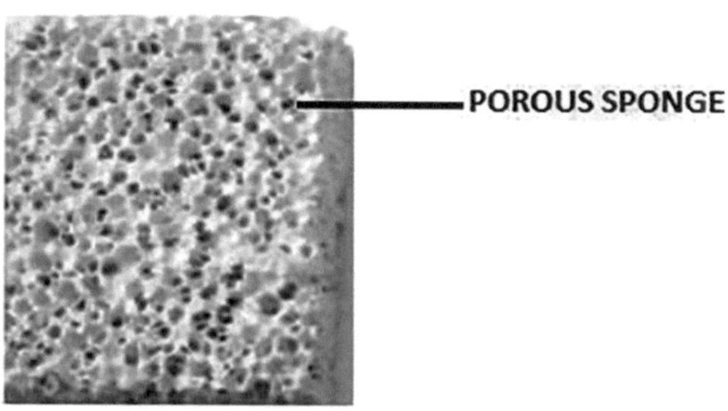

Another preparation included natural porous bioceramics from processing the cancellous bone. Calcined bovine bone was treated with sodium pyrophosphate and sintered to obtain HAP and was in turn converted to βTCP and BCP. This process was done to improve and increase the bioactivity of the ceramics when placed *in vivo* [40].

A newly evolved technique was prepared by using BCP with different HAP/βTCP ratios and was analyzed for its bioactivity with SBF solution and osteoconductivity in rabbits. The study found that BCP with a HAP/TCP ratio of 60:40 was found to be best in showing the bioactivity and osteoconductivity compared to pure HAP and other BCP ratios. A newly developed implant was created using a coating material for orthopedic metal implants. In this study, a new bioglass was prepared and coated on Ti-based and Co-Cr alloys. This was done to enhance the cell adhesion when placed *in vivo* as a dental implant. This coated metal implant was prepared for dental applications [41].

Another novel implant was prepared by using composite material consisting of poly-L-lactide (PLLA) and bioactive glass by solvent evaporation technique. The composite was bathed and soaked in SBF for 3 days for allowing the HAP deposition on the composite. The dried composite was subjected to various characterization techniques. The study found that the bioactivity of the composite was highly increased and it, in turn, supported the composite to promote bone integration when placed *in vivo* [42].

3.4.3 Chitosan-HAP composite

Another group of researchers synthesized a composite containing chitosan, HAP, and bioglass. Chitosan-HAP composite was prepared using calcium nitrate and orthophosphoric acid in SBF. The novel prepared composite bioactive glass was added to this preparation. *In vitro* bioactivity was determined for the composite and the study found that the addition of bioactive glass improved the compression strength of the material [43]. A prepared HAP-bioglass composite was developed to improve the compression strength of the composite compared to pure HAP. In this study, HAP was synthesized and combined with a varying percentage of bioglass and was pelletized. The biocomposite dental implanting material was characterized using various techniques and the study found that HAP with 10% bioglass was having increased bioactivity and compression strength (**Figure 2**) [44].

3.4.4 Vitamin E

Another implant was prepared with a bioglass composite film consisting of poly (3-hydroxybutyrate) and vitamin E. The incorporation of vitamin E was done to increase the protein adsorption and hydrophilicity on the surface of the film. This

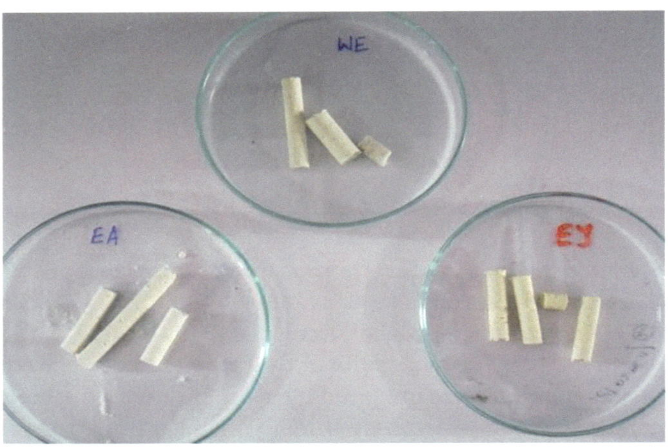

Figure 2.
Cassia occidentalis.

composite film was subjected to various characterized studies and the results reported that they can be applied [45] in tissue engineering as a better matrix material for cell adhesion [46]. Chin et al. worked on preparing a novel multi-component skin substitute by using collagen as a matrix material which typically depicts the normal architecture of the skin. This implanting material has a main advantage in producing a cost-effective bone substitute. A novel prepared magnetic fibrin incorporated with nanoparticles and characterized those nanoparticles by various physicochemical techniques using Saos 2 cells, the cell viability, adhesion, and alkaline phosphatase assay. The study revealed that the [47] material exhibited good osteogenic property and hence it can be used in bone tissue engineering .

3.4.5 Collagen

Auxenfans et al. [48], a researcher investigated a scaffold that contains collagen and glycosaminoglycans (GAG). The matrix was seeded with fibroblast and the study found that it forms a typical reconstructed skin or hemicornea once epithelialization completes. Another study analyzed the rate of degradation of pure collagen and collagen–HAP beads using collagenase enzyme. This enzyme was able to digest pure collagen quickly compared to collagen-HAP gel beads. The HAP provides resistance for quick degradation and the matrix structure could be maintained for a greater period and it supports the cell to adhere, proliferate, and then differentiate [49].

3.4.6 Gluataraldehyde and barium sulfate

Another research study reported the collagen type II scaffolds by cross-linking with glutaraldehyde and scaffold without cross-linking with glutaraldehyde. The study explained that the scaffolds were seeded with chondrocytes and observed the interaction of cells with the scaffold. The cell adherence on the surface of the scaffold was high which was confirmed by SEM analysis [50]. Another implant using used barium sulfate and zirconia as additives to implant as a bone cement was created to enhance the visualization through X-ray imaging. The incorporation of these additives in bone cement helps to locate the material placed in the bone defect areas [51]. Brown et al. [52, 53] formulated a bone cement consisting of tetra calcium phosphate (TTCP) and dicalcium phosphate (DCPA or DCPD) with a P/L ratio of 4:1 and mixed with water. The mixture was allowed to set for 30 min which formed calcium-deficient HAP. The formed material was hardened and molded and has wide applications in craniofacial surgery. Yamaguchi et al. [54] suggested the inclusion of zinc along with bone cement which induces osteoblast formation at the localized area and eventually new bone formation happens. Another material was developed where Co-Cr alloy was coated with bioactive glass by a process of enameling. The coated alloy was immersed in SBF for 30 days to observe the deposition of HAP on its surface which eventually increases the bioactivity of the material. This has also had wide applications in the tissue engineering field [55].

3.4.7 Agarose and BSA

Another new fabrication was created using a porous scaffold containing foam-like bioglass and poly (lactide-co-glycolide) PLGA. The scaffold showed high microporosity and also the material was favorable for cell adhesion and hence this scaffold was widely applied in tissue engineering [56]. Another researcher [57] also developed a scaffold containing BCP and agarose gel. He analyzed the compression behavior of the scaffold and found that agarose improved the property of BCP by imparting elasticity, ductility, and toughness to the material. Hence, this scaffold could be used in the tissue engineering process. Another researcher [58] too prepared a scaffold comprising of two proteins namely bovine serum albumin and alpha casein by a cold gelation process. The developed scaffold can perform better in its porosity, cytotoxicity, and swelling ratio and the pH changes unalters the scaffold performance. An Indian researcher [59] also prepared bone grafts containing fibrin functionalized graphene oxide (FGO) and graphene oxide (GO) on to which HAP was grown by wet precipitation method. An *in vitro* analysis was performed to study its biocompatibility, cell viability, alkaline phosphatase activity, and protein expression studies. The graft containing FGO–HAP showed a better osteoconductive compared to the GO–HAP graft and the results clearly indicated that FGO–HAP can be used in repairing bone defects.

3.4.8 Terminalia arjuna bark

Another Indian scientist team [60] prepared a bone substitute with the incorporation of the extracts of *Terminalia arjuna* bark. The bark extracts were collected, added with BCP, casein gel, and cast into cylindrical bone grafts. The grafts were immersed in SBF for 21 days and analyzed using conventional techniques. The graft was subjected to *in vitro* cell studies to observe its ossification property. The plant bark extract was traditionally used in fracture healing and hence its incorporation in the graft to enhance the osteogenic property of the graft which was evident in *in vitro* studies. Santhosh et al. [61] synthesized a bone graft containing BCP, biocompatible casein, and the extracts of *Myristica fragans*. The prepared graft was analyzed for *in vitro* bioactivity and subjected to *in vitro* cell analysis. The results revealed the deposition of apatite on the graft after immersing in SBF and also the ALP activity was high when treated with MG-63 cells, NIH-3 T3, and Saos 2 cell lines. This study indicates that the inclusion of plant extract enhances the osteogenic property of the graft.

4. Conclusion

The widely used dental implants are known for their unique characteristics. Recently, novel dental implants incorporated with herbal composites were evaluated by research scientists and revealed abundant evidence on such materials. These implants developed enhanced bone healing and strengthens the bone, accelerates osseointegration, inhibits osteopenia, and inhibits inflammation. These novel implants allow good biocompatibility, viability and shorten the rehabilitation time for the patients. The application of herbal composite inclusion in dentistry and its applications has a greater potential to improve the success rate of dental implant and allows the implications of biotechnology in implant dentistry.

Author details

Gopathy Sridevi[1]* and Seshadri Srividya[2]

1 Department of Physiology, Saveetha Dental College and Hospital, Saveetha Institute of Medical and Technical Sciences, Tamil Nadu, India

2 Department of Biochemistry, Sathyabama Dental College and Hospital, Tamil Nadu, India

*Address all correspondence to: sridevig.sdc@saveetha.com

References

[1] https://www.healthline.com/health/deciduous-teeth

[2] https://my.clevelandclinic.org/health/articles/11179-teeth-eruption-timetable

[3] https://www.who.int/news-room/fact-sheets/detail/oral-health

[4] Loesche WJ. Microbiology of dental decay and periodontal disease. In: Baron S, editor. Medical Microbiology. 4th ed. Galveston (TX): University of Texas Medical Branch at Galveston; 1996. Chapter 99. Available from: https://www.ncbi.nlm.nih.gov/books/NBK8259/

[5] https://www.who.int/oral_health/media/en/orh_report03_en.pdf

[6] Al-Maskari AY, Al-Maskari MY, Al-Sudairy S. Oral manifestations and complications of diabetes mellitus: A review. Sultan Qaboos University Medical Journal. 2011;**11**(2):179-186

[7] http://www.ada.org/~/media/ADA/Publications/Files/ADA_PatientSmart_Tooth_Replacement.ashx

[8] Osman RB, Swain MV. A critical review of dental implant materials with an emphasis on titanium versus zirconia. Materials. 2015;**8**(3):932-958. DOI: 10.3390/ma8030932

[9] John WN. Titanium alloys for dental implants: A review. PRO. 2020;**2**:100-116. DOI: 10.3390/prosthesis2020011

[10] Ong JL, Chan DCN, Bessho K. HA coatings on dental implants. In: Wise DL, Trantolo DJ, Lewandrowski KU, Gresser JD, Cattaneo MV, Yaszemski MJ, editors. Biomaterials Engineering and Devices: Human Applications. Totowa, NJ: Humana Press; 2000. DOI: 10.1007/978-1-59259-197-8_3

[11] Saini M, Singh Y, Arora P, Arora V, Jain K. Implant biomaterials: A comprehensive review. World Journal of Clinical Cases. 2015;**3**(1):52-57. DOI: 10.12998/wjcc.v3.i1.52

[12] Kasemo B, Lausmaa J. Biomaterial and implant surfaces: A surface science approach. The International Journal of Oral & Maxillofacial Implants. 1988;**3**:247-259

[13] Heydecke G, Kohal R, Gläser R. Optimal esthetics in single-tooth replacement with the Re-Implant system: A case report. The International Journal of Prosthodontics. 1999;**12**(2):184-189

[14] Kohal RJ, Klaus G. A zirconia implant-crown system: A case report. The International Journal of Periodontics & Restorative Dentistry. 2004;**24**(2):147-153

[15] Sennerby L, Dasmah A, Larsson B, et al. Bone tissue responses to surface-modified zirconia implants: A histomorphometric and removal torque study in the rabbit. Clinical Implant Dentistry and Related Research. 2005;**7**(Suppl 1):S13-S20

[16] Depprich R, Zipprich H, Ommerborn M, et al. Osseointegration of zirconia implants compared with titanium: An in vivo study. Head & Face Medicine. 2008;**4**:30

[17] Piconi C, Maccauro G. Zirconia as a ceramic biomaterial. Biomaterials. 1999;**20**(1):1-25

[18] Williams DF. Implants in dental and maxillofacial surgery. Biomaterials. 1981;**2**(3):133-146

[19] Craig RG. Restorative Dental Materials. 9th ed. St. Louis, MO, USA: C.V. Mosby; 1993. p. 169

[20] Lemons JE. In: Lin OCC, Chao EYS, editors. Perspectives on Biomaterials. New York, NY: Elsevier; 1986. pp. 1-13

[21] Burkhardt F, Harlass M, Adolfsson E, Vach K, Spies BC, Kohal R-J. A novel zirconia-based composite presents an aging resistant material for narrow-diameter ceramic implants. Materials. 2021;**14**(9):2151

[22] Glantz PO. The choice of alloplastic materials for oral implants: Does it really matter? The International Journal of Prosthodontics. 1998;**11**(5):402-407

[23] Lemons JE. Dental implant biomaterials. Journal of the American Dental Association (1939). 1990;**121**(6):716-719

[24] Carvalho TL, Araujo CA, Teofilo JM, et al. Histologic and histometric evaluation of rat alveolar wound healing around polyurethane resin implants. International Journal of Oral and Maxillofacial Surgery. 1997;**26**(2):149-152

[25] Meijer GJ, Starmans FJ, de Putter C, van Blitterswijk CA. The influence of a flexible coating on the bone stress around dental implants. Journal of Oral Rehabilitation. 1995;**22**(2):105-111

[26] Meijer GJ, Dalmeijer RA, de Putter C, et al. A comparative study of flexible (polyactive) versus rigid (hydroxyapatite) permucosal dental implants II. Histological aspects. J Oral Rehabil. 1997;**24**(2):93-101

[27] Meena M, Figueiredo NR, Trivedi K. *Aloe vera* – An Update for Dentistry. Journal of Dentofacial Sciences. 2013;**2**(4):1-4

[28] Phyllis B, James B. Prescription for nutritional healing, 3rd ed. Vol. 1. Avery Publishing; 2000. p. 94

[29] Burrow A, Eccles R, Jones AS. The effects of camphor, eucalyptus and menthol vapour on nasal resistance to airflow and nasal sensation. Acta Oto-Laryngologica. 1983;**96**(1-2): 157-161

[30] Crowell PL. Prevention and therapy of cancer by dietary monoterpenes. The Journal of Nutrition. 1999;**129**(3): 775S-7758S

[31] Chainani-Wu N. Safety and antiinflammatory activity of curcumin: A component of turmeric (Curcuma longa). Journal of Alternative and Complementary Medicine. 2003;**9**:61-68

[32] Wang Q, Wang X, Xu X. Icariin: Can an herbal extract enhance dental implant outcomes? Dental Hypotheses. 2012;**3**(4):133-137

[33] Das S, Dholam K, Gurav S, et al. Accentuated osseointegration in osteogenic nanofibrous coated titanium implants. Scientific Reports. 2019;**9**:17638

[34] Mohammed M, Aboki MA, Saidu HM, Victor O, Tawakalitu A, Maikano SA. Phytochemical and Some Antmicrobial Activity of *Cassia occidentalis* L. (Caesalpiniaceae). Int J Sci Technol. 2012;**2**(4)

[35] Lee SU, Shin HK, Min YK, Kim SH. Emodin accelerates osteoblast differentiation through phosphatidylinositol 3-kinase activation and bone morphogenetic protein-2 gene expression. International Immunopharmacology. 2008;**8**:741-747

[36] Nayar S, Guha A. Waste utilization for the controlled synthesis of nanosized

hydroxyapatite. Materials Science and Engineering C. 2009;**29**:1326-1329

[37] Rajkumar M, Meenakshi Sundaram N, Rajendran V. In-situ preparation of hydroxyapatitenanorod embedded poly (vinyl alcohol) composite and its characterization. International Journal of Engineering Science and Technology. 2010;**2**(6):2437-2444

[38] Nasr-Esfahani M, Mehrabanian M. Production of Bone-like 40% nylon 6,6-Nano Hydroxyapatite Scaffold via Salt-Leaching/Solvent Casting Technique. 2nd International Conference on Chemistry and Chemical Engineering IPCBEE, Barcelona, Spain. Vol. 14; 2011. pp. 40-44

[39] LeGeros RZ, Lin S, Rohanizadeh R, et al. Biphasic calcium phosphate bioceramics: Preparation, properties and applications. Journal of Materials Science: Materials in Medicine. 2003;**14**:201-209. DOI: 10.1023/A:1022872421333

[40] Lin EK, Kolb R, Satija SK, Wu W-L. Reduced polymer mobility near the polymer/solid interface as measured by neutron reflectivity. Macromolecules. 1999;**32**:3753-3757

[41] Lopez-Estebana S, Saiza E, Fujinob S, Okuc T, Suganumac K, Tomsiaa AP. Bioactive glass coatings for orthopedic metallic implants. Journal of the European Ceramic Society. 2003;**23**:2921-2930

[42] Zhou G, Li Y, Zhang L, Zuo Y, Jansen JA. Preparation and characterization of nano-hydroxyapatite/chitosan/konjac glucomannan composite. Journal of Biomedical Research. 2007;**83**(4):931-939. DOI: 10.1002/jbm.a.31427

[43] Liu A, Hong Z, Zhuang X, Chen X, Cui Y, Liu Y, et al. Surface modification of bioactive glass nanoparticles and the mechanical and biological properties of poly(L-lactide) composites. Acta Biomaterialia. 2008;**4**:1005-1015

[44] Kapoor S, Batra U. Preparation and bioactivity evaluation of bone like hydroxyapatite – bioglass composite. International Journal of Chemical and Biological Engineering. 2010;**3**(1):24-28

[45] Chin CD, Khann K, Samuel K. Biomed microdevices: A microfabricated porous collagen-based scaffold as prototype for skin substitutes. Biomaterials. 2008;**10**:456-454

[46] Misra SK, Ansari T, Mohn D, Valappil SP, Brunner TJ, Stark WJ, et al. Effect of nanoparticulate bioactive glass particles on bioactivity and cytocompatibility of poly(3-hydroxybutyrate) composites. J R Soc Interface. 2010;7(44):453-465. DOI: 10.1098/rsif.2009.0255

[47] Periyathambi P, Vedakumari WS, Baskar SK, Bojja S, Sastry TP. Osteogenic potency of magnetic fibrin nanoparticles - a novel perspective in bone tissue engineering. Materials Letters. 2014;**139**:108-111

[48] Auxenfans BV, Andre CA, Lequeux S, Rose F, Braye J, Fradette, et al. Porous matrix and primary-cell culture: A shared concept for skin and cornea tissue engineering. Pathologie et Biologie. 2009;**57**(4):290-298

[49] Wu TJ, Huang HH, Lan CW, Lin CH, Hsu FY, Wang YJ. Studies on the microspheres comprised of reconstituted collagen and hydroxyapatite. Biomaterials. 2004;**25**:651-658

[50] Shields KJ, Beckman MJ, Bowlin GL. Mechanichal properties and cellular proliferation of electrospun collagen type II. Tissue Engineering. 2004;**10**:1510-1517

[51] Gillani R, Ercan B, Qiao A, Webster TJ. Nanofunctionalized zirconia and barium sulfate particles as bone cement additives. International Journal of Nanomedicine. 2010;**5**:1-11

[52] Brown WE, Chow LC. Dental restorative cement pastes. U.S. Patent No. 4,518, 430, May. 1985

[53] Brown WE, Chow LC. A new calcium phosphate water setting cement. In: Brown PW, editor. Cements Research Progress. Westerville, USA: American Ceramic Society; 1986. pp. 352-379

[54] Yamaguchi M, Oishi H, Suketa Y. Stimulatory effect of zinc on bone formation in tissue culture. Biochemical Pharmacology. 1987;**36**(22):4007-4012

[55] Fujino S, Tokunaga H, Saiz E, Tomsia AP. Fabrication and characterization of bioactive glass coatings on Co-Cr implant alloys. Materials Transactions. 2004;**45**(4):1147-1151

[56] Boccaccini AR, Maquet V. Bioresorbable and bioactive polymer/ Bioglass® composites with tailored pore structure for tissue engineering applications. Composites Science and Technology. 2003;**63**:2417-2429

[57] Puertolas JA, Vadillo JL, Sanchez-Salcedo S, Nieto A, Gomez-Barrena E, Vallet-Regi M. Compression behavior of biphasic calcium phosphate-agarose scaffolds for bone regeneration. Acta Biomaterialia. 2011;**7**:841-847

[58] Novaes AB Jr, Scombatti de Souza SL, Martins de Barros RR. Influence of implant surfaces on osseointegration. Brazilian Dental Journal. 2010;**21**(6):471-481

[59] Deepachitra R, Nigam R, Purohit SD, Kumar BS, Hemalatha T, Sastry TP. In vitro study of hydroxyapatite coatings on fibrinfunctionalized/pristine graphene oxide for bone grafting. Mater. Manufact. Process. 2015;**30**:804-811. DOI: 10.1080/10426914.2014.994758

[60] Krithiga G, Jena A, Selvamani P, Sastry TP. In vitro study on biomineralization of biphasic calcium phosphate biocomposite crosslinked with hydrolysable tannins of Terminalia chebula. Bulletin of Materials Science. 2011;**34**(3):589-594

[61] Santhosh Kumar B, Muthukumar T, Deepachitra R, Charumathy RK, Hemalatha T, Sastry TP. In-vitro evaluation of biphasic calcium phosphate/casein incorporated with Myristica fragrans for bone tissue engineering. Ceramics International. 2014;**41**(1):1725-1734

Chapter 8

New Trends in Bioactive Glasses for Bone Tissue: A Review

Petrică Vizureanu, Mădălina Simona Bălțatu, Andrei Victor Sandu, Dragos Cristian Achitei, Dumitru Doru Burduhos Nergis and Manuela Cristina Perju

Abstract

Bioactive glasses are very attractive materials, used for tissue engineering materials, usually to fill and restore bone defects. This category of biomaterials, show considerable potential for orthopaedic surgery because they can promote bone tissue regeneration. Many trace elements have been incorporated in the glass network, an example is metallic glasses to obtain the desired properties. Because of tolerable mechanical properties, and because they are able to bond to living bone and stimulate its regeneration, this bioactive glasses have a particular interest and are in a continuous research and improvement. The chapter presents the history of bioactive glasses, classification, include a summary of common fabrication methods, applications, surface coatings, applications and future trends in relation to human bone. This review highlight new trends and areas of future research for bioactive glasses.

Keywords: bioactive glasses, bioactivity, glass-ceramics, biodegradable, melt-derived glasses, bone, applications, tissue engineering

1. Introduction

Research in the field of materials science and engineering has expanded greatly in recent decades, especially in the field of biocompatible materials. This is because, on the one hand, medicine is constantly looking for solutions to remedy many health problems, and on the other hand, certain classes of materials have already proven useful in alleviating or even curing certain human suffering [1, 2].

The development of biocompatible materials research is an evolving process driven by the increase in the number of accidents and many health problems, but also by the desire to increase the average life expectancy in humans. As research in the field of biomaterials science advances at the laboratory level, the incidence of serious diseases is increasing in the global human community. The World population is getting larger and the percent of elder persons is increasing and influencing the increase of chronic illness, like cancer or cardiovascular diseases. Next to this on large scale other infectious diseases are getting more common like: HIV/AIDS, tuberculosis or gastrointestinal issues. On this reason the focus of the research in the field of medical materials and instruments should prepare for the request on the market [3].

While traditional biomaterials were based on polymers, ceramics and metals, now the latest generation of biomaterials incorporates biomolecules, therapeutic drugs and even living cells. At present, biomaterials are a special category of materials, indispensable for raising the quality of human life and extending its duration [4].

Biomaterials are generally intended to be implanted in a living organism to restore the shape and function of a part of a tissue destroyed by disease or trauma.

The introduction of a biomaterial into the human body determines an implant versus tissue interaction, which can generate conflicting reactions. They can be toxic, mechanical, and electrochemical biological. It can even lead to serious damage to the bone or adjacent tissue, or assembly used. Due to these phenomena, depending on the quality of the biomaterial, the place of implantation and other causes, corrosion occurs on the surface of the implant, with loss of quality his.

Depending on the medical application for which it is suitable, a biomaterial must have one or more of the properties presented in **Figure 1**. These factors are very important and have a close correlation between them: to be biologically compatible with the host tissue (for example, it does not have to causes rejection, inflammation and immune responses); Easily achieve direct bio-chemical attachment to the host tissue; The biodegradation time must be adjusted to suit the time of natural bone formation; Degradation mode: Surface or depth erosion; Ability to support the growth of germinal capillaries, tissues perivascular mesenchymal and osteoprogenitor cells from host in the three-dimensional structure of the graft that acts as a support; Needed to maximize space for grip and growth cellular, revascularization, proper nutrition and oxygen supply; For support in the process of cell growth and in the transport of nutrients and oxygen [5].

A material suitable for use in medicine must have, where appropriate, certain characteristics special and offer a number of advantages: mechanical integrity of the tissues acting as a support for growth living tissue; control of the biological response, by promoting dynamic interactions with tissues surrounding; behaving as a space for the survival of host cells, facilitating the transport of nutrients and metabolites, by maximizing the biological and / or pharmaceutical response; good biocompatibility / biodegradability, with adequate degradation kinetics; new tissue formation, thus minimizing both tissue and response toxicity systemic; feasibility in production [6, 7].

Of all the factors, biocompatibility is the most important feature to be taken into account consideration in the clinical applications of a biomaterial and which is related to

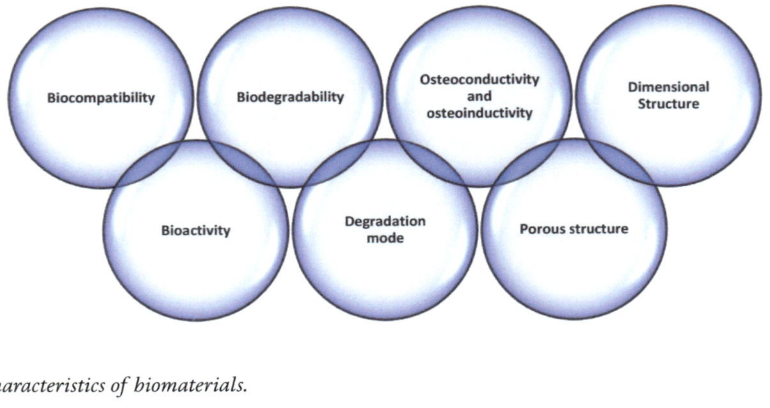

Figure 1.
The main characteristics of biomaterials.

behavior biomaterials in various contexts. Biocompatibility is correlated with the appearance of a response weak immune system in contact with a particular biomaterial [8, 9].

The most complex unit is the human body, having many levels of tissues, organs and systems. If we speak about tissues these can be soft or hard, after that being classified in ones in contact with blood or not, in contact with the biomaterials or not [10].

On biomaterials the classification can vary, according to the composing materials and their use; the origin – natural or synthetic, simple or mixed composite and so on. Regarding the composition these can be metallic, ceramic, polymeric, composite and of natural origin.

According to every biomaterial, the advantages and disadvantages can influence their use, being induced by the characteristics of biomaterials and by the functional requirements of implants.

Bioglass (BGs) is a chemical compound that is part of a compositional family known to have the best bioactivity properties. This are osteoconductive and osteoinductive as well biocompatible and highly bioactive, as demonstrated by the connection with living tissues in a short time to just a few hours [11].

This new class of biomaterials, based on an amorphous mixture of oxides (SiO_2-Na_2O-K_2O-CaOMgO-P_2O_5), was patented in 1968 by Larry Hench by preparing the well-known Bioglass 45S5.

Depending on the percentage of SiO_2 mainly, these biomaterials can be bioinert, bioactive or bioresorbable. Hench and Clark were the first researchers to observe the bioactivity of this material in vitro and in vivo and demonstrated its osteointegrative potential [12].

At the same time, the antimicrobial and anti-inflammatory properties and the possibility to easily control the crystallinity by applying heat treatments corresponding to the glassy phase present in the bioglass structure were noted. All these are additional arguments for this class of biomaterials to be a first objective in research in the field [13].

L.L. Hench developed the concept of using a material based on silicon dioxide, calcium oxide and phosphorus pentoxide, in a proportion similar to that of natural bone, to make implants, which have the property of developing a bond with the bone. In **Figure 2** is presented the Hench Diagram. The level of biocompatibility of a material can be correlated with the time in which it was performed bone binding for more than 50% of implant surface ($t_{0.5bb}$) [15].

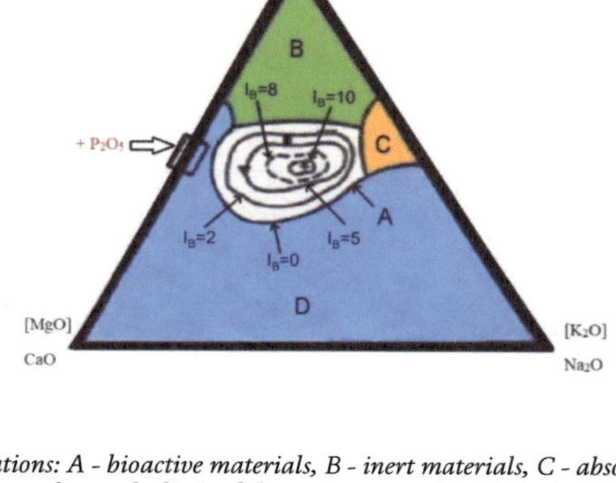

Figure 2.
*Hench diagram [14]. *notations: A - bioactive materials, B - inert materials, C - absorbable materials, D - cannot be obtain bioglasses, la = 0 the limit of the compositions that allow the binding to the hard tissues, l_a = 8 is the limit of the compositions that allow the binding of soft tissues.*

The bioactivity index is defined by the following formula:

$$I_B = \frac{100}{t_{0.5bb}} \quad (1)$$

Because some studies show that the GBs are fragile and exhibit poor mechanical properties, this limiting the involvement in load-bearing applications, another way to represent a feasible solution, is to incorporate the bioactive glasses into gelatine matrices and to fabricate composites [16, 17].

2. History - current level of development

Although 40 years have passed since the patenting of this material, until now it has been intensively used only in the form of large diameter particles (~ 100 μm), grouped in blocks with different geometries, with applications in regenerative orthopedic surgery (bone fillers).

Enamel-glazing and flame / plasma spray are used as commercial methods to obtain bioglass thin films at the commercial level, and in recent years' intensive research has been carried out in many biomaterials research laboratories to find alternative methods to the traditional ones, which lead to thick coatings with low mechanical strength.

Although their superficial properties are interesting, their development is limited due to: high fragility and reduced mechanical resistance to static fatigue. However, they are used to make middle ear bones, alveolar reconstructions, dental implants, films for total coverage of prostheses (alumina or titanium alloy), for modern cancer treatments.

For all these applications, the bioglasess have seen a spectacular development, as shown in **Table 1**.

Due to the high fragility and low mechanical strength of bioglasses as well as the toxicity of metal ions that can occur from metal alloys used in internal prostheses, the study of metal orthopedic prostheses coated with thin bioglasses films was studied.

Their use is motivated, among other things, by the porosity characteristics of the bioglasses, which allow a very intimate propagation of the tissues, thus ensuring a perfect connection with the implant. Thus, these structures have the advantage of combining the bioactive properties of the coating material with the mechanical strength of the support (**Figure 3**).

Bioglasses are superficially active, they have the property of binding mechanically or biochemically to bone tissue or collagen fibers in contact with soft, living tissue.

It has been shown that the connection between the bioglass and the bone is achieved by the formation of a superficially active interface based on hydroxyapatite, which further determines the reconstruction action of the tissue cells; such a mechanism is stimulated by a slightly basic pH, caused by ion exchanges between the bioglass and the tissue.

Materials with limited reactivity, such as dense hydroxyapatite, have a weaker effect than biosticles in the healing process of bone tissue.

All classes of the biomaterials are used throughout the human body, for this purpose, physical, chemical and biological properties of materials are exploited, often new or improved properties, and the resulting structures can interact faster at the biomolecular level, both on the surface and inside the cell.

Year	Stage/Achievement/Application
1969	Highlighting the binding (binding) of the bone with the help of bioglass and bioglass-ceramics
1973	Specification of the interaction mechanism at the bone-bioglass interface
1973	Binding of bone to active biovitroceram
1976	Measurement of the profiles of compositions in the bioglass-bone connection area
1976	Successful introduction of bioglass into the dental implant
1980	Comparative histology of variable bioactivity implants
1981	Ultrastructure analysis of biovitroceram and bone
1981	Toxicology and biocompatibility tests of biostycles and evidence of soft tissue binding
1981	Clinical use of vitroceram (Ceravital) in the middle ear prosthesis
1982	Comparison between the glass implant and other inert implants instead of the middle ear bone
1982	High mechanical strength vitroceram (apatite and wollastonite) for vertebral prostheses
1983	Mechanically machinable vitroceram based on apatite and fluoroflogopite
1984	The FDA approves the sale of bioglasses and prostheses for the middle ear
1986	Clinical trial of bioglasses for alveolar ridges
1993	PerioGlas approved by FDA (45S5 Bioglass® for bone and dental repair)
1998	Peripheral nerve repair
1999	Radioactive glasses approved by FDA (TheraSphere®) for cancer treatment
2000	Wound healing
2002	Medpor®-PlusTM approved by FDA (polyethylene/45S5 Bioglass® composite porous orbital implants).
2003	Antibacterial (Zn-containing) bone/dental cements
2004	Lung tissue engineering
2004	Use of mesoporous bioactive glass (MBG) as a drug delivery system
2005	Skeletal muscle and ligament repair
2005	Treatment of gastrointestinal ulcers
2010	Cardiac tissue engineering
2011	Commercialization of a cotton-candy borate bioactive glass for wound healing in veterinarian medicine. FDA approval was pending.
2012	Embolization of uterine fibroids
2012	Spinal cord repair
2018	Use of radioactive glasses (TheraSphere®) in patients with metastatic colorectal carcinoma of the liver

Table 1.
Stages of development of bioglass and glass-ceramics [4, 5, 15].

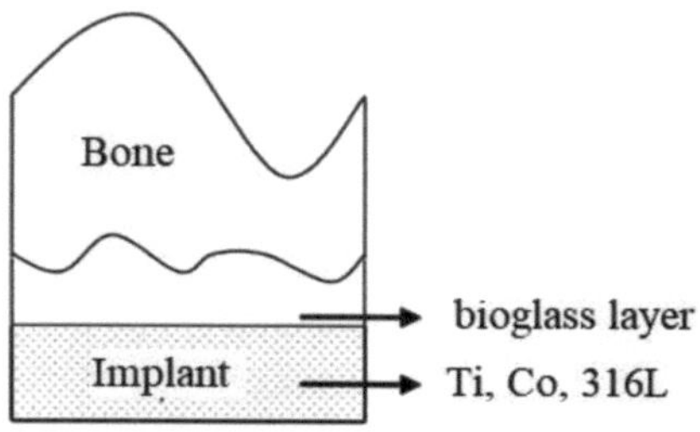

Figure 3.
Multilayer structure [9].

3. Relevant studies

Most of the commercial biomaterials (glass, ceramics, glass-ceramics and composites) are known that bind to bones, being called bioactive ceramics. Also other strictly specialized compositions of bioactive glasses bind to soft tissues. A common feature of bioactive glasses and ceramics is the change of the material surface after time-dependent implantation. On the surface it is formed a biologically active layer of hydroxycarbonate apatite (HCA), which provides the tissue-binding structure [4].

Many studies have shown bone-related bioactive implants with sufficient adhesion to the interface to withstand mechanical fracture. A failure never occurs at the interface, but either in the implant or in the bone.

Bone binding was initially demonstrated for some compositional domains of bioactive glasses, containing SiO_2, Na_2O, CaO and P_2O_5, in the proportions specified in **Table 2**.

During the years many types and variations of the composition were approved by FDA and named Bioglass.

When introducing a material into the living organism, a series of very complex interactions can appear, being able to identify four specific phenomena that are unitary in the so-called "concept of biocompatibility", namely:

1. initial processes that take place at the biomaterial interface ÷ living tissue and that are closely related to the physico - chemical processes that take place in the first minutes of the contact between the biomaterial and the living tissue;

2. the effect induced by presence of biomaterial as a foreign body in the living tissue surrounding the implant, which can be measured at any time, from a few minutes to years;

3. the effect that living tissue has on the biomaterial through the changes observed in the biomaterial, effect described in the form of corrosion or degradation;

4. consequences of the reaction at the interface that are systematically seen on the surface of the body or in certain specific areas, medically recognized as the development of specific allergies, the initiation of tumors or the appearance of infectious processes [5].

Chemical interactions that occur at the surface are:

- Rapid exchange of Na + and Ca2 + ions with H + and HO- ions in solution, leading to hydrolysis of silica groups, with the formation of silanol groups;

$$Si-O-Na^{+}+H^{+}+HO^{-}\rightarrow Si-OH+Na^{+}+HO^{-} \tag{2}$$

- The cation exchange increases the concentration of hydroxyl ions in the solution, which leads to the attack of the silica network;

- Condensation and repolymerization of a SiO_2-rich layer on the glass surface, depleted in alkaline and alkaline-earth cations;

Component	45S5 Bioglass®	45S54F Bioglass®	45B15S5 Bioglass®	52S4.6 Bioglass®	55S4.3 Bioglass®	KGC Ceravital®	KGS Ceravital®	KGy213 Ceravital®	A/W Glass–ceramic	MB Glass–ceramic	S45P7
SiO_2	45	45	30	52	55	46.2	46	38	34.2	19–52	45
P_2O_2	6	6	6	6	6				16.3	4–24	7
CaO	24.5	14.7	24.5	21	19.5	20.2	33	31	44.9	9–3	22
$Ca(PO_3)_2$						25.5	16	13.5			
CaF_2		9.8							0.5		
MgO						2.9			4.6	5–15	
MgF_2											
Na_2O	24.5	24.5	24.5	21	19.5	4.8	5	4		3–5	24
K_2O						0.4				3–5	
Al_2O_3								7		12–33	
B_2O_3			15								2
Ta_2O_5/ TiO_2								6.5			
Structure	Glass and glass–ceramic	Glass	Glass	Glass–ceramic	Glass–ceramic	Glass–ceramic	Glass–ceramic	Glass–ceramic	Glass–ceramic	Glass–ceramic	Glass–ceramic

Table 2.
Composition of bioactive glass and glass ceramics (% weight) [18].

- Migration of Ca^{2+} and PO_4^{3-} cations to the surface through the SiO_2-rich layer, forming above it an amorphous CaO-P_2O_5-rich film, which grows by incorporating calcium and phosphates from the solution;
- Crystallization of the amorphous film rich in CaO-P_2O_5 by incorporation from the solution of OH- and CO_3^{2-} anions, with the formation of a mixed layer containing carbonated hydroxyapatite (HCA).

The biomaterial versus tissue interface, which is established by implantation, is almost inevitably a blood ÷ material interface and the initial events are dominated by the absorption of blood proteins on the implant surface. At this contact it was established that a series of biological processes: Adsorption and desorption of biological growth factors, in the HCA layer, which determines the activation of stem cell differentiation; The action of macrophages, which phagocytose local residues, allowing cells to grow; Attachment to the bioactive surface of stem cells; Differentiation of stem cells with the formation of bone growth cells, called osteoblasts; Osteoblasts generates extracellular matrix with bone formation; Crystallization of the phosphate inorganic matrix by embedding bone cells in a living composite structure (**Figure 4**) [19].

The chemical and topological properties of the implant surface strongly influence the properties of the biolayer and this influence must be understood and controlled in order to optimize the biocompatibility of the material used. Relevant in the study of biocompatibility is the fact that proteins and cells have nano- and micrometer sizes, which requires extremely delicate approaches. Of equal importance are the properties of cells, for example, their ability to communicate via the extracellular matrix with signal molecules (molecules used in the process of living cell synthesis). During tissue healing, numerous bioactive signaling molecules control tissue formation, and some proteins have demonstrated the ability to stimulate healing near the implant. All these mechanisms contribute to the response of the tissues to the implant and can determine whether the body accepts the implant or not, whether it is biocompatible.

Japanese researchers have tested the effect of surface area on bone proliferation. Three types of biomaterials were compared: bioactive glass, dense hydroxyapatite and glass ceramics. Each material was implanted in a 6 mm diameter hole, which was drilled into the bone of an adult rabbit's leg. Bioactive glass has been found to produce

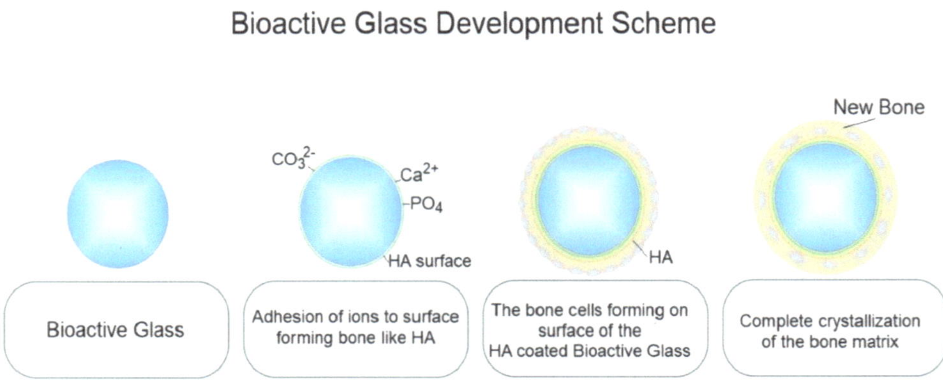

Figure 4.
Bioactive glass surface reaction [19, 20].

bone tissue and is subsequently resorbed much faster than the other two materials, both of which have a lower surface reactivity than glass.

The rate of bone growth around an implanted material depends in part on the rate of dissolution of the silica network and therefore it is very good to determine as accurately as possible the system in which the oxide composition of the bioglass.

Alkaline content plays an important role in the stability of bioglass. From this point of view, two categories are distinguished: bioglass with rich alkaline content and bioglass with poor alkaline content. The latter are characterized by a high degree of decomposition over time, during bone reconstruction. This type of bioglass has been used in maxillofacial applications and in the chaining of the inner ear bones.

Most determinations were made with glasses based on 6 oxides: SiO_2-Na_2O-K_2OCaO-MgO-P_2O_5, as it was found that the bone binds to materials with a wide range of compositions in this system. Soft tissue binding occurs for a much smaller range of compositions.

There are three basic compositional requirements for silico-chalco-sodium glasses to bind to hard tissue. These are: less than 60% SiO_2 (mol), high content of Na_2O and CaO, high CaO / P_2O_5 ratio. The level of bioactivity is strongly dependent on the relative concentrations of ions.

The most successful bioactive glass is the one that contains P_2O_5 between 6 and 15%.

In the diagram of the SiO_2-CaO-Na_2O ternary system (6% P_2O_5), some materials form a bond with the bone in 30 days. Other glasses bind to the soft tissue, some of the glasses are almost chemically inert and others are resorbable and dissolve in 10 to 30 days.

Bioglasses from another part of diagrams, from a technological point of view, are not forming glass and have not been tested as implant materials. Until now, it has been considered that in order to be bioactive, glasses and glass-ceramics must contain both CaO and P_2O_5, which are the component oxides of hydroxyapatite.

Ohura and collaborators have shown that glasses in the CaO-SiO_2 system without P_2O_5, as well as those containing very small amounts of P_2O_5, form a layer of hydroxyapatite on their surface when immersed in simulated body fluid (SBF). In contrast, under the same conditions, the glasses in the SiO_2-free CaO-P_2O_5 system do not form the hydroxyapatite layer. It follows that bioactive compositions can be obtained in the CaO-SiO_2 system rather than in the CaO-P_2O_5 system.

Bioactive glasses usually have weak strength and resilience properties, which is why they are reinforced with metal fibers made of stainless steel, titanium and Co-Cr alloys. As a result of the reinforcement with metal fibers, the volume of defects and the residual tensions decrease, and the microcracks produced are below the critical length and have rounded extremities.

4. Methods of obtaining

The most methods used for bioglass nanoparticles obtain are: quenching method, sol–gel, flame synthesis, microwave irradiation and microemulsion. Two main process that can synthesize the biomaterial are the melt quenching method and sol–gel.

4.1 Quenching method

The melt queching method can synthesize bioglass in a short time, by heating the initial precursors to high temperatures and following special rules. The preparation process proposed by Hench by melting is based on the following steps:

- Melting of the mixture of high purity raw materials, in Pt-10% Rh crucibles, covered, in order to prevent the volatilization of the components.
- The melt is loosened for at least 2 hours, without removing the lid.
- The glass is poured into graphite molds. If the sample diameter is larger than 1 cm then the mold is preheated to 300°C.
- The glass is annealed at different temperatures depending on the composition, for 4 hours (see **Table 3**)
- The glass is cooled slowly in the oven for 16 hours.

The role of annealing is to create the conditions for the formation of microcrystals, thus obtaining a bioactive glass–ceramic.

The melt quenching method synthesis was also carried out by Shams et al. in 2018. Bioglass nanoparticles were prepared from analytical grade SiO_2, Na_2CO_3, $CaCO_3$, and P_2O_5 precursors. As an example from the literature [21]: the precursors were mixed in 53.0 SiO_2:23.0 Na_2CO_3:20.0 $CaCO_3$:4.0 P_2O_5 molar ratios followed by milling in an agate mortar [22]. The blend was mixed in a jar for several hours and then pressed into discs with 10 mm in diameter using a hydraulic press apparatus. Than the samples were placed in an alumina crucible and heat treated in the furnace [21].

In **Figure 5** we can see the thermal program: melting at 1400°C for 3 hours - resulting molten material, then quenched in distilled water to produce glass frit. The glass frit was than dried in an oven at 80°C for 5 hours. The dried glass frit was milled in a Retch PM400 milling machine using zirconia cups for 6 h to obtain the bioglass powder [21]. FESEM micrograph of bioglass nanoparticles, includes spherical particles with a wide size distribution from 100 to 800 nm [21].

Although the melt technique is a fast method, the resulting glass usually has a low specific surface area value. According to previous research, the specific surface area value is a key factor affecting bioglass bioactivity. Increasing the specific surface area can increase the surface reaction between the artificial material and the physiological environment, thereby increasing the formation of the HA layer.

4.2 Sol–gel method

One of the most common method - the sol–gel process is well known for obtaining synthetic materials, like silicate and oxide systems and respectively thin films, coatings, nanoparticles, and fibers. The sol–gel reactions takes place at low temperatures and involves the synthesis of a solution (sol), usually consisting of metal–organic and/or metal salt precursors followed by gelling by chemical reactions, or

Type	45S5	45B15S5	KLP1	KZS3020	45S5N	45S5-L	45S5-F
Tmelting [°C]	*1350*	*1150*	*1350*	*1500*	*1350*	*1350*	*1200*
T annealing [°C]	*500*	*375*	*550*	*700*	*550*	*550*	*350*

Table 3.
Heat treatment temperatures for Hench glasses.

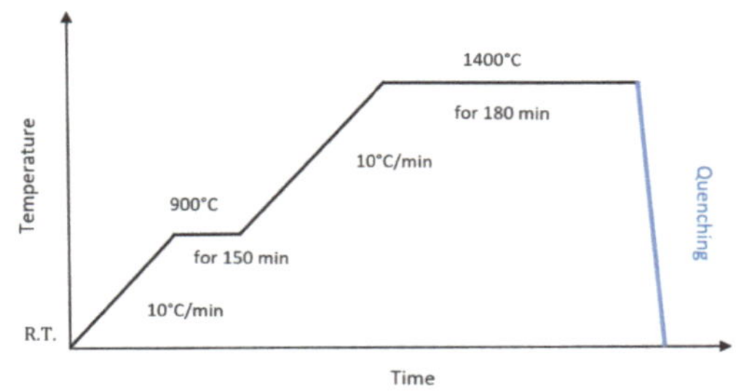

Figure 5.
The furnace temperature programming. Image adopted from [21].

aggregation, and finally thermal treatment for drying, removal of organic substances, and sometimes crystallization and cooling. Some ions (magnesium, zirconium, zinc, silver, titanium, boron) can be also added to the bioactive glass in order to enhance glass functionality and bioactivity. However, bioactive glass is difficult to synthesize on a nanoscale with the addition of ions [22].

The sol–gel method can synthesize bioglass at lower temperatures, has a porous structure, and a high specific surface area value which can increase the bioactivity of synthetic materials.

The raw materials used in the sol–gel method are alkoxide precursors or soluble inorganic salts derived from the oxide components of the glasses.

If a glass is prepared in the SiO_2-CaO-P_2O_5 ternary system, the precursors used may be:

- TEOS - tetraethylorthosilicate ($C_8H_{20}O_4Si$)
- Calcium nitrate ($Ca(NO_3)_2 \cdot 4H_2O$)
- PET - triethylphosphate ($C_6H_{15}O_4P$)

The following factors are considered: the raw materials are added dropwise, under continuous stirring; the pH is adjusted with nitric acid to 2–3 thus taking place an acid catalysis; the soil thus obtained is left to gel for a few hours in an oven at 60° C.

The advantages of the sol–gel method are:

- Low obtaining temperature;
- High purity;
- Improved homogeneity;
- Variation of the composition in order to maintain bioactivity;
- Modification of structural characteristics, by controlling hydrolysis and condensation reactions;
- Powders of nanometric dimensions;
- Nanostratified porous materials.

Kumar et al. [23] synthesizing bioglass nanoparticles (SiO_2 (60%)-CaO (30%) -P_2O_5 (10%)) through the sol–gel method. The synthesis of bioglass nanoparticles was carried out by mixing TEOS (4.054 g) with ethanol using a magnetic stirrer for one hour at room temperature. In separate containers, calcium nitrate tetrahydrate (2.372 g) and phosphate pentoxide (0.267 g) were dissolved in distilled water and stirred each with a magnetic stirrer for 30 minutes at room temperature as well. After one hour, the solution containing calcium was added dropwise to the solution containing TEOS, as well as the solution containing the phosphate. After that, ammonia solution was added to the mixture to maintain pH 11. The mixture was then put in an incubator for 48 hours to obtain the gel. The obtained gel was placed in an oven at 100°C to dry [23]. The result of TEM analysis shows that the shape of the bioglass nanoparticles is irregular at the nano and micro scales due to the presence of agglomeration, the particle size varies from 200 to 500 nm, average surface area of the bioglass nanoparticles measured using BET with N2 was 10.4 m^2/g. The larger the particle size, the smaller the surface area.

Another study made by Durgalakshmi et al., by mixing tertraethyl orthosilicate (TEOS) and HNO_3 as an acid medium, then added alcohol to help the hydrolysis process. Gel formation occurred after 30 minutes of mixing. At 20 minute intervals, other reagents are added to the mixture such as phosphoric acid, calcium nitrate, and sodium hydroxide. The solution was mixed for 4 hours to obtain a homogeneous gel. After the hydrolysis process is complete, the sol is stored at 70°C for 24 hours, and then the dry white powder is taken at 600°C for 2 hours [24]. Scanning electron microscope analysis shows that the particles do not have a well-defined shape, having less than 100 nm in length [24]. The large particles of over 200 nm could be formed due to particle agglomeration during sintering [25].

5. Applications

From ancient times there has been an interest in repairing and replacing parts of the human body that present problems and this has been done using various materials more or less suitable depending on the information available at that time [26].

Due to the evolution of science and equipment today, the medical world is in a period of transition from the healing of existing organs to their replacement with synthetic materials obtained in high-performance laboratories [27].

Bone replacement is in the 2nd place as a tissue replacement procedure, in the first place being the blood transfusion. Yearly are done more than 2 million bone reconstructions in orthopedics, neurosurgery and dentistry.

A wide variety of biomaterials are used in restorative medicine. The choice of material for a practical application in medicine remains a key factor in the design and development of medical implants and devices. Currently, more than 50 biomaterials (BIOGLASS 45S5®, CERABONE A-W®, TheraSphere®, Corglaes®, NovaBone®, NovaMin® etc.) of synthetic or natural origin are used in medicine, covering a wide variety of applications. The tables below (**Tables 4** and **5**) show some of the applications of bioactive glass and glass ceramics due to their well-defined bioactive properties [28].

Figure 6 illustrate some examples of commercially glasses, available on the market. All research leads to a great potential of BGs in medicine but it is not fully exploited yet and the next years a rapid growth is expected.

Composition	Form	Application	Function
Bioglass 45S5	Solid body	Reconstruction of the alveolar margin	Filling the space and tying the tissue
	Solid body	Middle ear prosthesis	Reconstruction of the ear canal by replacing part of the bone chain
	Powder	Reconstruction of defects caused by periodontitis	Replacing lost bone and preventing gum retraction
	Powder	Fixation of hip implants	Replacement of lost bone due to a defective fixed implant

Table 4.
Applications for BIOGLASS 45S5.

Composition	Form	Application	Function
Cerabone A-W glass–ceramic	Solid body	Iliacal ridge prosthesis	Replacement of extracted bone for autograft
		Vertebral prosthesis	Replacement of a vertebra lost during surgical removal of a tumor
	Deposition	Fixing hip prostheses	Provides bioactive binding of the implant

Table 5.
Applications for CERABONE A-W.

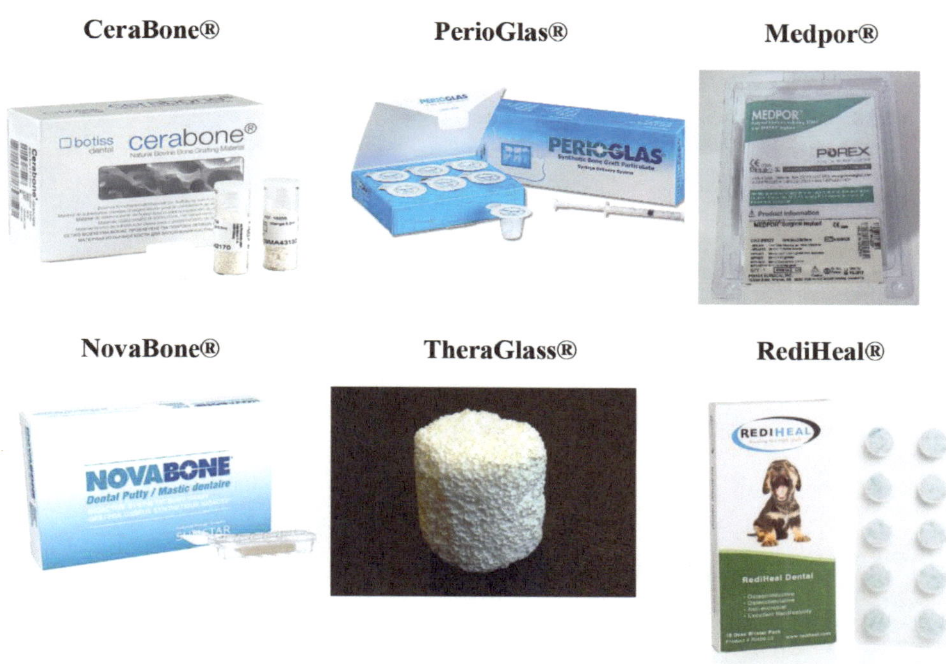

Figure 6.
Examples of commercially produced glasses, available on the market [29–33].

6. Future trends

It is hard to say which is the most feasible bioglass. So the focus of the research is now on optimisation of the materials with deposition techniques, influenced by the parameters of the coatings and the composition of the bioglass, in order to obtain a multi-functional coatings, that will give long-term qualitative implants without side effects and ensuring regeneration.

Figure 7 shows the challenges and future trends for bioactive glasses (BGs)in medicine promoted by researchers which will lead to better implants. The properties of a biomaterial are decisive in ensuring the biocompatibility of an implant:

- from a chemical (compositional) point of view, a biomaterial must not contain elements that generate adverse and / or inflammatory reactions upon implantation. An important aspect is also related to the possible formation on the implant surface, in in vivo conditions, of new structures and compositions, dependent on the interactions that are manifested between the biomaterial and the environmental conditions specific to the implantation area. Their nature and physico - chemical characteristics can affects the long-term reliability of the implant.

- from a structural point of view, a biomaterial must have a density and a porosity corresponding to the structural function that the implant is to fulfill in the organism in which the implantation is made. Of particular importance is the microscopic nature of the implant surface.

- mechanical properties - a biomaterial, depending on the function that the implant must perform in the living organism, must have adequate mechanical strength, hardness and reliability.

- in the case of ocular, dermatological and dental applications, biomaterials must also have appropriate optical properties.

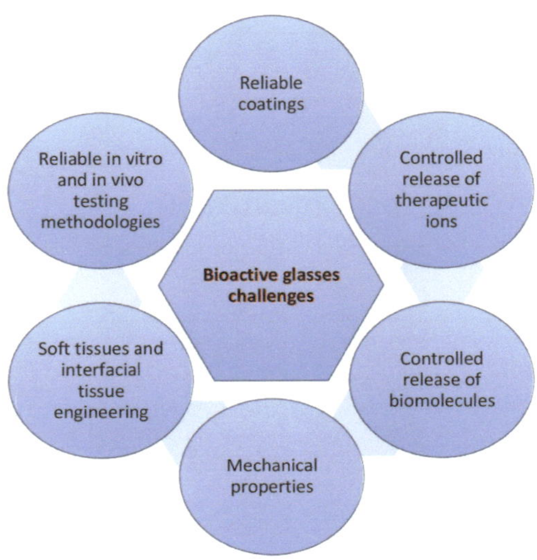

Figure 7.
Challenges and future trends for bioactive glasses (BGs)in medicine [34].

- another important aspect is related to the machinability of the biomaterial, this influencing the engineering of the implant itself.

Reliable Coatings with BGs on the mettalic implants are the oldest challenge but still researched. Thanks to their excellent mechanical properties and corrosion resistance, some metals are used as passive substitutes for the replacement of hard tissues (total hip and knee implants), as well as fracture implants (plates and rods), column fixing devices, and implantology. Dental. Other metal alloys have more active roles in implantology, such as vascular stents, catheter guidewires, orthodontic wires, and cochlear implants.

However, the biocompatibility of metal implants creates considerable concerns due to the fact that they can corrode in an in vivo environment [6]. Weakening of the implant by disintegrating its actual material, respectively the harmful effects of the resulting chemical compounds on neighboring tissues and organs are among the consequences of corrosion.

Pure metals are less commonly used, their alloys being used more often due to the fact that they improve some of their properties, such as corrosion resistance and hardness. Three groups of materials dominate the group of metallic biomaterials: 316 L stainless steels, cobalt and pure titanium alloys or titanium alloys.

Every material and class of materials works differently after the implantation, like some metals encapsulate fibrous tissue. The great advantage of the coatings on bioglass is that is not releasing toxic ions in the human body due to the potential to improve the implant stability by bonding it to the host bone and protect the implant from corrosion resistance.

The technologies involved for the surface modification of metallic implants with bioglass are: thermal spraying, sol–gel, chemical and electrochemical treatment. Unfortunately, not all technologies are suitable, some of them show many disadvantages like poor bonding strength between implants and coatings, the induction of phase transformation, modifications in the properties of coating or metallic implant, or both, and presence of impurities. **Table 6** present a synthesis of different glass coatings obtained through various methods [57].

Another perspective and future tendince of biomaterials is nanomedicine. Nanomedicine can be defined as an application of nanotechnology in the field of health in order to maintain and / or improve the health of the population using knowledge about the human body at the molecular level, as well as tools / nanoscale structures [22].

For this purpose, physical, chemical and biological properties of nanoscale materials are exploited, often new or improved properties, and the resulting nanostructures (nanoparticles or nanodevices), having the same size as biological entities, can interact more rapidly at the biomolecular level. on the surface as well as inside the cell [22].

So, in the near future, nanomedicine will seek to provide the tools and devices for research and practice, useful in the medical clinic, which could revolutionize the current way of thinking (prevention and diagnosis) and action (applied therapies) in the medical field.

By using nanoengineering, artificial tissues can be obtained and used to replace affected organs (kidneys, liver) or to regenerate nerves or produce implants that restore lost senses, such as sight or hearing. A major contribution is expected to nanomedicine could be brought about in areas such as: the definition and classification of diseases, their diagnosis and treatment, and the improvement of the structure and functioning of the human body [22].

Coating material	Substrate	Technique	Coatings' characteristics	Ref.
Biovetro®	Ti6Al4V	Atmospheric plasma spraying (APS)	Surface with wide superficial area of microcavities with round grains	[35]
45S5	Pure Titanium	APS	Bonding strength of BG + bond coat average 27.18 ± 2.24 MPa, and of BG average 8.56 ± 0.57 MPa.	[36]
P1, P2	AISI 316 L	APS	Microhardness of the coating 4.7–5.2 GPa; thickness of M1 389.8 ± 5.4 μm, M2 91.2 ± 8.2 μm, M3 262.6 ± 5.4 μm, and M4 80.8 ± 6.5 μm; adhesion strength of M1 2.7 ± 0.5 MPa, M2 3.7 ± 0.2 MPa, M3 3 ± 0.007 MPa, M4 4.4 ± 0.1 MPa	[37]
P0, P2	AISI 316 L & Ti6Al4V	Flame spraying (FS)	Microstructure consists of melted particles, pores and both vertical and parallel cracks. Thickness 126–275 μm; fracture toughness 5–7 $MPa/m^{1/2}$; Vickers hardness 4–5 HV	[38]
45S5	AISI 304	Solution precursor plasma spraying (SPPS)	Uniform coating average thickness 35 μm	[39]
Bio-K	Titanium	High velocity suspension flame spraying HVSFS	Coatings are entirely glassy. Tensile adhesion strength without bond coat: BioK-1 7 N/mm^2, BioK-2 3.8 N/mm^2, BioK-3 5 N/mm^2, BioK-4 9.8 N/mm^2 BioK-5 8 N/mm^2. With bond coat BioK-1 4 N/mm^2, BioK-2 5 N/mm^2, BioK-3 3 N/mm^2, BioK-4 9.8 N/mm^2 BioK-516 N/mm^2	[40]
BG-Ca/Mix	Grade 2 Titanium	HVSFS and suspension plasma spraying (SPS)	HVSFS coating very dense and thin. Hardness 396–516 HV; elastic modulus 61–95 GPa. Thickness 20–50 μm. SPS coatings thickness 50 μm	[41]
BG_Ca/HA	316 L Stainless Stell	SPS	Coatings compact and with continuous thickness with limited presence of pore	[42]
BG_Ca glass	Ti6Al4V	SPS	Coatings continuous and homogeneous thickness 31–40 μm; hardness 34–98 HV; elastic modulus 16–23 GPa and critical load 18–21 N	[43]
45S5, Bio K	Alumina	Enameling technique	Bio K completely amorphous, 45S5 some crystalline phases; both compact coatings. Vickers hardness 157 ± 39 HV, 146 ± 28 HV 45S5	[44]
RKKP, AP40	Zirconia	Enameling technique	Coatings with good mechanical properties and improved biocompatibility. ALP activity 1d 3.91 ± 1.15 μm AP40, 4.69 ± 2.10 μm RKKP. 9.98 ± 0.80 μm AP40 and 9.94 ± 2.90 μm RKKP at 5 and 10 days	[45]

Coating material	Substrate	Technique	Coatings' characteristics	Ref.
BG_Ca, BG_Ca/Mix BG_Ca_K	Ti6Al4V	Enameling technique	Uniform and well distributed coatings. Thickness BG_Ca 108 μm, BG_Ca/Mix 113 μm, BG_Ca_K 121 μm; Vickers hardness BG_Ca 232.1 ± 76.8 HV, BG_Ca/Mix 329.0 ± 81.0 HV, BG_Ca_K 317.9 ± 48.8 HV	[46]
LY-B0, LY-B1, LY-B2, LY-B3, LY-B4, LY-B5	Ti6Al4V	Enameling technique	Thickness 90–100 μm; critical strain energy release 6.56–14.61 J/m^2	[47]
6P61, 6P55	Ti6Al4V	Enameling technique	Some small pores. Thickness 86.0 ± 11.5 μm	[48]
Bioglass©, 6P44-a, 6P44-b, 6P44-c, 6P53-a, 6P53-b, 6P55, 6P57, 6P61, 6P68	Titanium, Ti6Al4V, Vitallium ©, Co-Cr alloy	Sol–gel method	Coatings without cracks or delamination. Hardness 5.3–6.3 GPa; density 2.5–2.7 g/cm^3	[49]
57.44CaO-35.42SiO_2-7.15P_2O_5 (mol.%)	CrCoMo alloy, Ti6Al4V, AISI 316 L	Sol–gel method	Glassy matrix with some defects and cracks. Thickness 1.5–3 _μm	[50]
45S5 BCG	AZ31 magnesium alloy	Sol–gel method	Integrated coatings with some asperities. Thickness 1.1 μm	[51]
Ag-BG	Titanium	Sol–gel method	Homogeneous and without macro and micro cracks	[52]
45S5	Ti6Al4V	Electrophoretic deposition (EPD)	Coatings with good adhesion without cracks. Rough surface in which the initial powder particles are still visible. Thickness 50–250 μm	[53]
Bioglass®	NiTi Alloy	EPD	Homogeneous microstructure without cracks or pores with uniform topography. Thickness 5–15 μm	[54]
45S5	Ti6Al4V	Pulsed laser deposition (PLD)	Coatings uniform without microcracks and pores. Thickness 1 μm; surface roughness 6 nm	[55]
T1, T2, T3, T4, T5, T6	Titanium	Radio-frequency magnetron sputtering (RF-MS)	Amorphous coatings with some crystalline phases. Thickness 1.8–2.4 μm	[56]

Table 6.
Summary of bioactive glass coatings on different metallic substrate.

In recent years, nanotechnology has found countless applications in the medical field, in the fields of: pharmaceutical (in targeted drug therapy), regenerative medicine (making nano-robots and devices used in cell regeneration), disease prevention, diagnosis (including by methods high-performance imaging) and nano-technology-based therapy.

The future of the field stays in the nanotechnology, being the most effective on cell and tissue level, mainly on the integration and regeneration, but also the identification of effective ways to trigger and control the regenerative process. The "nano-biomimetic" strategy depends on the following elements: intelligent biomaterials, bioactive signaling molecules and cells. Biomaterials are designed to react positively to changes in the proximity environment, stimulating specific regenerative events at the molecular level, directing cell proliferation and then differentiation, as well as the production and organization of the extracellular matrix.

A huge impact will also have the ability to implant cells, intelligent bioactive materials, which trigger the process of self-healing through the patient's own stem cells [22].

The field of nanotechnologies has established itself in recent years as one of the most topical fields, with a sustained pace of development and application and a revolutionary impact on industry and society. The global emergence of government investment programs in the field of nanotechnology is clear evidence of global interest in this field.

The potential evolutions of the research - development in the field of nanotechnologies, in the following years, are the following:

- half of the new materials that will appear will be obtained with the help of nanotechnologies, in sectors such as: electronics, chemical industry, heavy industry, pharmaceutical industry and aeronautical industry;

- the development of nanobiosystems science and engineering will allow a better understanding of living systems, the development of new solutions in health care and better biocompatible materials, the understanding of processes inside the cell or nervous system;

- application and integration of nanotechnology in fields of activity such as biology, electronics, medicine, etc., fields that include artificial organs, prolonging life, creating

- new systems by using biological principles, the laws of physics and the properties of different materials;

- tracking biocompatibility when creating new products;

- learning and education, based on nanoscale [22].

- In the future, the rapid development of nanomedicine could also be stimulated by better multidisciplinary collaboration between sectors of activity, such as industry, scientific research in general and medical research in particular.

7. Conclusions

In conclusion, bioglass is a chemical compound that belongs to a compositional family known to have the best bioactivity properties, as demonstrated by the connection with living tissues in a short time to only a few hours.

It is also known that the generation of artificial bone tissue would be very useful in cases of massive fractures. Based on bioactive glass, three-dimensional bioactive matrices have also been developed for tissue regeneration using the deposition of human osteoblasts on the 3D matrix for tissue creation in vitro.

The results obtained so far qualify the bioglasses for widespread use in medical interventions and the ongoing research currently underway increases the hope of success of the intervention and also increases confidence in this material.

Conflict of interest

"The authors declare no conflict of interest."

Author details

Petrică Vizureanu*, Mădălina Simona Bălţatu, Andrei Victor Sandu, Dragos Cristian Achitei, Dumitru Doru Burduhos Nergis and Manuela Cristina Perju
Faculty of Materials Science and Engineering, Department of Technologies and Equipments for Materials Processing, "Gheorghe Asachi" Technical University of Iaşi, Mangeron, Iasi, Romania

*Address all correspondence to: peviz2002@yahoo.com; peviz@tuiasi.ro

References

[1] Bombac D.M., Brojan M., Fajfar P., Kosel F., Turk R.: Review of materials in medical applications. Materials and Geoenvironment. 2007; 54(4): 471-499.

[2] Popa C., Cândea V., Șimon V., Lucaciu D., Rotaru O. Știința biomaterialelor. Ed. U.T. Press; 2008. 59 p.

[3] Antoniac I., Biomateriale metalice utilizate la executia componentelor endoprotezelor totale de sold. Ed. Printech; 2007. 94 p.

[4] Hench L.L., Wilson J., An Introduction to Bioceramics, Advanced Series in Ceramics. World Scientific Publishing. 1993; 1: 23 p. https://doi.org/10.1142/2028

[5] Hench L.L.: Bioceramics. J. Am. Cer. Soc. 1998; 81 (7): 1705-1728 p. doi:10.1111/j.1151-2916.1998.tb02540.x

[6] Hench L.L., Wilson J.: Bioceramics. MRS Bulletin. 1991; 62-74 p.

[7] Osborn J.F., Weiss T.: Hydroxylapatite ceramics - a bone-like biomaterial. Preliminary report. SSO Schweiz Monatsschr Zahnheilkd. 1978; 88 (10): 1166-1172 p.

[8] Gibson L.J.: The mechanical behaviour of cancellous bone. J. Biomechanics. 1985; 18 (5): 317-328 p. https://doi.org/10.1016/0021-9290(85)90287-8

[9] Vallet-Regi M., Arcos D. Biomimetic Nanoceramics in Clinical Use - From Materials to Applications. RSC Publishing. 2008; 100-120 p.

[10] Fetner A.E., Low S.B., Wilson J., Hench L.L: Histologic evaluation of bioglass particulates in gingival tissue. J Dent Res. 1987; 66: 298-398 p.

[11] Wilson J., Low S.B: Bioactive ceramics for periodontal treatment – comparative studies in the Patus monkey. J Appl Biomater. 1992; 3:123-129 p. DOI: 10.1002/jab.770030208

[12] Schepers E.J.G., Ducheyne P: Bioactive glass particles of narrow size range for the treatment of oral bone defects: a 1-24 months experiment with several materials and particle sizes and size ranges. J Oral Rehabil. 1997; 24: 171-181 p. https://doi.org/10.1111/j.1365-2842.1997.tb00311.x

[13] Low S.B., King C.J., Krieger J. An evaluation of bioactive ceramic in the treatment of periodontal osseous defects. Int J Periodontol Rest, Dent. 1997; 17: 359-367 p.

[14] Wers E. Elaboration d'un biomatériau poreux à base d'une matrice vitreuse présentant le phénomène d'ostéoconduction. 2014; 50-80 p.

[15] Kokubo T.: Bioactive glass-ceramics – properties and applications. Biomaterials. 1991; 12: 155-163 p. DOI: 10.1016/0142-9612(91)90194-f

[16] Hench L.L., Polak J.M.: Third-generation biomedical materials. Science. 2002; 295: 1014-1017 p. DOI: 10.1126/science.1067404

[17] Rahaman M.N., Day D.E., Bal B.S., Fu Q., Jung S.B., Bonewald L.F., et al.: Bioactive glass in tissue engineering. Acta Biomater. 2011; 7: 2355-2373 p. DOI: 10.1016/j.actbio.2011.03.016

[18] Drago L., Toscano M., Bottagisio M.: Recent Evidence on Bioactive Glass Antimicrobial and Antibiofilm Activity: A Mini-Review. Materials. 2018; 11(2): 326. DOI: 10.3390/ma11020326

[19] Rabiee S.M., Nazparvar N., Azizian, M., Vashaee D., Tayebi L.: Effect of ion substitution on properties of bioactive glasses: A review. Ceramics International. 2015; 41 (6): 7241-7251 p. DOI:10.1016/j.ceramint.2015.02.140

[20] https://en.wikipedia.org/wiki/Bioglass_45S5 [Internet] [Accessed: 2021-06-22]

[21] Shams M., Karimi M., Ghollasi M., Nezafati N., Salimi A.: Electrospun poly-l-lactic acid nanofibers decorated with melt-derived S53P4 bioactive glass nanoparticles. the effect of nanoparticles on proliferation and osteogenic differentiation of human bone marrow mesenchymal stem cells in vitro. Ceramics International. 2018; 44(16): 20211-20219 p. DOI: 10.1016/j.ceramint.2018.08.005

[22] Widiyanti S., Faradisa E., Mubarok A.M., Fauziyyah N., Triadi H.A., Nawawi M.R., Nandiyanto A.B.D. REVIEW: SYNTHESIS OF NANO BIOACTIVE GLASS OR BIOGLASS. Green and Applied Chemistry. 2020; 10: 01-32 p. ISSN: 2605-6895.

[23] Kumar P., Dehiya B.S., Sindhu A., Kumar V.: Synthesis and Characterization of Nano Bioglass for the Application of Bone Tissue Engineering. Journal of Nanoscience and Technology. 2018; 471-474 p. https://doi.org/10.30799/jnst.127.18040503

[24] Durgalakshmi D., Subhathirai S. P., Balakumar S.: Nano-bioglass. a versatile antidote for bone tissue engineering problems. Procedia Engineering. 2014; 92: 2-8 p. https://doi.org/10.1016/j.proeng.2013.08.288

[25] Liu Z., Peng R.: Inorganic nanomaterials for tumor angiogenesis imaging, European Journal of Nuclear Medicine and Molecular Imaging. 2010; 37(1): S147-163 p. DOI: 10.1007/s00259-010-1452-y

[26] Sculean A., Barbe G., Chiantella G.C., Arweiler N.B., Berakdar M., Brecx M.: Clinical evaluation of an enamel matrix protein derivative combined with a bioactive glass for the treatment of intrabony periodontal defects in humans. J Periodontol. 2002; 73: 401-408 p. https://doi.org/10.1902/jop.2002.73.4.401

[27] Mengel R., Soffner M., Flores-De-Jacoby L.: Bioabsorbable membrane and bioactive glass in the treatment of intrabony defects in patients with generalized aggressive periodontitis: results of a 12-month clinical and radiological study. J Periodontol. 2003; 74: 899-908 p. DOI: 10.1902/jop.2003.74.6.899

[28] Sergi R., Belluci D., Cannillo V., A review of bioactive glass/natural polymer composites: State of the Art. Materials. 2020; 13: 5560. DOI: 10.3390/ma13235560

[29] http://www.keydent.net/cerabone [Internet] [Accessed: 2021-06-22]

[30] http://rontis.ro/divisions-business-units/consumer-healthcare/novabone/?lang=en [Internet] [Accessed: 2021-06-22]

[31] https://theraglass.co.uk/ [Internet] [Accessed: 2021-06-22]

[32] https://avalonmed.com/product/rediheal-dental-care-10-pod-blister-pack/ [Internet] [Accessed: 2021-06-22]

[33] https://www.dotmed.com/listing/disposables-general/porex/medpor-surgical-implant-ref%3A-8322-titan-%26-barrier/chin-two-piece-large-9mm-projection-56-x-38-x-9mm-exp.-10.2019/3369310 [Internet] [Accessed: 2021-06-22]

[34] Francesco B., Sepideh H., Saeid K.: Bioactive Glasses: Where Are We and Where Are We Going?. Journal of Functional Biomaterials. 2018; 9: 25. DOI: 10.3390/jfb9010025

[35] Gabbi C., Cacchioli A.: Bioactive glass coating: Physicochemical aspects and biological findings. Biomaterials. 1995; 16: 515-520 p. https://doi.org/10.1016/0142-9612(95)91123-G

[36] Goller G. The effect of bond coat on mechanical properties of plasma sprayed bioglass-titanium coatings. Ceram. Int. 2004; 30: 351-355 p. DOI: 10.1016/S0272-8842(03)00107-X

[37] Monsalve M., Ageorges H., Lopez E., Vargas F., Bolivar F.: Bioactivity and mechanical properties of plasma-sprayed coatings of bioglass powders. Surf. Coat. Technol. 2013; 220: 60-66 p. https://doi.org/10.1016/j.surfcoat.2012.11.075

[38] Monsalve M., Lopez E., Ageorges H., Vargas F.: Bioactivity and mechanical properties of bioactive glass coatings fabricated by flame spraying. Surf. Coat. Technol. 2015; 268: 142-146 p. https://doi.org/10.1016/j.surfcoat.2014.08.041

[39] Cañas E., Orts M.J., Boccaccini A.R., Sánchez E.: Solution precursor plasma spraying (SPPS): A novel and simple process to obtain bioactive glass coatings. Mater. Lett. 2018; 223: 198-202 p. DOI: https://doi.org/10.1016/j.matlet.2018.04.031

[40] Bellucci D., Bolelli G., Cannillo V., Gadow R., Killinger A., Lusvarghi L.: High velocity suspension flame sprayed (HVSFS) potassium-based bioactive glass coatings with and without TiO_2 bond coat. Surf. Coat. Technol. 2012; 206: 3857-3868 p. DOI:10.1016/j.surfcoat.2012.02.041

[41] Bolelli G., Bellucci D., Cannillo V., Gadow R., Killinger A., Lusvarghi L.: Comparison between suspension plasma sprayed and high velocity suspension flame sprayed bioactive coatings. Surf. Coat. Technol. 2015; 280: 232-249 p. https://doi.org/10.1016/j.surfcoat.2015.08.039

[42] Cattini A., Bellucci D., Sola A., Paw L., Cannillo V.: Suspension plasma spraying of optimised functionally graded coatings of bioactive glass/hydroxyapatite. Surf. Coat. Technol. 2013; 236: 118-126 p. DOI: 10.1016/j.surfcoat.2013.09.037

[43] Cattini A., Łatka L., Bellucci D., Bolelli G., Sola A., Lusvarghi L.: Suspension plasma sprayed bioactive glass coatings: Effects of processing on microstructure, mechanical properties and in-vitro behaviour. Surf. Coat. Technol. 2013; 220: 52-59 p. DOI:10.1016/j.surfcoat.2012.10.076

[44] Cannillo V., Sola A.: Different approaches to produce coatings with bioactive glasses: Enamelling vs. plasma spraying. J. Eur. Ceram. Soc. 2010; 30: 2031-2039 p. DOI:10.1016/j.jeurceramsoc.2010.04.021

[45] Bosetti M., Vernè E., Ferraris M., Ravaglioli A., Cannas M.: In vitro characterisation of zirconia coated by bioactive glass. Biomaterials. 2001; 22: 987-994 p. DOI: 10.1016/s0142-9612(00)00264-7

[46] Sola A., Bellucci D., Cannillo V.: Enamelled coatings produced with low-alkaline bioactive glasses. Surf. Coat. Technol. 2014; 248: 1-8 p. DOI:10.1016/j.surfcoat.2014.03.025

[47] Li Y., Matinmanesh A., Curran D.J., Schemitsch E.H., Zalzal P., Papini, M.: Characterization and fracture property of different strontium-containing borate-based glass coatings for Ti6Al4V substrates. J. Non-Cryst. Solids. 2017;

458: 69-75 p. https://doi.org/10.1016/j.jnoncrysol.2016.12.010

[48] Foppiano S., Marshall S.J., Saiz E., Tomsia A.P., Marshall G.W.: Functionally graded bioactive coatings: Reproducibility and stability of the coating under cell culture conditions. Acta Biomater. 2006; 2: 133-142 p. DOI: 10.1016/j.actbio.2005.12.003

[49] Lopez-esteban S., Saiz E., Fujino S., Oku T., Suganuma K., Tomsia A.P.: Bioactive glass coatings for orthopedic metallic implants. J. Eur. Ceram. Soc. 2003; 23: 2921-2930 p. DOI: 10.1016/S0955-2219(03)00303-0

[50] Durán A., Conde A., Gómez Coedo A., Dorado T., García C., Ceré S.: Sol-gel coatings for protection and bioactivation of metals used in orthopaedic devices. J. Mater. Chem. 2004; 14: 2282-2290 p. https://doi.org/10.1039/B401370K

[51] Huang K., Cai S., Xu G., Ye X., Dou Y., Ren M.: Preparation and characterization of mesoporous 45S5 bioactive glass-ceramic coatings on magnesium alloy for corrosion protection. J. Alloys Compd. 2013; 580: 290-297 p. DOI:10.1016/j.jallcom.2013.05.103

[52] Pouraghaei S., Moztarzadeh F., Nezafati N., Rahmanian F.: Synthesis and characterization of silvercontaining sol-gel derived bioactive glass coating. Prot. Met. Phys. Chem. Surf. J. 2016; 52: 285-290 p. DOI: https://doi.org/10.1134/S2070205116020246

[53] Luis J., Manrique E.: Processing and characterisation of bioglass® coating on Ti6Al4V substrates. Supl. Rev. Latinoam. Metal. Mater. 2009; S1: 77-90 p.

[54] Boccaccini A.R., Peters C., Roether J.A., Eifler D., Misra S.K., Minay E.J.: Electrophoretic deposition of polyetheretherketone (PEEK) and PEEK/Bioglass® coatings on NiTi shape memory alloy wires. J. Mater. Sci. 2006; 41: 8152-8159 p. https://doi.org/10.3390/ma13153251

[55] Zhao Y., Song M., Chen C., Liu, J.: The role of the pressure in pulsed laser deposition of bioactive glass films. J. Non-Cryst. Solids. 2008; 354: 4000-4004 p. DOI: 10.1016/j.jnoncrysol.2008.05.019

[56] Stuart B., Gimeno-Fabra M., Segal J., Ahmed I., Grant D.M.: Preferential sputtering in phosphate glass systems for the processing of bioactive coatings. Thin Solid Films. 2015; 589: 534-542 p. DOI 10.1016/j.tsf.2015.05.072

[57] Sergi R., Bellucci D., Cannillo V.: A Comprehensive Review of Bioactive Glass Coatings: State of the Art, Challenges and Future Perspectives. Coatings. 2020; 10: 757. DOI: 10.3390/coatings10080757

Chapter 9

Surface Modification of Titanium Orthodontic Implants

Abdulqadir Rampurawala and Amol Patil

Abstract

Orthodontic miniscrews have had a considerable impact on modern orthodontic treatment, not only by providing a new source of anchors for anchorage-demanding cases, but also for force management and control. Whilst miniscrews need to be mechanically stable during treatment to provide sufficient anchorage and predictable force control, as temporary anchorage devices they need also be easy to remove after orthodontic treatment. These requirements differentiate orthodontic miniscrews from dental implants - which once placed, are not to be removed - and dictate the approach as to how their clinical performance can be optimized. Over the past decade, various titanium surface modifications and improvements in implant surface topography have shown to enhance osseointegration of endosseous dental implants. Some of these techniques have helped provide a similar enhancement of the biomechanical potential of orthodontic miniscrews as well. In this perspective, we present a brief discussion on all such reported techniques followed by a detailed account of the most recently proposed ultraviolet photofunctionalization technique - a novel chair-side surface modification method.

Keywords: anchorage, stability, surface modification, osseointegration, biomechanical potential, photofunctionalization, miniscrews

1. Introduction

Anchorage control plays an important role in orthodontic treatment. Nevertheless, in clinical practice, this was a typically difficult and unpredictable challenge for many years. In the 1990s, temporary anchorage devices (TADs) called mini-implants were the first implants used to provide absolute and compliance-free intraoral anchorage [1]. Subsequently, these implants became smaller in size and are today used as 'orthodontic miniscrews' (**Figure 1**). They have the advantages of low cost, simple surgical placement, and ease of removal. Miniscrews have, therefore, found applications in the treatment of a variety of malocclusions. However, as with any other implanted material in the human body, the stability of orthodontic miniscrews is paramount to their clinical acceptability. The clinical stability of miniscrews has proven to be exceptionally high (**Table 1**). A few studies have reported success rates higher than 90% [2, 3], while others have reported slightly lower success rates [4, 5]. Notwithstanding such a high rate of clinical success, various surface modification techniques have been

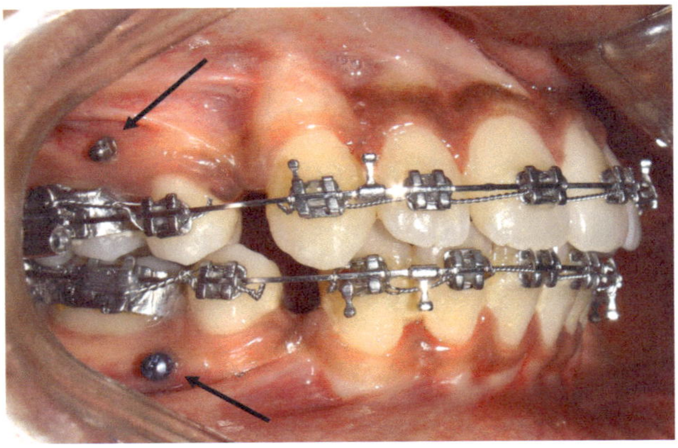

Figure 1.
Miniscrews used as temporary anchorage devices (TADs) in fixed orthodontic treatment of malocclusions (black arrows).

Study	Result
Antoszewska et al. (2009) [2]	Success rate of 93.43%
Park et al. (2006) [3]	Success rate of 91.6%
Papageorgiou et al. (2012) [4]	Failure rate of 13.5%
Alharbi et al. (2018) [5]	Failure rate of was 13.5%

Table 1.
Clinical stability of orthodontic miniscrews.

proposed to further enhance the stability of miniscrews, thereby allowing the orthodontist to optimize and expand its clinical use.

2. Surface modification of orthodontic miniscrews

The use of commercially pure titanium or titanium alloy (Ti-6Al-4 V) as an implant material has made it possible to predictably secure miniscrews into the maxilla and/or mandible by facilitating direct bone apposition to the implant surface and creating a unique bone-implant interface. This process is termed as "osseointegration" [6]. It is this intimate relationship between living bone and the titanium miniscrew surface that is responsible for its high degree of stability. Various surface treatments of titanium implants have been known to modify both the surface composition as well as its topography, thereby increasing the implant surface roughness and area, which might lead to enhanced bone-screw contact (BSC) [7–12]. Surface modification also enhances the interactions with biological fluids and cells, and thereby accelerates peri-implant bone healing as well as improves osseointegration at sites that lack sufficient quantity and/or quality of bone [7, 11–14]. Evaluation of BSC and removal torque (RT) can, therefore, be used as reliable measures of osseointegration of implants [4]. The improved osseointegration by surface modification is a characteristic exhibited by all titanium surfaces and hence, it applies equally to titanium orthodontic miniscrews [15].

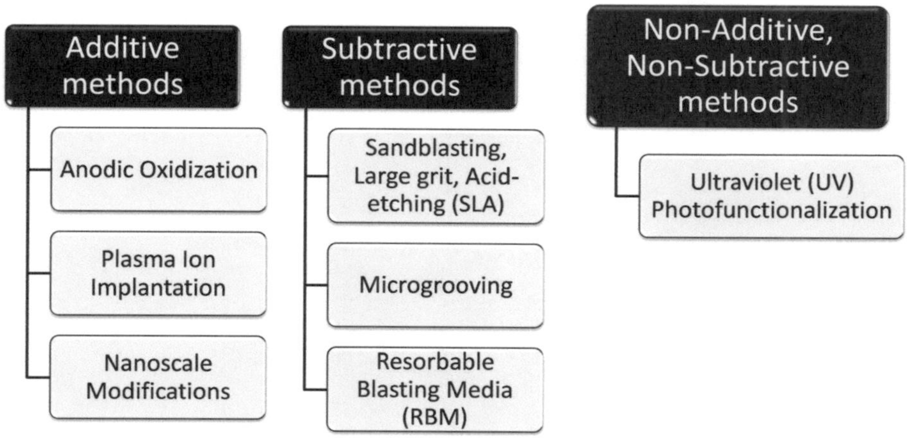

Figure 2.
Different types of surface modification techniques available for orthodontic miniscrews.

Since the advent of titanium dental implants as prosthetic tooth replacements in the 1990s and titanium mini-plates and miniscrews as skeletal anchorage devices later in the same decade, a considerable amount of research has been done on surface treatments and modifications of these titanium devices. Broadly, these surface modifications can be categorized as either subtractive or additive methods (**Figure 2**). The subtractive methods are machining/turning, sandblasting, acid-etching, sandblasting (large-grit) combined with acid-etching (SLA), dual acid-etching and laser treatment. The additive methods are anodization (also known as anodic oxidization), fluoride surface treatment, plasma spraying (titanium or hydroxyapatite), sol–gel coating, sputter deposition, electrophoretic deposition, biomimetic precipitation (Ca-P) and most recently, nanoscale modifications with or without drug incorporation [16, 17]. Many of these techniques have been used to augment the biomechanical potential of orthodontic miniscrews and have proven to be experimentally as well as clinically effective. Following is an account of all the surface modification techniques that have been used to enhance the biomechanical potential of orthodontic miniscrews.

2.1 Sandblasting, large-grit, acid-etching

One of the earliest methods for surface treatment that was introduced, and one that has stood the test of time, is sandblasting with or without acid-etching. In this technique, alumina (Al_2O_3) particles at high pressures are blasted onto the implant surface, after which it may be treated with acidic solutions. The alumina particles are essentially large-grit particles with sizes ranging from approximately 250–500 μm, and the solutions used are highly concentrated acids like hydrochloric acid (HCl), nitric acid (HNO_3) and sulfuric acid (H_2SO_4). This process creates the desired roughness on the implant surface. The application of sandblasting using large-grit alumina particles followed by acid-etching is collective known as the SLA method (**Figure 3**). Wehrbein et al. was one of the first to study the effects of SLA surface treatment on orthodontic implants in humans. Histomorphometric findings revealed that the SLA technique was able to achieve up to 70–80% of BSC, which was remarkably high [18].

Animal studies have routinely been carried out in this regard and have shown successful results. Various experimental studies conducted in rabbit tibiae and

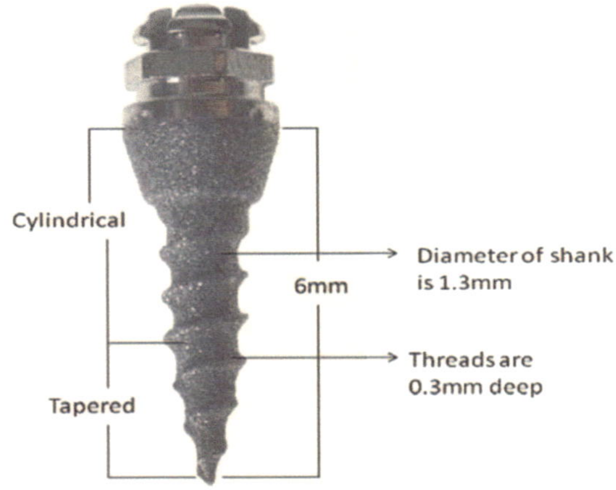
Cylindrical
Diameter of shank is 1.3mm
6mm
Threads are 0.3mm deep
Tapered

Figure 3.
Miniscrew surface modified with large-grit sand-blasting and acid-etching (SLA) (Taken from: Yadav et al. [20].)

femurs that have compared smooth (machined or untreated) and SLA miniscrews have reported greater RT values and BSC in the surface treated miniscrews [19–22]. These results are suggestive of higher miniscrew stability especially in the early stages of healing thereby allowing immediate/early loading, and of an enhanced biological response due to increased osseointegration potential. Chang *et al.* compared conventional smooth miniscrews with SLA as well as alkaline-etched (SL/NaOH) miniscrews in rabbit tibiae and found that both SLA and SL/NaOH groups had greater RT and BSC values than the conventional group [15]. However, as per a scanning electron microscope (SEM) analysis, the SLA surface showed roughness at two levels: (i) small micro-pits produced by the acid-etching procedure and (ii) microscopic pits superimposed on a sandblasted macro-rough texture, whereas the SL/NaOH surface showed only macroscopic surface properties. This indicates that alkaline-etching might not be as effective as acid-etching for surface treatment of miniscrews. Sirisa-Ard et al. reported that despite an increase in BSC values of SLA miniscrews over 8 weeks of healing in New Zealand rabbits, there was no significant increase of RT values as compared to machined miniscrews over a similar period, suggesting that SLA surface preparation did not have any added benefit in enhancing miniscrew stability [23].

Similar comparative studies between SLA and machined miniscrews have been carried out in other animals such as beagle, foxhound and mongrel dogs. Histomorphometric and micro-computed tomographic (micro-CT) analyses from those studies have revealed greater BSC values with SLA miniscrews indicating their increased osseointegration potential [24, 25]. Some studies have also reported variable torque values for SLA miniscrews at both insertion and removal, essentially indicating equal or improved stability when compared to machined miniscrews [25, 26]. Kim et al. used a digital device to measure the total energy at removal of miniscrews and found that the SLA group had greater values, thus indicating an enhanced biomechanical potential [26]. On the contrary, a similar torque analysis by Vilani et al.

concluded that since there was no significant difference between mobility and insertion torque (IT) or RT of the SLA and machined miniscrew groups, their stability was nearly comparable [27].

The aforementioned positive effects of SLA surface treatment have been validated by a few *in vivo* studies on humans as well. Schätzle et al. compared the stability of standard SLA treated palatal implants with those modified by rinsing under nitride (N_2) protection following SLA treatment to enhance their wettability [28]. Resonance frequency analysis (RFA) at various time points over a period of 12 weeks showed that the implant stability quotient (ISQ) for both groups was similar at the beginning but gradually increased significantly for the experimental group by the end of the study period. This suggests that chemical modification of SLA miniscrews can positively influence their biologic potential and decrease healing time. While most of the research has been focused on evaluating BSC and individual implant stability, some authors have also reported the effect of SLA surface modification on the anchorage ability of miniscrews under orthodontic loads. Calderón et al. used a method of angular measurements on occlusal radiographs for evaluation of positional mini-implant stability and subsequently confirmed those readings on a cone-beam computed tomography (CBCT) occlusal view of just one patient from the study group [29]. As per their calculations, 65% mini-implants showed a $\leq$ 1degree shift, whereas 35% mini-implants showed a $\geq$ 2 degree shift. Kim et al. conducted a comprehensive 3-dimensional CBCT analysis of SLA treated mini-implants inserted in the posterior maxillary buccal alveolar region and found that there was no significant change in implant position over 9 months of en-masse retraction [30]. Both of these studies indicate that SLA modification of miniscrews may provide stable and stationary anchorage for orthodontic considerations. However, a couple of studies have reported that despite their relatively greater success rates and better IT values, SLA miniscrews do not have any significant advantage over conventional machined miniscrews in terms of initial stability or overall success [31, 32].

Results from clinical studies hold greater value if they are supplemented by similar proofs from experiments carried out at cellular and/or molecular levels, and vice-versa. In an *in vitro* study, Proff et al. compared three groups: airflow treated, SLA treated and machined miniscrews, incubated in a fibroblast cell culture [33]. Using the AlamarBlue assay and fluorescence microscopy, they reported a slight reduction in metabolic cell activity after 24 hours in the airflow group but fibroblast survival and rate of cell proliferation were identical in all the three groups. In an *ex vivo* study of the peri-implant tissue surrounding SLA miniscrews obtained from beagle dogs after 1 and 4 weeks of healing, Nahm et al. carried out gene profiling analyses to reveal that genes encoding extracellular matrix (ECM) constituents were upregulated at the early stage of healing and that genes associated with bone mineralization, ossification, stem-cell fate regulation were upregulated at the later stage of healing [34]. Kim et al. attempted to study the chemical integration mechanism between human bone and titanium miniscrew surfaces at a nanoscale level [35]. A single SLA treated miniscrew was analyzed after 2 months of healing. High-resolution transmission electron microscopy (TEM) and energy dispersive X-ray spectroscopy (EDS) showed evidence of crystalline hydroxyapatite and intermixing of bone with the oxide layer of the miniscrew surface. Scanning TEM (STEM) and electron energy loss spectroscopy (EELS) revealed that carbon existed in polysaccharides, calcium and phosphorus existed as tricalcium phosphate (TCP), and titanium existed in its oxidized form, all rather interesting results. Additionally, the oxygen energy loss near edge structures (ELNESs) showed a possibility of the presence of $CaTiO_3$. The possible existence of the osseohybridization area and the form of the carbon suggests that osseointegration is not purely a mechanical bone-implant interaction and therefore, reconsideration of the standard definition of osseointegration is necessary. In a most recent study on this topic, Kim et al. studied the molecular surface interaction of a titanium mini-implant (SLA treated) retrieved from a patient after 2 months of healing [36]. Layer profiling using atom probe tomography (APT) showed high concentrations of calcium (Ca) and phosphorus (P) in the bone, titanium oxide (TiO) in the interface, and titanium (Ti) in the implant. Such a nanoscale resolution showing atom-sharing zones at the implant-bone interface provides valuable insight into the process of osseointegration.

It is evident by now that SLA modification of the orthodontic miniscrew surface has some kind of positive biomechanical advantage over conventional machined miniscrews. One would think that this intimate bone-implant relationship comes at a cost of tissue damage to the surrounding bone while retrieval of miniscrews at the end of the treatment period. Studies have shown that despite SLA treated miniscrews having greater BSC and RT values on removal, there was no reported bone fracture or tissue destruction during unscrewing [30, 46]. Kim et al. recommended a non-loading period of fewer than 6 months before removal for optimal bone health and post-operative healing [37].

2.2 Microgrooving

Machining/turning is one of the most basic and simplest forms of implant surface treatment. In actuality, it is an essential part of the manufacturing process that gives shape to the cutting surface and determines the pitch of the screw, which in turn affects the cutting capacity and biomechanical properties of the implant (**Figure 4**). Kim et al. extended this concept of surface turning to a micro-scale level and prepared miniscrews with microgrooves (50 μm pitch, 10 μm depth) on 300 μm of the upper cutting surface [38]. This experimental group (MG) was compared against conventional non-microgroove (NMG) miniscrews in beagle dogs after 16 weeks of orthodontic loading. Histomorphometry revealed higher BSC values on the pressure side of the MG group. Further histological analysis showed that gingival connective tissue

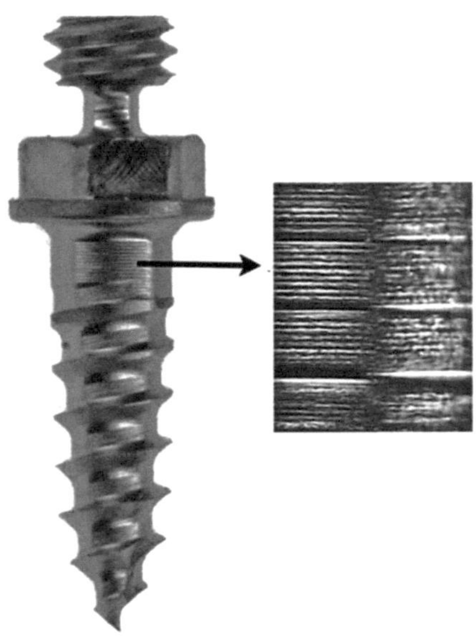

Figure 4.
Microgrooving technique of surface modification. The microgroove shown here is 50 μm pitch and 10 μm depth in 300 μm on the surface. (Taken from: Kim et al. [38].)

fibers (GCTF) in the MG group were oriented perpendicular to the miniscrew surface whereas in the NMG group they were parallel. Additionally, fluorescent microscopy showed more bone remodeling on the pressure sides in both groups as compared to the tension sides. This suggests that addition of microgrooves could exert some positive effects on the soft tissue adaptation and bone healing around orthodontic miniscrews.

2.3 Anodic oxidization

Another type of surface treatment reported in the past is anodic oxidization of titanium implants [39]. It is an electrochemical process wherein an oxide film is produced on a metallic substrate. Anodic oxidization of titanium orthodontic miniscrews produces a titanium dioxide (TiO_2) layer on the implant surface with a thickness ranging from 10 to 25 μm increasing from the neck of the implant to the apex (**Figure 5**). Ivanoff et al. conducted some of the first clinical studies to evaluate the effects of anodic oxidization on micro-implant osseointegration [40, 41]. With the help of an optical confocal laser profilometer and histomorphometric analysis, they showed that anodized micro-implants had an increased surface roughness and BSC value as compared to machined micro-implants. Omar et al. investigated the gene expression and cellular reaction around machined and anodized miniscrews in rabbit tibiae at 1, 3 and 6 days [42]. The quantitative polymerase chain reaction (qPCR) and immunohistochemistry results concluded that (i) the rapid recruitment of mesenchymal cells, (ii) the rapid triggering of gene expression crucial for bone remodeling and (iii) the transient nature of inflammation, probably constitute the biological mechanisms for osseointegration and high implant stability associated with anodically oxidized miniscrews. Karmarker et al. reported higher RT values for anodized miniscrews indicating their improved stability [43]. Choi et al. carefully studied the changes in surface roughness and characteristics of anodically oxidized miniscrews [44, 45]. Atomic force microscopy (AFM) revealed that anodized miniscrews had nanotubular open pores and increased roughness on the middle thread edges. Nonetheless, there were no differences in IT or RT

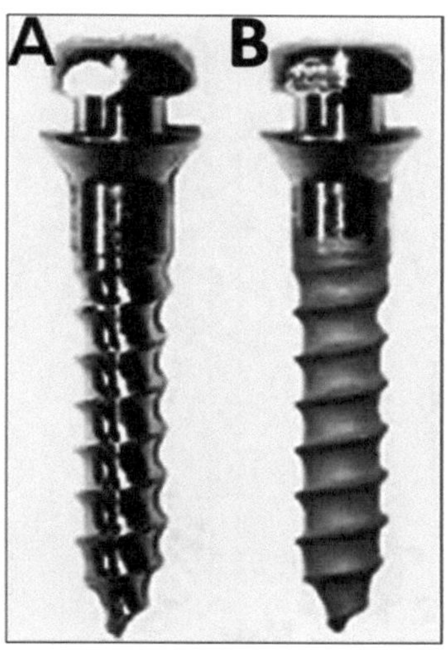

Figure 5.
Surface modification by anodic oxidization. (A) Machined surface miniscrew; (B) Anodic oxidized miniscrew. (Taken from: Choi et al. [44].)

values as well as BSC values of anodized miniscrews when compared to machined miniscrews. Conflicting results from the aforementioned studies suggest that the role of anodic oxidization in enhancing the biomechanical stability of orthodontic miniscrews might yet be questionable.

2.4 Plasma ion implantation

Attempts by some researchers to improve the corrosion and wear resistance of titanium implants have led to the development of a surface modification technique known as plasma ion implantation. In this technique, the surface of orthodontic mini-screws is coated with a thin film of titanium nitride (TiN) and/or zirconium nitride (ZrN) which acts as a protective layer (**Figure 6**). Kim et al. studied the mechanical and electrochemical changes on the surface of plasma ion implanted miniscrews [46]. Field emission SEM (FE-SEM) and EDS analysis showed that when compared to non-coated miniscrews, the TiN and ZrN coated miniscrews had a smoother surface owing to a decrease in the number of machined defects. Electrochemical tests revealed that coated miniscrews had a reduced corrosion current density. Later, on comparing the biologic stability of plasma ion implanted and SLA miniscrews in beagle dogs after a loading period of 3 and 12 weeks, Cho et al. concluded that since there was no difference in BSC, bone volume ratio or the number of osteoblasts around the miniscrews in both groups, they had similar biologic characteristics [47].

2.5 Resorbable blasting media

The previously described method of SLA surface modification of miniscrews consisted of sandblasting with alumina (Al_2O_3) particles. These particles do not resorb *in vivo* and therefore, are non-resorbable blasting media. However, sandblasting of implant surfaces with resorbable blasting media (RBM) such as hydroxyapatite or calcium phosphate particles has also been reported recently [48]. In an *in vitro* comparative evaluation of the physical characteristics of machined, acid-etched, RBM treated and hybrid (machined + acid-etched) orthodontic mini-implants, Kim et al. reported

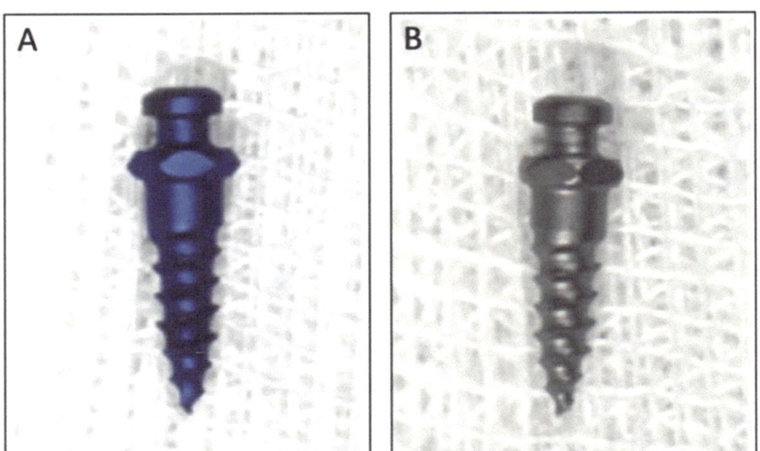

Figure 6.
Surface modification with plasma ion-implantation (A) and SLA treated miniscrew (B). (Taken from: Cho et al. [47].)

that all the surface treated groups had higher IT values, and the RBM and hybrid groups showed significantly higher surface roughness values [49]. *In vivo* studies on rabbit tibiae have also shown effective results. Gansukh et al. verified previous findings by reporting that after 4 weeks of healing, there was no difference in the IT, RT, and BSC values of machined and RBM treated mini-implants [50]. However, histomorphometric analysis showed an increased bone-area (BA) in the RBM group. In a similar study by Kim et al., the hybrid group consisted of partially RBM treated mini-implants i.e. lower 1/3rd of the cutting edge was left untreated [51]. Out of the four groups, the hybrid group showed the least reduction in bone cutting capacity, highest RT values at 4 and 8 weeks of healing, and the highest amount of tissue remnants on the mini-implant surface. Analysis by EDS showed that calcium and phosphorus were present only on the surface of the hybrid group implants, suggesting that partial RBM surface treatment was perhaps the most clinically effective one. All of these studies conclude that surface treatment of orthodontic mini-implants with RBM may provide good initial stability and has the potential to enhance osseointegration without negatively affecting their bone cutting capacity.

2.6 Nanoscale modifications

One of the latest techniques for surface modification of dental alloys and implants is their nanoscale modification. This involves the formation of nanotubular arrays mainly by anodization of the surface under specific voltages in various electrochemical solutions (**Figure 7**). Oh et al. combined multiple methods of surface treatment and studied its effect on the stability and osseointegration potential of orthodontic miniscrews in rat tibia [52]. This unique method involved anodization (TiO_2 nanotubular arrays) and cyclic pre-calcification (biomimetic Ca-P coating) of miniscrews followed by heat treatment. This method was called APH treatment. Results from mechanical torque testing and histological and SEM/EDS analysis showed that APH treated miniscrews had higher RT and BSC values after both 3 and 6 weeks of healing. Early deposition of densely mineralized bone around APH treated miniscrews was observed, implying good bonding to the treated surface. Jang et al. closely studied the effects of isolated nanoscale modifications on miniscrew biomechanical properties in rabbits [53]. Nanotubular arrays of TiO_2 (70 nm diameter, 5 μm length) were produced using a two-step anodization process. When compared to machined miniscrews, the experimental group showed higher BSC and bone-volume-ratio (BVR) values on histomorphometric and micro-CT analysis. Nanotubular arrays have also been used as drug-delivery systems to enhance the biologic potential of miniscrews. In a similar evaluation, Cha et al. used tunnel miniscrews with and without recombinant human bone morphogenetic protein – 2 (rhBMP-2) loaded

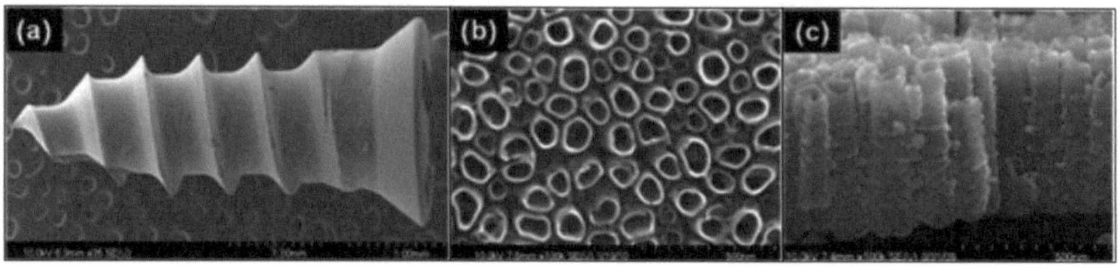

Figure 7.
SEM images of Ti_6Al_4V miniscrews: (A) untreated, and (B,C) nanotubes formed on the surface; (B) top and (C) cross-sectional views. (Taken from: Oh et al. [52].)

onto them and compared them against conventional machined miniscrews [54]. After 8 weeks of healing, BSC, BVR and bone-surface-ratio (BSR) values of tunnel miniscrews with nanotube arrays were considerably higher than machined miniscrews. The rhBMP-2-loaded miniscrews showed a slightly greater osseointegration potential than the non-loaded miniscrews. Jang et al. further studied the effects of drug-loaded nanotube arrays by comparing rhBMP-2-loaded and Ibuprofen-loaded miniscrews along with a machined and non-loaded nanotube array miniscrew group [55]. After 8 weeks of healing, the highest BSC values were recorded for the Ibuprofen-loaded miniscrews followed by the non-loaded, machined and rhBMP-2-loaded groups. In spite of their limited scope, these studies clearly suggest that nanoscale surface modifications of orthodontic miniscrews increase their biologic potential and the same nanotubular structures can also be used as drug-delivery systems to further enhance their osseointegration potential.

3. Ultraviolet photofunctionalization

Ultraviolet (UV) - mediated photofunctionalization is a method of surface modification for titanium that alters its physiochemical properties and enhances its biologic capability. It is characterized by remarkable efficacy, unique mechanisms, and a simple delivery method [56]. The effectiveness of UV treatment has been proven for all surface topographies tested. One of its unique features that set it apart from previously discussed surface modification techniques is that it does not alter the existing topography, roughness, or other morphologic features of miniscrews and is therefore categorized as neither an additive nor a subtractive method.

3.1 Physiochemical properties

For a very long time, it was assumed that the biologic properties of implant surfaces remained stable over time. It was later noted that over time, these surfaces underwent biologic degradation even when kept sterilized under optimal storage conditions. This is known as the time-dependent biologic degradation or biological aging of implant surfaces [57]. UV photofunctionalization affects these physiochemical changes via three key surface properties: i) the generation of superhydrophilicity; ii) a significant reduction of surface carbon, which unavoidably and unexceptionally accumulates on titanium surfaces; and iii) electrostatic conversion of surface charge from negative to positive.

3.1.1 Hydrophilic conversion

Titanium surfaces that have been sufficiently aged (i.e., more than 1 month after surface preparation) are hydrophobic; that is, the contact angle of water is greater than 60 degrees and close to or above 90 degrees on most surface types. Such a hydrophobic nature is common to all surface topographies of titanium and has been reported extensively [58, 59]. Water dropped on these surfaces does not spread and stays in a hemispherical form. Very intriguingly, after treatment with UV light, these titanium surfaces become remarkably wettable to water, with a contact angle of 0 degrees, which is referred to as being superhydrophilic (**Figures 8** and **9**) [56, 58, 59–63]. The superhydrophilic surfaces were obtained after UV treatment at

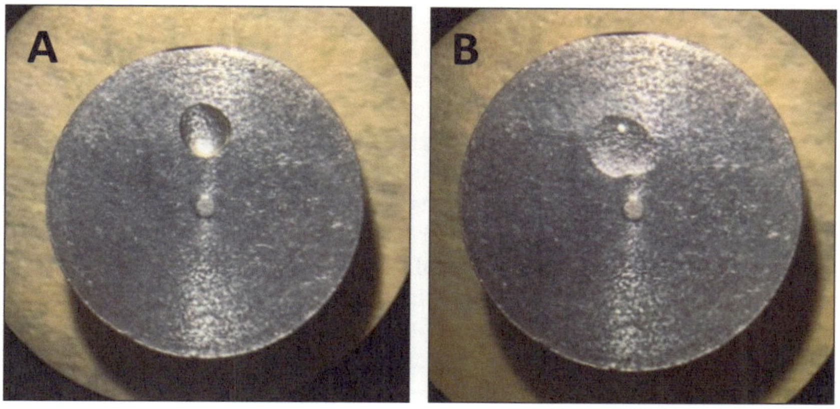

Figure 8.
(A) Untreated titanium surface showing lack of droplet spread. (B) UV-treated titanium surface showing complete spread of water droplet. (Taken from: Rampurawala et al. [105].)

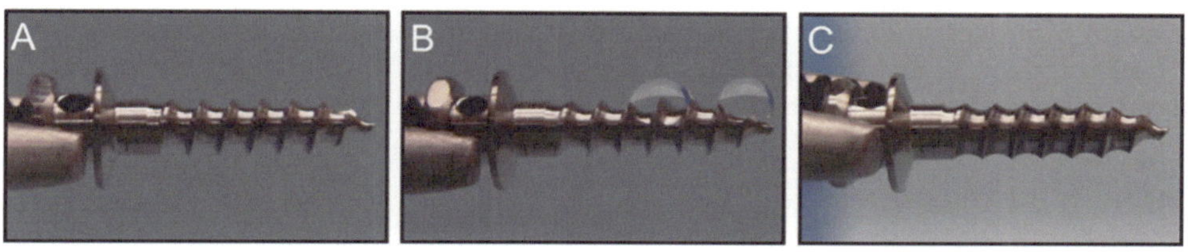

Figure 9.
Hydrophilic conversion by photofunctionalization: (A) miniscrew; (B) untreated miniscrew with 2 drops (1 μL each); (C) photofunctionalized miniscrew with 2 drops (Taken from: Tabuchi et al. [103].)

an intensity of 0.1 mW/cm2 (λ = 360 ± 20 nm) and 2 mW/cm2 (λ = 250 ± 20 nm) for varying durations of time ranging from as little as 20 minutes to as much as 48 hours.

3.1.2 Carbon reduction

Another notable change affected by UV modification is seen in the chemical composition of implant materials. Titanium surfaces, which become titanium dioxide surfaces as soon as they are exposed to the atmosphere, are covered by carbon-containing molecules to a significant degree because of the unavoidable constant accumulation of carbonyl moiety, particularly hydrocarbons, from the atmosphere and surrounding environment during surface preparation and storage [56, 57]. Similarly, presently used titanium implants are also contaminated with hydrocarbons. The amount of carbon varies depending upon the age of the surface. X-ray photoelectron spectroscopy (XPS) studies have revealed that the atomic percentage of carbon increases from 20% up to 60% after 4 weeks of aging. UV photofunctionalization of these surfaces reduces the atomic carbon percentage to 20–35% depending on the wavelength of UV light used [58]. Thus, photofunctionalization of titanium has proven to be effective in reducing the atomic percentage of carbon, thereby cleaning such carbon-contaminated surfaces [56, 57, 60–62, 64–66].

3.1.3 Electrostatic conversion

At an ionic level, ordinary titanium surfaces, viz. titanium surfaces without UV treatment, require inorganic bridges for protein adsorption and cell surface interaction, thus making titanium a bioinert material. In contrast, UV-treated titanium enables a direct cell-surface protein-titanium interaction without the aid of any inorganic bridges, thereby converting it into a bioactive surface (**Figure 10**). Albumin adsorption examined under different electrostatic environments revealed that adsorption on UV-treated surfaces at pH 7.0 was considerably greater than that on untreated surfaces (6-fold after 3 hrs of incubation and 2.5-fold after 24 hrs). Albumin adsorption on untreated control titanium surfaces increased after treating these surfaces with divalent cations but not after treating them with monovalent cations [66]. These findings suggest that the distinctly induced electropositive charge on UV-photofunctionalized titanium surfaces was responsible for the substantially increased efficiency of and capacity for protein adsorption on these titanium surfaces. Conversely, UV-enhanced cell adhesion was eliminated when the UV-treated titanium surfaces were electrostatically neutralized by either removing the electric charge or masking with monovalent anions, while the surfaces maintained their superhydrophilicity [67]. This unique electrostatic status of UV-treated titanium surfaces serves as a chemo-attractant for proteins, superseding the effect of the hydrophilic status, and may, therefore, be a critical regulatory factor in determining its subsequent bioactivity.

3.2 *In vitro* effects

The *in vitro* effects of UV-treated titanium have been studied extensively. A majority of these studies have been aimed at the discovery and explanation of the interaction between living cells and implant material after UV treatment. The key findings of these studies are that UV photofunctionalization leads to: i) increased protein adsorption, ii) increased osteogenic cell attachment and facilitated cell spread, iii) increased retention of cells, iv) increased cell proliferation, and v) enhanced osteoblastic differentiation.

The affinity between biomaterials and cells is determined initially by the interaction between cells as well as proteins adsorbed on material surfaces. Protein adsorption to titanium implant surfaces plays a crucial role in cell attachment and subsequently regulates the spread, proliferation, and other cell functions [56, 60, 63, 66, 68–70]. UV-mediated enhancement of protein adsorption has been reported with different surface topographies of titanium as well as with different proteins. The amount of albumin and fibronectin adsorbed to titanium surfaces after 3 to 6 hrs of incubation was 6-fold greater for UV-treated surfaces in the initial few hours and remained up to 3-fold greater after 24 hrs [56, 66]. Iwasa et al. reported that the protein adsorption levels on the UV-treated 4-week-old titanium surface were equivalent to that on the new surfaces after 3 and 24 hrs of incubation [63]. Qin *et al.* reported that UV photofunctionalization increased adsorption of fibrinogen along with albumin but had no influence on competition between the two proteins [68]. Even though most studies have reported increased protein adsorption following UV treatment, Areid et al. found no qualitative differences in protein adsorption between UV and non-UV treated surfaces, but found that platelet adhesion was increased after UV treatment and that might suggest UV-enhanced thrombogenicity of nanostructured titanium [70].

Various behaviors and responses of osteogenic/osteoblastic cells have been compared in cultures on UV-treated and untreated titanium surfaces. Osteogenic cell

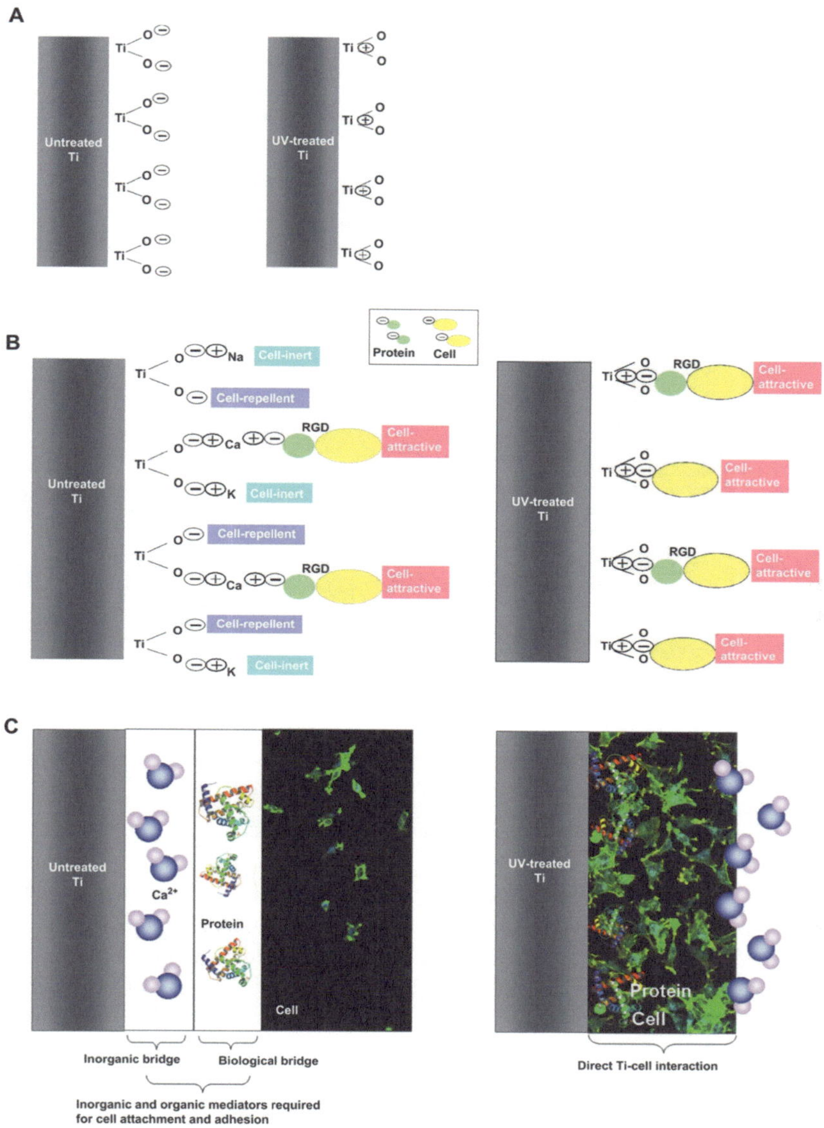

Figure 10.
Schematic description of the proposed mechanism of electrostatic interactions underlying the UV-photofunctionalization of titanium dioxide surfaces: UV-mediated conversion of titanium surfaces from bioinert to bioactive. (A) Hypothetical electric status of untreated and UV-treated TiO2 surfaces. As known and understood, ordinary TiO2 surfaces are electronegative, whereas UV-treated TiO2 surfaces are electropositively charged because of exited electrons from valence bands to conduction bands. (B) Electrostatic interaction of TiO2 surfaces with ions, proteins and cells. The untreated titanium surface (left) largely involves cell-inert terminals consisting of competitive binding of monovalent cations to negatively charged TiO2 surface. When cations are insufficient, this titanium surface remains electronegative and protein- and cell-repellent. The surface attracts proteins and cells only with an aid of divalent cations, such as Ca^{2+}. In contrast, the UV-treated titanium surface (right) is full of cell-attracting terminals consisting of the RGD sequence of proteins or positively charged TiO2 surface, which serve as direct chemo-attractants to cells without divalent cations such as Ca^{2+}. Proteins, that are negatively charged, adsorb directly to the positively charged the TiO2 surface. Cells, that are negatively charged, also attach directly to the positively charged the TiO2 surface. (C) A distinct interfacial layer formation at UV-photofunctionalized titanium surfaces. Based on the mechanisms in panel B, UV-induced bioactive titanium surfaces enable direct titanium–cell interaction, as opposed to untreated titanium surfaces that are bioinert and require inorganic and biological bridges for cell attachment and adhesion. (Taken from: Iwasa et al. [67].)

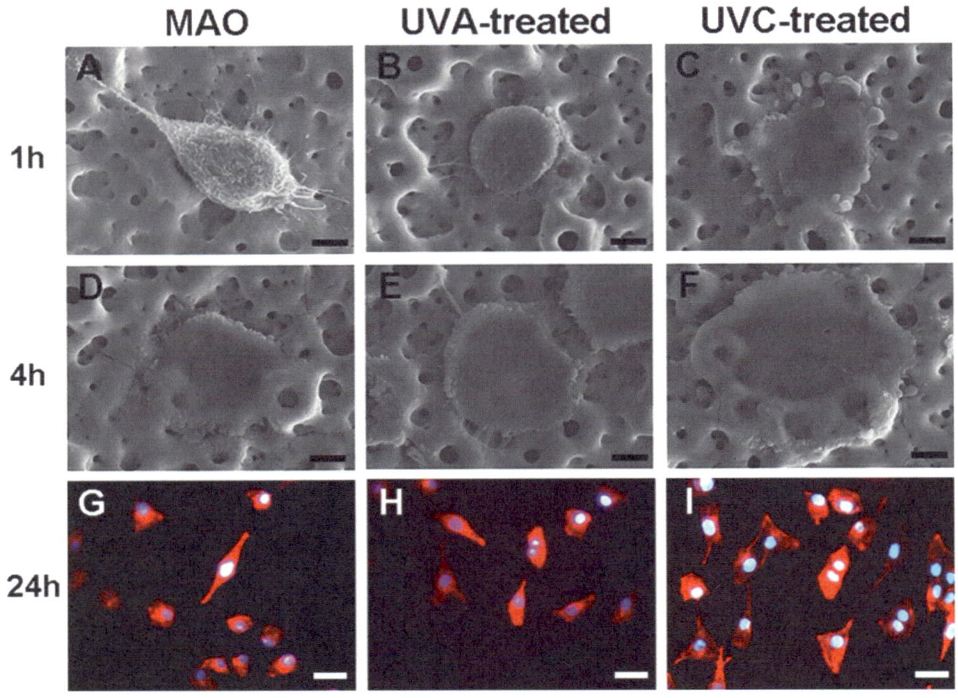

Figure 11.
Initial morphologies of the MG-63 osteoblasts on the titanium surface. (3000X, bar = 10 mm) SEM images of cells on the micro-arc oxidized (MAO), UVA-treated and UVC-treated surfaces after (A–C) 1 h and (D–F) 4 h incubation; (400X, bar = 50 mm) Fluorescence microscopy images of cells on the MAO, UVA-treated and UVC-treated surfaces after (G–I) 24 h incubation. (Taken from: Gao et al. [60].)

attachment and spread is one such behavior that may indicate the responsiveness of implant materials towards UV pre-treatment. Different surface topographies, including but not limited to acid-etched, sandblasted, machined, and nano-featured surfaces, have been investigated [56, 57, 59, 60, 63, 67, 69, 71–76]. The number of osteoblasts attached to UV-treated surfaces was reported to be 3 to 5-fold higher after 3 hrs of incubation, and 2 to 3-fold higher after 24 hrs of incubation [56, 67, 74]. It is evident from these studies that UV photofunctionalization increases the capacity of osteoblastic cells to attach to and spread along titanium surfaces (**Figure 11**).

The degree and nature of osteogenic cell settlement on implant surfaces is important. For instance, lack of adequate attachment and spread of osteogenic cells fails to induce their functional phenotypes or even their differentiation [69, 71]. Further, considering that implant materials are subjected to functional loading which causes mechanical stress and friction at the interface, the initial settlement and retention of osteogenic cells is crucial. Iwasa et al. studied the retentive capacity of osteoblasts cultured on titanium surfaces for 3 and 24 hrs [67]. Cell detachment was attempted mechanically by vibrational force and enzymatically by trypsin treatment. Retention of the cells, as evaluated by the percentage of cells remaining after the detachment procedures, was substantially enhanced on UV-treated titanium surfaces compared to untreated surfaces (110–120% greater for cells incubated for 3 hrs and 50–60% greater for cells incubated for 24 hrs). Miyauchi et al. and Yamada et al. used a special biomechanical setup monitored under phase-contrast microscopy to assess the retention capacity of cultured osteoblasts [73, 77]. Their results showed that after incubation of 3 hrs, the mean critical shear force required to initiate detachment of a single osteoblast and the total energy required to complete the detachment was much greater for UV-treated TiO_2 surfaces as compared to untreated surfaces. Such substantial increases in single-cell adhesion were also observed for osteoblasts cultured for 24 hrs.

Cell retention and adhesion can also be assessed by studying the cytoskeletal structure and proteins on the osteoblasts. It was observed by Iwasa et al. that during the initial stage of cell culture, osteoblasts on UV-treated surfaces were larger, with elongated cytoplasmic projections (filopodia and lamellipodia) and increased formation of cytoskeleton [67]. Vinculin, a focal adhesion protein involved in cell linkage serving a key role in initiating and establishing cell adhesion, has also been used to evaluate cell retention capacity. Studies using image-based densitometry as well as western blot test revealed that the extent of vinculin expression in an individual osteoblast was substantially higher on UV-treated surfaces than on untreated surfaces after incubation with rat-derived osteoblasts (up to 5-fold higher at 3 hrs and 2.5-fold higher at 24 hrs). However, the increased vinculin expression was observed only when standardized with the total protein and not when standardized with the cell area [63, 67, 69, 73, 77]. Iwasa et al. found that expression of other focal adhesion proteins such as paxillin and phosphorylated paxillin was higher on UV-treated surfaces [63]. Thus, the increased retention of the cells may be caused by the expedited and efficient settlement as well as reinforced adhesion of cells on UV-treated titanium surfaces.

The proliferation and differentiation of osteogenic cells determine the amount and speed of bone formation, respectively. The rate of proliferation of osteoblasts evaluated by BrdU incorporation assay, which targets the S phase of the cell cycle, has been reported to increase by up to 50–80% after UV-treatment of titanium [71]. The rate of osteogenic differentiation can be examined using multiple assays for various biologic markers. Alkaline phosphatase activity, calcium ion deposition, expression of collagen I, osteopontin, osteocalcin, and expression of other osteoblastic genes are some parameters which have been consistently evaluated on UV-treated titanium surfaces [67, 71, 72, 77]. Cell mineralization assays have reported increased alkaline phosphatase activity as well as increased calcium ion deposition for all UV-treated surfaces with different topographies. Studies with RT-PCR analysis showed an upregulation of the expression of collagen I, osteopontin and osteocalcin by up to 70%. As much as adhesion behavior varies with surface properties of implant materials, it is also regulated by the Rho-family GTPase enzymes. These enzymes are controlled by the Rac, Rho and Cdc42 genes. Gene expression analysis by Iwasa et al. revealed that for UV-treated titanium surfaces cultured with rat-derived osteoblasts, expression of Rac was upregulated by 1.5-fold after 3 hrs and 1.7-fold after 24 hrs of incubation, expression of Cdc42 was upregulated by 2-fold after 3 hrs and 1.5-fold after 24 hrs, but expression of Rho was not altered significantly [63]. Harder et al. studied the changes in pro-inflammatory gene expression in human whole blood after initial contact with UV-conditioned implant surfaces and found that there was suppression of IL-1β expression whereas there was no change in TNF-α expression [78]. All of the above *in vitro* studies have been confirmed with both animal and human-derived osteoblasts, as well as periosteum-derived osteogenic cells [63, 67, 68].

Microbial attachment on implant surfaces, especially at the implant-tissue interface is the primary cause of peri-implant inflammation and subsequent implant failure. UV photofunctionalization has been shown to have a considerable effect on bacterial accumulation around implants. The UV-induced physiochemical changes in titanium surfaces were reported to be responsible for the reduced bacterial attachment and biofilm formation. Yamada et al. reported via fluorescence microscopic quantification that attachment of bacterial pathogens such as *Staphylococcus aureus* or *Streptococcus pyogenes* on titanium surfaces (irrespective of their topography) was reduced following UV treatment [61]. Denaturing gradient gel-electrophoresis (DGGE) and DNA sequencing analyses by de Avila et al. revealed that while bacterial community profiles appeared different between UV-treated and untreated titanium in the initial attachment phase, this difference vanished as biofilm formation progressed [79]. Jain et al. reported that despite the reductive effect of UV pre-irradiation on bacterial attachment, cell viability was not affected adversely as 50% of bacterial killing capacity was maintained [80]. This suggests that UV-photofunctionalization of titanium has a strong potential to improve the outcome of implant placement by creating and maintaining antimicrobial surfaces.

A few authors sought to explain the effect of implant photofunctionalization from a technical perspective. Ohyama et al. carried out finite element analyses to understand how the photofunctionalization-led increase in BSC affected the peri-implant mechanical stress distribution. They reported that the simulated increase in BSC from 53–98% improved distribution and diffusion of peri-implant stress more effectively than using longer implants [81]. Another such study by Ohyama et al. concluded that under vertical loading, photofunctionalization had a greater effect than increased implant diameter on stress reduction [82]. Thus, UV treatment of implants may potentially reduce peri-implant stress and counteract the stress-induced marginal bone loss.

3.3 *In vivo* effects

It is important to correlate the results from *in vitro* studies with the results of *in vivo* studies to help understand and validate the biologic processes and mechanisms behind them. *In vivo* establishment of implant fixation in bone is a pertinent variable that reflects the clinical capacity of implants to bear loading. There has been extensive documentation regarding the strength of osseointegration and implant stability as determined by the histomorphometric assessment of BSC, biomechanical testing, and ISQ measurements.

Photofunctionalization substantially increases the strength of bone-implant integration by enabling near-complete coverage of bone around the implant. Various studies have reported the degree of osseointegration as evaluated by micro-CT, SEM and EDS analyses to be considerably higher when implants were pre-treated with UV light [56, 64, 71, 72, 83–85]. Pyo et al. evaluated the bone-implant interface of UV-treated implants using static and dynamic histological techniques, and when compared to UV-untreated implants, they reported an intensive mineralized layer in marginal bone which improved marginal bone seal and support, and expedited robust interfacial bone deposition (**Figure 12**) [83]. Studies have also shown that new bone formation occurs extensively around UV-treated implants, with little intervention by soft tissue (less than 1%), while the bone tissues around untreated implants are fragmentary and localized with intervening soft tissue (up to 21%) [71]. Yamazaki et al. reported increased peri-implant bone volume (1.5–2 fold) after UV treatment at the early and late stages without deterioration of bone mineral density [84]. In addition to bone volume studies, Hirota et al. used EDS mapping to determine the mineral content of new bone. Their results showed elemental peaks of calcium and phosphorus on various parts of UV-treated implants but the treated, as well as untreated implants, comprised the same Ca/P ratio, indicating bone tissue. However, the Ca/Ti ratios of the UV-treated implant surfaces were approximately 20 times greater than those of the control group (**Figure 13**) [72]. It is noteworthy that UV photofunctionalization maintains its advantage during later stages of healing, unlike other surface modification techniques which are effective only initially, indicating that UV photofunctionalization does not merely accelerate the process of osseointegration but also increases the level/degree of osseointegration [71].

RT values for UV-treated implants were reported to be 50–60% than those of untreated implants [83]. The osseointegration speed index (OSI) calculated as the difference between two ISQ readings at different intervals was reported to be 2–3 times higher for UV-treated implants [86–89]. The biomechanical push-in values assessed for UV-treated implants using a rat model were 2.5–3 times greater than those of untreated implants [63, 64, 71, 90]. In most of the studies the level of osseointegration seen at week 2 around UV-treated implants was equivalent to that seen around the untreated implants at week 8, indicating that UV treatment may have the potential to accelerate the process of osseointegration 4-fold [71]. These results suggest that UV photofunctionalization may be effective in enhancing the anchoring capability of titanium implants.

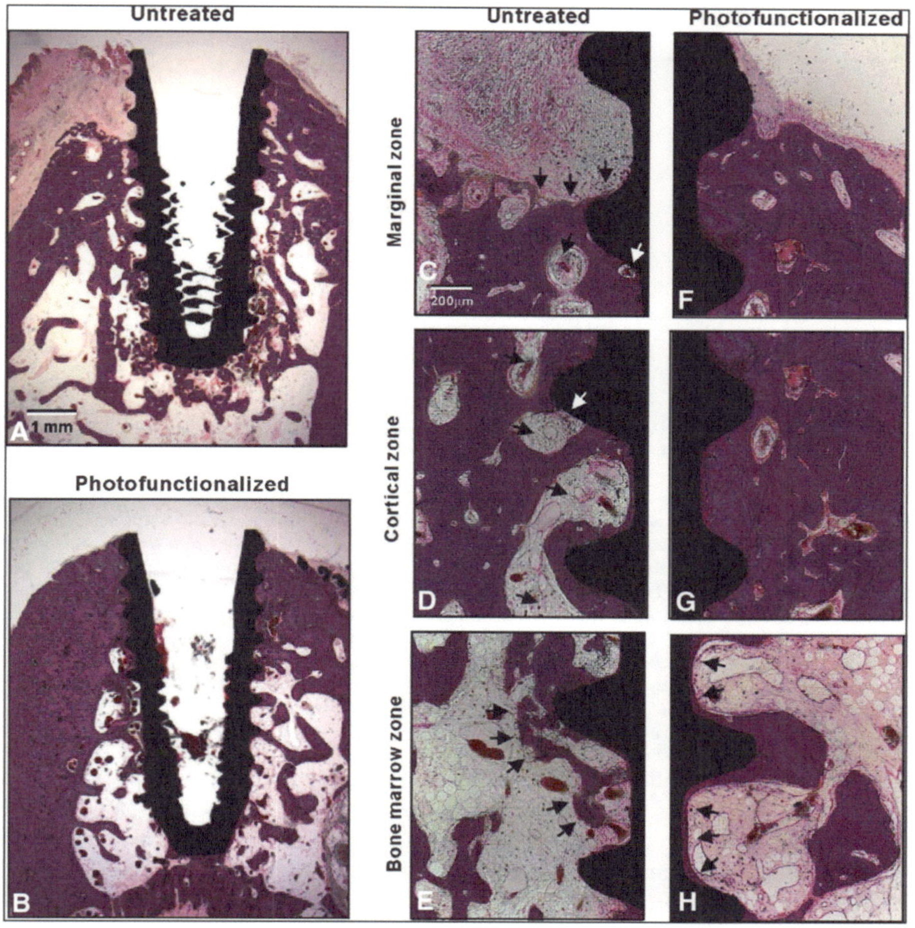

Figure 12.
Peri-implant bone morphogenesis enhanced by photofunctionalization. Low magnification microscopic images of peri-implant tissues around untreated implants (A) and photofunctionalized implants (B). High magnification images of untreated implants (C–E) and photofunctionalized implants (F–H), zooming up the portions in (A) and (B) in each of marginal, cortical, and bone marrow zones. (Taken from: Pyo et al. [83].)

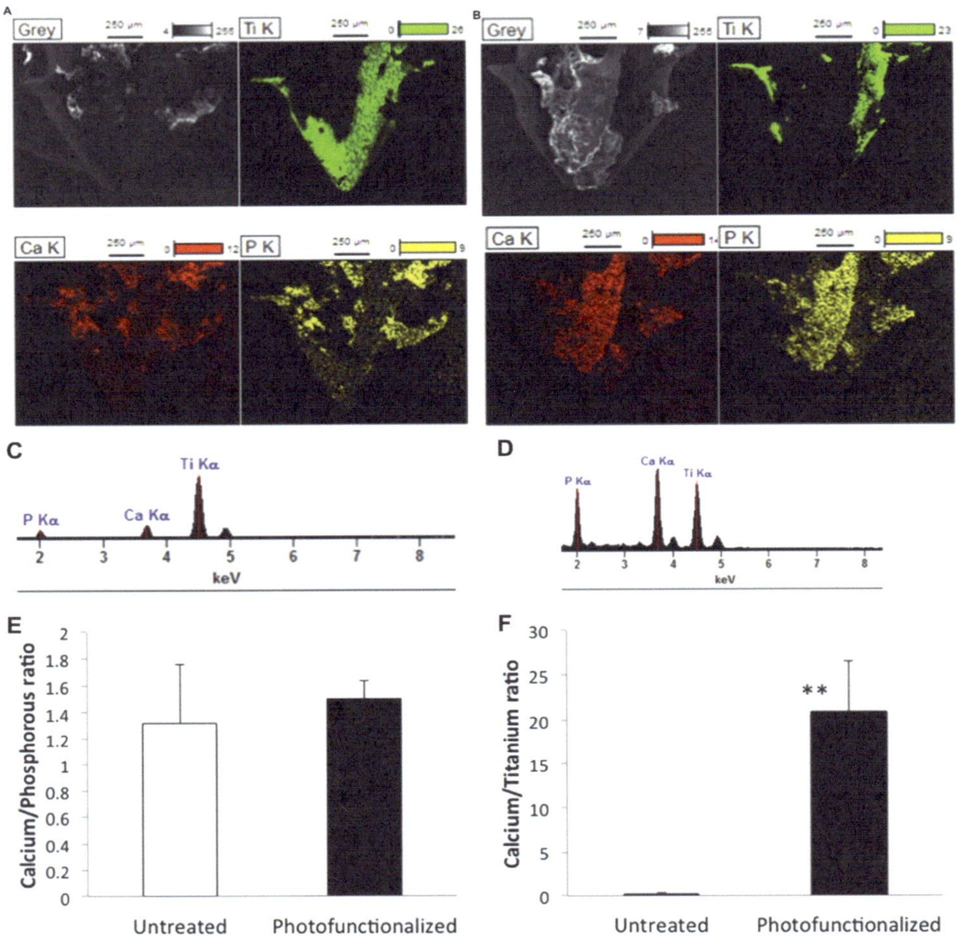

Figure 13.
*Scanning electron microscopy images showing energy dispersive x-ray spectroscopy (EDX) mapping (A,B) and EDX spectrum (C,D) of the apical part of the screw at 4 weeks. The Ca/P ratio shows that the mineralized tissue attached to the surface on the screw is bone. Titanium (Ti) was mainly detected in the mapping of the untreated group (A). However, much more bone tissue had attached to the screws in the photofunctionalized group, and mapping showed more Ca and P than Ti, indicating that the surface was more greatly covered by bone tissue than in the untreated group (B). Ca/P ratio (E) and Ca/Ti ratio (F) of the surface of the apical part of the screw at 4 weeks. Both Ca/P ratios were equal and consistent with bone tissue. The Ca/Ti ratio in the photofunctionalized group was extraordinarily greater compared with that of the untreated group, indicating dense and rich bone tissue covering the screw surface (**P < .01). (Taken from: Hirota et al. [72])*

The effects of UV photofunctionalization of implants have been studied in challenging host conditions for osseointegration to simulate clinical situations [64, 65, 66, 69, 91–94]. Ueno et al. reported greater strength of osseointegration in a rat model at both early and late healing stages for UV-treated shorter implants as compared to untreated regular length implants [91]. This suggests that UV photofunctionalization may overcome the loss of anchoring capacity due to reduced length of implants and may allow the use of shorter implants in certain clinical situations. Kim et al. reported enhanced osseointegration in UV-treated implants placed near critical one-wall defects in beagle dogs [85]. Kitajima et al. reported that photofunctionalized implants placed with low, extremely low, or even absent primary stability showed a high success rate eventually

[92]. Kim et al. and Lee et al., through their studies in rabbit calvarial defects, showed that UV-treatment promoted *de novo* osteogenesis as well as enhanced bone regeneration in critical rabbit calvarial defects [93, 94]. Thus, there is enough evidence to suggest that UV photofunctionalization may play a major role in mitigating challenging/compromised host conditions and aid in enhanced implant integration.

However, of all the studies which have reported the effects of photofunctionalization, only Mehl et al. reported this surface modification technique to be ineffective in enhancement of implant biologic activity [95]. Their *in vivo* study in edentulous minipig jaws revealed that the BSC value for UV-treated implants after 9 months of healing was about 64% only, which is similar to what many studies have reported for conventional UV-untreated implants, suggesting that photofunctionalization had no significant effect in enhancing osseointegration.

3.4 Effects on other implant materials

A majority of published literature on UV photofunctionalization is based on titanium as the implant material as it is most commonly used. However, there are some studies which have reported the effect of UV treatment on other implant materials as well. *In vitro* analyses of zirconia disks showed that their UV pre-treatment resulted in a physiochemical alteration of surface properties similar to those seen in UV-treated titanium surfaces [96, 97]. Brezavšček et al. showed that osteoconductive capacity of zirconia-based implant materials in a rat model was enhanced by their UV pre-treatment [98]. Shahramian et al. reported that UV treatment of zirconia disks (TiO_2-coated and non-coated) promoted platelet activation and thereby hastened blood coagulation [99]. This suggests that UV treatment has the potential to expedite wound healing around plain as well as coated zirconia implants.

Decco et al. reported that UV treatment of sandblasted chromium-cobalt-molybdenum (Cr-Co-Mo) alloy disks resulted in physiochemical alteration of surface properties similar to that of UV-treated titanium [100]. A recent study by Elkhidir et al. on rat-derived mesenchymal stem cells (MSCs) showed that UV treatment of gold nanoparticles increased its osteogenic capabilities by enhancing cell functions as well as osteogenic gene expression (Col-1, osteoprotegerin, osteocalcin) and mineralization [101]. All of these studies suggest that photofunctionalization of non-titanium implant materials also enhances their bioactivity and can have varied applications in the future.

3.5 Effects on orthodontic miniscrews

Despite this technique having been proven effective for all sizes and topographies of titanium implants, its clinical use with orthodontic miniscrews has not yet been investigated thoroughly. An *in vivo* study by Tabuchi et al. in rat femurs evaluated the osseointegration potential of photofunctionalized orthodontic miniscrews [102]. Via biomechanical push-in tests, it was found that displacement of untreated screws was 1.5–1.7 times greater than that of UV-functionalized screws (**Figure 14**). Surface evaluation showed robust bone formation around UV-treated screws with strong elemental peaks of calcium and phosphorus, whereas the tissue around untreated miniscrews appeared thin and showed no clear peak of calcium. In a similar comparative study, the maximum IT and RT values were measured. While the IT values were similar for both groups, the RT values were considerably higher for UV-treated miniscrews. This implied that implant strength at insertion was similar whereas, at removal, the strength of UV-treated miniscrews was much greater. SEM analysis

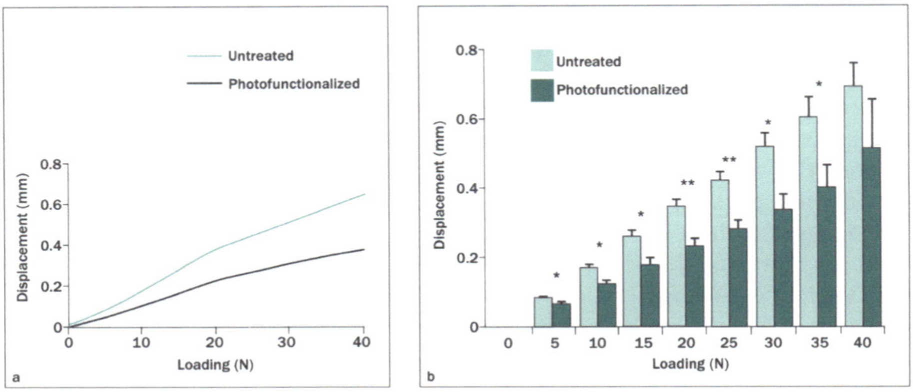

Figure 14.
*The anchorage strength of orthodontic miniscrews with and without photofunctionalization. (a) Representative load–displacement curves for untreated and photofunctionalized miniscrews subjected to a lateral tipping load. (b) The amount of miniscrew horizontal displacement under various levels of load; *P < .05; **P < .01. (Taken from: Tabuchi et al. [102].)*

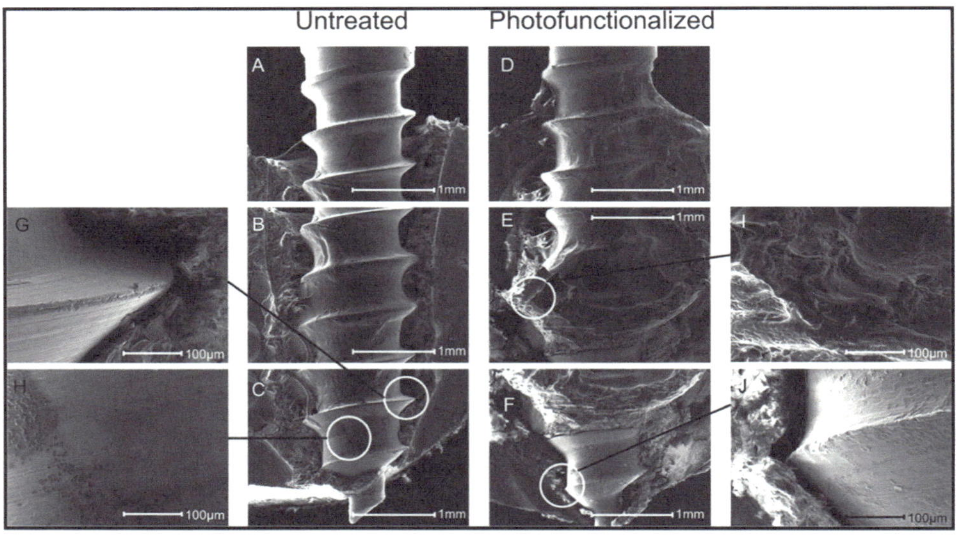

Figure 15.
Scanning electron micrograms of the miniscrews at week 3: (A-J) miniscrews with and without photofunctiolization were compared. (Taken from: Tabuchi et al. [103].)

revealed that regenerated bone tissue was more intact and contiguous around the UV-treated miniscrews than around the untreated ones, and the miniscrew-bone complex seemed to produce interface failure, and not cohesive fracture (**Figure 15**) [103]. Takahashi et al. studied the stability of UV-functionalized orthodontic miniscrews under immediate loading in growing rats [104]. A significantly less (almost 1/2) screw mobility was observed with the UV-treated miniscrews in both, the unloaded as well as immediately loaded groups. Once again SEM analysis revealed an increased BSC (1.8 times) in the UV-treated miniscrew groups.

Recently, the authors conducted a split-mouth *in vivo* human study for the first time using photofunctionalized miniscrews [105]. They studied the effect of UV

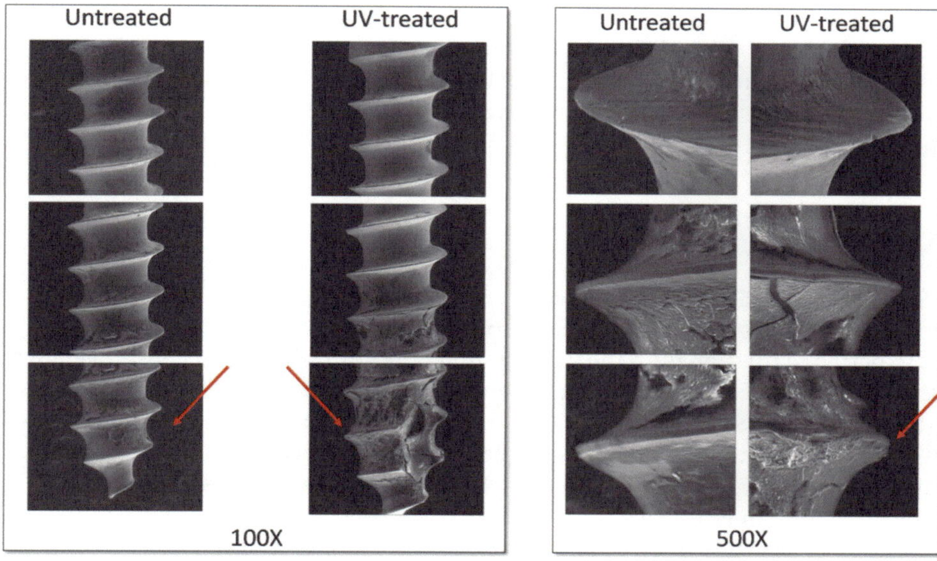

Figure 16.
Representative SEM images of untreated and UV-treated groups from upper, middle and lower regions of miniscrews: **A**, *images taken at 100X magnification,* **B**, *images taken at 500X magnification. (Taken from: Rampurawala et al. [105].)*

Comparison	M_1-M_2	sd	t-value	p-value	Inference
Ca/Ti Ratio					
Upper region of untreated v/s UV-treated group	0.08	0.4199	0.70	0.75619	NS
Middle region of untreated v/s UV-treated group	-0.05	0.2683	-0.701	0.24853	NS
Lower region of untreated v/s UV-treated group	-0.75	2.4915	-0.998	0.16978	NS
Ca/P Ratio					
Upper region of untreated v/s UV-treated group	-0.03	0.8025	-0.153	0.4415	NS
Middle region of untreated v/s UV-treated group	-0.07	0.7978	-0.393	0.34946	NS
Lower region of untreated v/s UV-treated group	0.19	0.8616	0.912	0.81202	NS

Table 2.
Comparison of Ca/Ti and Ca/P ratios between surfaces of untreated and UV-treated miniscrews in the upper, middle and lower regions.

photofunctionalization on orthodontic miniscrews using SEM to evaluate the BSC and EDS to evaluate surface element deposition. It was observed that there was increased BSC in lower regions of miniscrews in the photofunctionalized group

(**Figure 16**), but this was not statistically significant. There was also no significant difference between the Ca/Ti and Ca/P ratios of UV-treated and untreated miniscrews (**Table 2**). The results of this study were in agreement with only one previous study that reported a lack of improvement in the biomechanical potential of implants [95].

4. Conclusion

Surface modification of orthodontic miniscrews can serve to be an effective method for enhancement of the biologic potential of implant surfaces that could lead to better adaptation with the surrounding bone, as well as for the improvement of their mechanical capabilities thereby allowing better anchorage in more difficult intraoral sites. The SLA, microgrooving, anodization, plasma ion implantation, RBM and nanoscale modifications are techniques meant to be incorporated in the manufacturing process, whereas the UV photofunctionalization technique can be used as a chair-side method for surface treatment of miniscrews. All the aforementioned methods have shown to be effective in both experimental as well as clinical scenarios. The UV photofunctionalization technique is yet to be tested in a clinical situation with orthodontic miniscrews, and it may take a few more years of research before any or some of these techniques can be substantiated to become a standard operating procedure.

Conflict of interest

The authors declare no conflict of interest.

Author details

Abdulqadir Rampurawala[1*] and Amol Patil[2]

1 Private Practice, Mumbai, India

2 Bharati Vidyapeeth Deemed to be University Dental College and Hospital, Pune, India

*Address all correspondence to: aqrampura@gmail.com

References

[1] Kanomi R. Mini-implant for orthodontic anchorage. J Clin Orthod. 1997;31(11):763-767.

[2] Antoszewska J, Papadopoulos MA, Park HS, Ludwig B. Five-year experience with orthodontic miniscrew implants: A retrospective investigation of factors influencing success rates. Am J Orthod Dentofac Orthop. 2009;136(2):158.e1-10.

[3] Park HS, Jeong SH, Kwon OW. Factors affecting the clinical success of screw implants used as orthodontic anchorage. Am J Orthod Dentofac Orthop. 2006;130(1):18-25.

[4] Papageorgiou SN, Zogakis IP, Papadopoulos MA. Failure rates and associated risk factors of orthodontic miniscrew implants: A meta-analysis. Am J Orthod Dentofac Orthop. 2012;142(5):577-595.

[5] Alharbi F, Almuzian M, Bearn D. Miniscrews failure rate in orthodontics: systematic review and meta-analysis. *Eur J Orthod.* 2018;40(5):519-530.

[6] Brånemark PI, Hansson BO, Adell R, Breine U, Lindström J, Hallén O, Ohman A. Osseointegrated implants in the treatment of the edentulous jaw. Experience from a 10-year period. Scand J Plast Reconstr Surg Suppl. 1977;16:1-132.

[7] Buser D, Schenk RK, Steinemann S, Fiorellini JP, Fox CH, Stich H. Influence of surface characteristics on bone integration of titanium implants. A histomorphometric study in miniature pigs. J Biomed Mater Res. 1991;25(7):889-902.

[8] Buser D, Broggini N, Wieland M, Schenk RK, Denzer AJ, Cochran DL, Hoffmann B, Lussi A, Steinemann SG. Enhanced bone apposition to a chemically modified SLA titanium surface. J Dent Res. 2004;83(7):529-533.

[9] Giavaresi G, Fini M, Cigada A, Chiesa R, Rondelli G, Rimondini L, Aldini NN, Martini L, Giardino R. Histomorphometric and microhardness assessments of sheep cortical bone surrounding titanium implants with different surface treatments. J Biomed Mater Res A. 2003;67(1):112-120.

[10] Bagno A, Di Bello C. Surface treatments and roughness properties of Ti-based biomaterials. J Mater Sci Mater Med. 2004;15(9):935-949.

[11] Germanier Y, Tosatti S, Broggini N, Textor M, Buser D. Enhanced bone apposition around biofunctionalized sandblasted and acid-etched titanium implant surfaces. A histomorphometric study in miniature pigs. Clin Oral Implants Res. 2006;17(3):251-257.

[12] Tavares MG, de Oliveira PT, Nanci A, Hawthorne AC, Rosa AL, Xavier SP. Treatment of a commercial, machined surface titanium implant with H2SO4/H2O2 enhances contact osteogenesis. Clin Oral Implants Res. 2007;18(4):452-458.

[13] Ogawa T, Nishimura I. Different bone integration profiles of turned and acid-etched implants associated with modulated expression of extracellular matrix genes. Int J Oral Maxillofac Implants. 2003;18(2):200-210.

[14] Ogawa T, Ozawa S, Shih JH, Ryu KH, Sukotjo C, Yang JM, Nishimura I. Biomechanical evaluation of osseous implants having different surface topographies in rats. J Dent Res. 2000;79(11):1857-1863.

[15] Chang CS, Lee TM, Chang CH, Liu JK. The effect of microrough surface treatment on miniscrews used as orthodontic anchors. Clin Oral Implants Res. 2009;20(10):1178-1184.

[16] Fouziya B, Uthappa MA, Amara D, Tom N, Byrappa S, Sunny K. Surface modifications of titanium implants - The new, the old, and the never heard of options. J Adv Clin Res Insights. 2016;3:215-219.

[17] Le Guéhennec L, Soueidan A, Layrolle P, Amouriq Y. Surface treatments of titanium dental implants for rapid osseointegration. Dent Mater. 2007;23(7):844-854.

[18] Wehrbein H, Merz BR, Hammerle CH, Lang NP. Bone-to-implant contact of orthodontic implants in humans subjected to horizontal loading. Clin Oral Implants Res. 1998;9(5):348-353.

[19] Jeon MS, Kang YG, Mo SS, Lee KH, Kook YA, Kim SH. Effects of surface treatment on the osseointegration potential of orthodontic mini-implant. Korean J Orthod. 2008;38(5):328-336.

[20] Yadav S, Upadhyay M, Roberts WE. Biomechanical and histomorphometric properties of four different mini-implant surfaces. Eur J Orthod. 2015;37(6):627-635.

[21] Espinar-Escalona E, Bravo-Gonzalez LA, Pegueroles M, Gil FJ. Roughness and wettability effect on histological and mechanical response of self-drilling orthodontic mini-implants. Clin Oral Investig. 2016;20(5):1115-1120.

[22] Maino BG, Di Blasio A, Spadoni D, Ravanetti F, Galli C, Cacchioli A, Katsaros C, Gandolfini M. The integration of orthodontic miniscrews under mechanical loading: a pre-clinical study in rabbit. Eur J Orthod. 2017;39(5):519-527.

[23] Sirisa-Ard A, Woodroffe Michael SN, Ahmed K, Dunstan CR, Pearce SG, Bilgin AA, Dalci O, Darendeliler MA. Histomorphological and torque removal comparison of 6mm orthodontic miniscrews with and without surface treatment in New Zealand rabbits. Eur J Orthod. 2015;37(6):578-583.

[24] Park SH, Kim SH, Ryu JH, Kang YG, Chung KR, Kook YA. Bone-implant contact and mobility of surface-treated orthodontic micro-implants in dogs. Korean J Orthod. 2008; 38(6):416-426.

[25] Ikeda H, Rossouw PE, Campbell PM, Kontogiorgos E, Buschang PH. Three-dimensional analysis of peri-bone-implant contact of rough-surface miniscrew implants. Am J Orthod Dentofac Orthop. 2011;139(2):e153-163.

[26] Kim SH, Lee SJ, Cho IS, Kim SK, Kim TW. Rotational resistance of surface-treated mini-implants. Angle Orthod. 2009;79(5):899-907.

[27] Vilani GNL, Ruellas AC deO, Elias CN, Mattos CT. Stability of smooth and rough mini-implants: clinical and biomechanical evaluation - an in vivo study. Dent Press J Orthod. 2015;20(5):35-42.

[28] Schätzle M, Männchen R, Balbach U, Hämmerle CHF, Toutenburg H, Jung RE. Stability change of chemically modified sandblasted/acid-etched titanium palatal implants: a randomized-controlled clinical trial. Clin Oral Implants Res. 2009;20(5),489-495.

[29] Calderón JH, Valencia RM, Casasa AA, Sánchez MA, Espinosa R, Ceja I. Biomechanical anchorage

evaluation of mini-implants treated with sandblasting and acid etching in orthodontics. Implant Dent. 2011;20(4):273-279.

[30] Kim SH, Choi JH, Chung KR, Nelson G. Do sand blasted with large grit and acid etched surface treated mini-implants remain stationary under orthodontic forces? Angle Orthod. 2012;82(2):304-312.

[31] Chaddad K, Ferreira AF, Geurs N, Reddy MS. Influence of surface characteristics on survival rates of mini-implants. Angle Orthod. 2008;78(1):107-113.

[32] Park HJ, Choi SH, Choi YJ, Park YB, Kim KM, Yu HS. A prospective, split-mouth, clinical study of orthodontic titanium miniscrews with machined and acid-etched surfaces. Angle Orthod. 2018;89(3):411-417.

[33] Proff P, Kauschke E, Rumpel E, Bayerlein T, Dietze S, Fanghänel J, Gedrange T. The survival and proliferation of fibroblasts on orthodontic miniscrews with different surface treatment: an in vitro study. Folia Morphol (Warsz). 2006;65(1):78-80.

[34] Nahm KY, Heo JS, Lee JH, Lee DY, Chung KR, Ahn HW, Kim SH. Gene profiling of bone around orthodontic mini-implants by RNA-sequencing analysis. Biomed Res Int. 2015;2015:538080.

[35] Kim JS, Kang SM, Seo KW, Nahm KY, Chung KR, Kim SH, Ahn JP. Nanoscale bonding between human bone and titanium surfaces: osseohybridization. Biomed Res Int. 2015:960410.

[36] Kim JS, Ahn JP, Kim YH, Seo KW, Zadeh H, Kim SH. Atomic layout of an orthodontic titanium mini-implant in human tissue: Insights into the possible mechanisms during osseointegration. Angle Orthod. 2019;89(2):292-298.

[37] Kim SH, Cho JH, Chung KR, Kook YA, Nelson G. Removal torque values of surface-treated mini-implants after loading. Am J Orthod Dentofac Orthop. 2008;134(1):36-43.

[38] Kim TW, Baek SH, Kim JW, Chang YI. Effects of microgrooves on the success rate and soft tissue adaptation of orthodontic miniscrews. Angle Orthod. 2008;78(6):1057-1064.

[39] Hall J, Lausmaa J. Properties of a new porous oxide surface on titanium implants. Appl Osseointegration Res. 2000;1:5-8.

[40] Ivanoff CJ, Hallgren C, Widmark G, Sennerby L, Wennerberg A. Histologic evaluation of the bone integration of TiO_2-blasted and turned titanium microimplants in humans. Clin Oral Implants Res. 2001;12(2):128-134.

[41] Ivanoff CJ, Widmark G, Johansson C, Wennerberg A. Histologic evaluation of bone response to oxidized and turned titanium micro-implants in human jawbone. Int J Oral Maxillofac Implants. 2003;18(3):341-348.

[42] Omar O, Svensson S, Zoric N, Lennerås M, Suska F, Wigren S, Hall J, Nannmark U, Thomsen P. In vivo gene expression in response to anodically oxidized versus machined titanium implants. J Biomed Mater Res A. 2010;92(4):1552-1566.

[43] Karmarker S, Yu W, Kyung HM. Effect of surface anodization on stability of orthodontic microimplant. Korean J Orthod. 2012;42(1):4-10.

[44] Choi SH, Cha JY, Joo UH, Hwang CJ. Surface changes of anodic oxidized orthodontic titanium

miniscrew. Angle Orthod. 2012;82(3): 522-528.

[45] Choi SH, Jang SH, Cha JY, Hwang CJ. Evaluation of the surface characteristics of anodic oxidized miniscrews and their impact on biomechanical stability: an experimental study in beagle dogs. Am J Orthod Dentofac Orthop. 2016;149(1):31-38.

[46] Kim SJ, Moon YP, Park GH, Jo HH, Kim WG, Son MK, Choe HC. Surface characteristics and electrochemical behaviors of TiN and ZrN coated orthodontic miniscrew. J Korean Inst Surf Eng. 2008;41(5):232-239.

[47] Cho YC, Cha JY, Hwang CJ, Park YC, Jung HS, Yu HS. Biologic stability of plasma ion-implanted miniscrews. Korean J Orthod. 2013;43(3):120-126.

[48] Coelho PG, Granjeiro JM, Romanos GE, Suzuki M, Silva NR, Cardaropoli G, Thompson VP, Lemons JE. Basic research methods and current trends of dental implant surfaces. J Biomed Mater Res B Appl Biomater. 2009;88(2):579-596.

[49] Kim SC, Kim HY, Lee SJ, Kim CM. Influence of surface treatment on the insertion pattern of self-drilling orthodontic mini-implants. Korean J Orthod. 2011;41(4):268-279.

[50] Gansukh O, Jeong JW, Kim JW, Lee JH, Kim TW. Mechanical and histological effects of resorbable blasting media surface treatment on the initial stability of orthodontic mini-implants. Biomed Res Int. 2016;2016:7520959.

[51] Kim HY, Kim SC. Bone cutting capacity and osseointegration of surface-treated orthodontic mini-implants. Korean J Orthod. 2016;46(6):386-394.

[52] Oh EJ, Nguyen TDT, Lee SY, Jeon YM, Bae TS, Kim JG. Enhanced compatibility and initial stability of Ti6Al4V alloy orthodontic miniscrews subjected to anodization, cyclic precalcification, and heat treatment. Korean J Orthod. 2014;44(5):246-253.

[53] Jang I, Shim SC, Choi DS, Cha BK, Lee JK, Choe BH, Choi WY. Effect of TiO_2 nanotubes arrays on osseointegration of orthodontic miniscrew. Biomed Microdevices. 2015;17(4):76.

[54] Cha BK, Choi DS, Jang I, Choe BH, Choi WY. Orthodontic tunnel miniscrews with and without TiO_2 nanotube arrays as a drug-delivery system: in vivo study. Biomed Mater Eng. 2016;27(4):375-387.

[55] Jang I, Choi DS, Lee JK, Kim WT, Cha BK, Choi WY. Effect of drug-loaded TiO_2 nanotube arrays on osseointegration in an orthodontic miniscrew: an in-vivo pilot study. Biomed Microdevices. 2017;19(4):94.

[56] Aita H, Hori N, Takeuchi M, Suzuki T, Yamada M, Anpo M, Ogawa T. The effect of ultraviolet functionalization of titanium on integration with bone. Biomaterials. 2009;30(6):1015-1025.

[57] Att W, Ogawa T. Biological aging of implant surfaces and their restoration with ultraviolet light treatment: a novel understanding of osseointegration. Int J Oral Maxillofac Implants. 2012;27(4):753-761.

[58] Att W, Hori N, Iwasa F, Yamada M, Ueno T, Ogawa T. The effect of UV-photofunctionalization on the time-related bioactivity of titanium and chromium-cobalt alloys. Biomaterials. 2009;30(26):4268-4276.

[59] Aita H, Att W, Ueno T, Yamada M, Hori N, Iwasa F, Tsukimura N, Ogawa T. Ultraviolet light-mediated

photofunctionalization of titanium to promote human mesenchymal stem cell migration, attachment, proliferation and differentiation. Acta Biomater. 2009;5(8):3247-3257.

[60] Gao Y, Liu Y, Zhou L, Guo Z, Rong M, Liu X, Lai C, Ding X. The effects of different wavelength UV photofunctionalization on micro-arc oxidized titanium. PLoS One. 2013;8(7):e68086.

[61] Yamada Y, Yamada M, Ueda T, Sakurai K. Reduction of biofilm formation on titanium surface with ultraviolet-C pre-irradiation. J Biomater Appl. 2014;29(2):161-171.

[62] Roy M, Pompella A, Kubacki J, Szade J, Roy RA, Hedzelek W. Photofunctionalization of titanium: an alternative explanation of its chemical-physical mechanism. PLoS One. 2016;11(6):e0157481.

[63] Iwasa F, Baba K, Ogawa T. Enhanced intracellular signaling pathway in osteoblasts on ultraviolet light treated hydrophilic titanium. Biomed Res. 2016;37(1):1-11.

[64] Hirota M, Ikeda T, Tabuchi M, Ozawa T, Tohnai I, Ogawa T. Effects of ultraviolet photofunctionalization on bone augmentation and integration capabilities of titanium mesh and implants. Int J Oral Maxillofac Implants. 2017;32(1):52-62.

[65] Shen J, Liu J, Chen X, Wang X, He F, Wang H. The in vivo bone response of ultraviolet-irradiated titanium implants modified with spontaneously formed nanostructures: an experimental study in rabbits. Int J Oral Maxillofac Implants. 2016;31(4):776-84.

[66] Hori N, Ueno T, Minamikawa H, Iwasa F, Yoshino F, Kimoto K, Lee MC, Ogawa T. Electrostatic control of protein adsorption on UV-photofunctionalized titanium. Acta Biomater. 2010;6(10):4175-4180.

[67] Iwasa F, Hori N, Ueno T, Minamikawa H, Yamada M, Ogawa T. Enhancement of osteoblast adhesion to UV-photofunctionalized titanium via an electrostatic mechanism. Biomaterials. 2010;31(10):2717-2727.

[68] Qin Z, Teng W. Effect of ultraviolet-photofunctionalization of titanium on protein adsorption and competition. Zhonghua Kou Qiang Yi Xue Za Zhi. 2015;50(7):428-432.

[69] Ishijima M, Hirota M, Park W, Honda MJ, Tsukimura N, Isokawa K, Ishigami T, Ogawa T. Osteogenic cell sheets reinforced with photofunctionalized micro-thin titanium. J Biomater Appl. 2015;29(10):1372-1384.

[70] Areid N, Kangasniemi I, Söderling E, Närhi TO. Ultraviolet photofunctionalization of nanostructured titanium surfaces enhances thrombogenicity and platelet response. J Mater Sci Mater Med. 2018;29(5):56.

[71] Ishijima M, Ghassemi A, Soltanzadeh P, Tanaka M, Nakhaei K, Park W, Hirota M, Tsukimura N, Ogawa T. Effect of UV photofunctionalization on osseointegration in aged rats. Implant Dent. 2016;25(6):744-750.

[72] Hirota M, Tanaka M, Ishijima M, Iwasaki C, Park W, Ogawa T. Effect of photofunctionalization on Ti6Al4V screw stability placed in segmental bone defects in rat femurs. J Oral Maxillofac Surg. 2016;74(4):861.e1-16.

[73] Miyauchi T, Yamada M, Yamamoto A, Iwasa F, Suzawa T, Kamijo R, Baba K,

Ogawa T. The enhanced characteristics of osteoblast adhesion to photofunctionalized nanoscale TiO_2 layers on biomaterials surfaces. Biomaterials. 2010;31(14):3827-3839.

[74] Tsukimura N, Yamada M, Iwasa F, Minamikawa H, Att W, Ueno T, Saruwatari L, Aita H, Chiou WA, Ogawa T. Synergistic effects of UV photofunctionalization and micro-nano hybrid topography on the biological properties of titanium. Biomaterials. 2011;32(19):4358-4368.

[75] Kim HS, Lee JI, Yang SS, Kim BS, Kim BC, Lee J. The effect of alendronate soaking and ultraviolet treatment on bone-implant interface. Clin Oral Implants Res. 2016;28(9):1164-1172.

[76] Henningsen A, Smeets R, Hartjen P, Heinrich O, Heuberger R, Heiland M, Precht C, Cacaci C. Photofunctionalization and non-thermal plasma activation of titanium surfaces. Clin Oral Investig. 2017;22(2):1045-1054.

[77] Yamada M, Miyauchi T, Yamamoto A, Iwasa F, Takeuchi M, Anpo M, Sakurai K, Baba K, Ogawa T. Enhancement of adhesion strength and cellular stiffness of osteoblasts on mirror-polished titanium surface by UV-photofunctionalization. Acta Biomater. 2010;6(12);4578-4588.

[78] Harder S, Quabius ES, Meinke F, Mehl C, Kern M. Changes in proinflammatory gene expression in human whole blood after contact with UV-conditioned implant surfaces. Clin Oral Investig 2019.

[79] de Avila ED, Lima BP, Sekiya T, Torii Y, Ogawa T, Shi W, Lux R. Effect of UV-photofunctionalization on oral bacterial attachment and biofilm formation to titanium implant material. Biomaterials. 2015;67:84-92.

[80] Jain S, Williamson RS, Marquart M, Janorkar AV, Griggs JA, Roach MD. Photofunctionalization of anodized titanium surfaces using UVA or UVC light and its effects against *Streptococcus sanguinis*. J Biomed Mater Res B Appl Biomater. 2017;106(6):2284-2294.

[81] Ohyama T, Uchida T, Shibuya N, Nakabayashi S, Ishigami T, Ogawa T. High bone-implant contact achieved by photofunctionalization to reduce periimplant stress: a three-dimensional finite element analysis. Implant Dent. 2013;22(1):102-108.

[82] Ohyama T, Yasuda H, Shibuya N, Tadokoro S, Nakabayashi S, Namaki S, Hara Y, Ogawa T, Ishigami T. Three-dimensional finite element analysis of the effects of implant diameter and photofunctionalization on peri-implant stress. J Oral Sci. 2017;59(2):272-278.

[83] Pyo SW, Park YB, Moon HS, Lee JH, Ogawa T. Photofunctionalization enhances bone-implant contact, dynamics of interfacial osteogenesis, marginal bone seal, and removal torque value of implants: a dog jawbone study. Implant Dent. 2013;22(6):666-675.

[84] Yamazaki M, Yamada M, Ishizaki K, Sakurai K. Ultraviolet-C irradiation to titanium implants increases peri-implant bone formation without impeding mineralization in a rabbit femur model. Acta Odontol Scand. 2015;73(4):302-311.

[85] Kim MY, Choi H, Lee JH, Kim JH, Jung HS, Kim JH, Park YB, Moon HS. UV photofunctionalization effect on bone graft in critical one-wall defect around implant: a pilot study in beagle dogs. Biomed Res Int. 2016;2016:4385279.

[86] Funato A, Ogawa T. Photofunctionalized dental implants: a case series in compromised bone. Int J

Oral Maxillofac Implants. 2013;28(6):1589-1601.

[87] Funato A, Yamada M, Ogawa T. Success rate, healing time, and implant stability of photofunctionalized dental implants. Int J Oral Maxillofac Implants. 2013;28(5):1261-1271.

[88] Suzuki S, Kobayashi H, Ogawa T. Implant stability change and osseointegration speed of immediately loaded photofunctionalized implants. Implant Dent. 2013;22(5):481-490.

[89] Hirota M, Ozawa T, Iwai T, Ogawa T, Tohnai I. Implant stability development of photofunctionalized implants placed in regular and complex cases: a case-control study. Int J Oral Maxillofac Implants. 2016;31(3):676-86.

[90] Soltanzadeh P, Ghassemi A, Ishijima M, Tanaka M, Park W, Iwasaki C, Hirota M, Ogawa T. Success rate and strength of osseointegration of immediately loaded UV-photofunctionalized implants in a rat model. J Prosthet Dent. 2017;118(3):357-362.

[91] Ueno T, Yamada M, Hori N, Suzuki T, Ogawa T. Effect of ultraviolet photoactivation of titanium on osseointegration in a rat model. Int J Oral Maxillofac Implants. 2010;25:287-294.

[92] Kitajima H, Ogawa T. The use of photofunctionalized implants for low or extremely low primary stability cases. Int J Oral Maxillofac Implants. 2016;31(2):439-447.

[93] Kim SY, Bark CW, Van Quy H, Seo SJ, Lim JH, Lee JM, Suh JY, Lee Y, Um HS, Kim YG. Photofunctionalizing effects of hydroxyapatite combined with TiO_2 on bone regeneration in rabbit calvarial defects. J Biomed Mater Res B Appl Biomater. 2019;107(6):1953-1959.

[94] Lee JE, Bark CW, Quy HV, Seo SJ, Lim JH, Kang SA, Lee Y, Lee JM, Suh JY, Kim YG. Effects of enhanced hydrophilic titanium dioxide-coated hydroxyapatite on bone regeneration in rabbit calvarial defects. Int J Mol Sci. 2018;19(11):e3640.

[95] Mehl C, Kern M, Neumann F, Bähr T, Wiltfang J, Gassling V. Effect of ultraviolet photofunctionalization of dental titanium implants on osseointegration. J Zhejiang Univ Sci B. 2018;19(7):525-534.

[96] Tuna T, Wein M, Swain M, Fischer J, Att W. Influence of ultraviolet photofunctionalization on the surface characteristics of zirconia-based dental implant materials. Dent Mater. 2015;31(2):e14-24.

[97] Roy M, Pompella A, Kubacki J, Piosik A, Psiuk B, Klimontko J, Szade J, Roy RA, Hedzelek W. Photofunctionalization of dental zirconia oxide: Surface modification to improve bio-integration preserving crystal stability. Colloids Surf B Biointerfaces. 2017;156:194-202.

[98] Brezavšček M, Fawzy A, Bächle M, Tuna T, Fischer J, Att W. The effect of UV treatment on the osteoconductive capacity of zirconia-based materials. Materials (Basel). 2016;9(12):e958.

[99] Shahramian K, Abdulmajeed A, Kangasniemi I, Söderling E, Närhi T. TiO_2 coating and UV photofunctionalization enhance blood coagulation on zirconia surfaces. Biomed Res Int. 2019;8078230.

[100] Decco O, Zuchuat J, Farkas N. Improvement of Cr-Co-Mo membrane surface used as barrier for bone regeneration through UV photofunctionalization: an in vitro study. Materials (Basel). 2017;10(7):e825.

[101] Elkhidir Y, Lai R, Feng Z. The impact of photofunctionalized gold nanoparticles on osseointegration. Heliyon. 2018;4(7):e00662.

[102] Tabuchi M, Ikeda T, Hirota M, Nakagawa K, Park W, Miyazawa K, Goto S, Ogawa T. Effect of UV photofunctionalization on biologic and anchoring capability of orthodontic miniscrews. Int J Oral Maxillofac Implants. 2015;30(4):868-879.

[103] Tabuchi M, Ikeda T, Nakagawa K, Hirota M, Park W, Miyazawa K, Goto S, Ogawa T. Ultraviolet photofunctionalization increases removal torque values and horizontal stability of orthodontic miniscrews. Am J Orthod Dentofac Orthop. 2015;148(2):274-282.

[104] Takahashi M, Motoyoshi M, Inaba M, Hagiwara Y, Shimizu N. Enhancement of orthodontic anchor screw stability under immediate loading by ultraviolet photofunctionalization technology. Int J Oral Maxillofac Implants. 2016;31(6):1320-1326.

[105] Rampurawala AH, Patil AS, Bhosale VI. Bone-miniscrew contact and surface element deposition on orthodontic miniscrews after ultraviolet photofunctionalization. Int J Oral Maxillofac Implants 2020;35(6):1090-1097.

Chapter 10

The Use of Cortical Bone Wedges from the Mandibular Ramus "Wedge Technique" for 3-Dimensional Bone Augmentation of the Atrophic Ridges

Fares Kablan

Abstract

Autogenous bone is still considered the gold standard in bone augmentation for implant insertion in atrophic ridges. However, augmentation of multiple edentulous atrophic segments usually necessitates the use of extraoral donor sites. This chapter introduces the Wedge Technique, as a new bone augmentation method that can augment multiple edentulous ridges with intraoral cortical bone grafts. Patients with moderate to severe ridge atrophy in different regions of the jaws were treated with the wedge technique (WT). Patients received a panoramic radiograph immediately after the surgery, and they were examined clinically and radiographically (periapical radiograph) every 2 weeks. At four months, CBCT was performed to evaluate the bone gain. Reentry was performed after 4 to 5 months to evaluate the new bone volume and quality and to insert implants. The follow-up period ranged from 30 to 120 months. The healing process was uneventful, with minimal morbidity. The success rate was 95%, the bone gain average was 3–6 mm vertically and 3–9 mm horizontally. The wedge technique can augment multiple segments of atrophic ridges with a small amount of autogenous graft. The achieved bone volume was satisfying, especially that the majority of the augmented areas were at posterior mandibular defects.

Keywords: bone augmentation, autogenous bone grafts, allogeneic bone substitute, donor site, space maintenance

1. Introduction

Alveolar bone loss as a result of teeth extractions, periodontal disease, dentoalveolar trauma, pathologic conditions, failed implants, and failed bone grafting procedures may provide poor bone quality in height, width, and angulation which may result in impaired intermaxillary relationships. Ridge augmentation is considered in such cases to enhance the insertion of dental implants with good diameter and length at a proper prosthetic position. Several augmentation methods and materials have been successfully used during the last decades, but much controversy still exists [1–10].

Autogenous bone grafts are still considered as the gold standard not only because of their osteogenic, osteoinductive, and osteoconductive biological activities but also due to their safety and their excellent incorporation in the recipient bed. Common extra donor sites such as iliac crest, rib, tibia, and cranium are used and provide large quantities of cortical and cancellous bone. However, extraoral donor sites have several disadvantages that include the need for hospitalization and general anesthesia, prolonged healing time of donor site, concomitant morbidities, and visible scars [11–17].

Different intraoral donor sites are widely used as bone blocks or particulate bone. The most common intraoral sites are the symphysis and ramus/retromolar area [18–22], they have different degrees of morbidities and complications [23–27]. Non-autogenous bone grafts such as allografts, xenografts, and synthetic bone substitutes are widely used either alone or in combinations [28–34]. They eliminate the potential complications associated with autogenous donor sites and their availability is unlimited, however, they have osteoconductive characteristics and lack of osteoprogenitor cells.

The incorporation of the autogenous bone graft at the recipient site depends mainly on the amount of revascularization together with remodeling and substitution of the graft, which leads to the integration of the graft at the recipient bed [35]. There is a solid connection between osteogenesis and revascularization inside and around the graft [36]. Revascularization of the bone graft starts when blood vessels sprouts grow and go through the bone block. They originate from two sources; first, from the bone at the recipient bed, and second from the surrounding soft tissue. Hammack and Enneking in 1960 found that penetration of the blood vessels to the cortical graft was observed on the sixth day [37]. De Marco et al. in 2005 reported the timing and the penetration rate of the blood vessels into the autogenous bone block in rats. New capillaries had migrated from the surface of the recipient bed and penetrated the graft to different degrees [38].

Graft fixation plays a crucial role in cortico-cancellous bone grafts survival. Fixation screws are usually used to prevent micromovement of the augmented bone blocks at the recipient site, preventing and minimizing early graft volume loss and infections [4, 39, 40]. This chapter introduces a new bone augmentation method, Wedge Technique (WT) as a biological approach that utilizes the main advantage of autogenic bone which is transferring living cells, and the main advantage of the allogenic bone as well which is the availability and the unlimited quantities. The surgical procedures of WT, including bone block harvesting, wedge preparation, recipient site preparation, and the augmentation methods are presented in this chapter. The biological rationale, the healing process, and the advantages of the WT are explained and discussed.

2. Patients and methods

Patients were referred by their surgeons due to different types and degrees of alveolar bone deficiencies, a lot of them result from failed implants or failed previous bone augmentation attempts. The majority of the cases had at least two sites at one or both jaws, and the majority of the sites were at the posterior mandible (**Table 1**). Inclusion criteria for the use of wedge-technique in the participants were: atrophic alveolar ridge

DOI: http://dx.doi.org/10.5772/intechopen.100099

Patient No.	Site's	Age	Sex	Augmented region	Available bone Height	Width	Donor side
1	1.1	48	F	44–47	4–5	1.2–2.4	RT
	1.2			35–36	5–7	2.5–3	
2	2.3	19	F	45–47	5.4–6.2	3.2–4.2	RT
	2.4			35–37	7–9	3–4.5	
3	3.5	28	F	13–23	10–12	1.5–2	RT
4	4.6	63	M	43–47	8–18	1.5–2.5	RT
	4.7			34–37	6–11	2–4	
5	5.8	29	F	32–42	9–12	1.5–3	RT
	5.9			44–47	6–10	2–6	
6	6.10		F	44–47	4.5–9	2–3.2	LT
	6.11	54		35–37	6–10	2.8–3.5	
7	7.12	54	F	44–47	6–10	3–4	LT
	7.13			35–37	6–8	4–6	
8	8.14	49	F	33–43	16–18	1.8–2.4	LT
	8.15			36–37	8–10	1–2	
9	9.16	63	M	35–37	7–9	2.5–5	LT
10	10.17	55	M	34–37	6–8	3–7	LT
11	11.18	47	F	34–37	5–7	2.4–4	RT
	11.19			45–47	5–8	2.8–4	
12	12.20	56	F	13–17	6–11	1.5–2.5	RT and LT
	12.21			23–27	7–12	1.5–3	
	12.22			43–47	8–18	1–3	
13	13.23	19	M	23–27	8–11	2.5–3.5	RT
14	14.24	39	F	43–47	5–7	6–8	LT
	14.25			34–37	5–7	6–8	
15	15.26	62	M	15–25	10–13	1–2	RT
16	16.27	67	M	34–36	5–7	2.4–4	LT
	16.28			44–47	5–8	2.9–4	
17	17.29	51	F	46–47	3–5	6	RT
	17.30			36–37	3.5–7	6	
18	18.31	30	F	12–15	8–11	2.5–3	RT
	18.32			33–43	14–18	2–3	
19	19.33	44	F	13–23	8–13	1.8–2.7	RT
	19.34			46–47	4–5	2–3	
	19.35			34–37	6–7	3–4.5	
20	20.36	54	F	44–47	3.5–4.8	4–5	RT
	20.37			35–37	4.6–5.2	3–6	
21	20.38	57	F	26–27	4–6	2–4	LT
22	22.39	53	M	35–37	8	2–4.5	LT

Table 1.
Patients demographics, augmented sites, and the donor sites.

with a bone deficit that needs vertical, horizontal or combined vertical and horizontal bone augmentation. The exclusion criteria were the severe atrophy of the mandibular retromolar area (the donor site); and patients with less than 3 mm bone over the inferior alveolar nerve at the posterior mandibular ridge.

Patients with informed consent underwent bone augmentation with the WT at least at one site in different arch regions. The retromolar/ramus area was the donor site of the bone cortical wedges of this technique. Post-operative instructions included a soft diet for six weeks, antibiotics for ten days, and meticulous oral hygiene. In addition, the use of removable appliances was not allowed.

Follow-up examinations were performed every 2 weeks. Four months after the surgery, the recipient site was evaluated clinically (to assess the contour and the volume of the augmented ridge), and radiographically (by computed tomography) to examine the bone gain and the new available bone for dental implant placement. Reentry was performed after 4 to 5 months to evaluate the new bone volume, to obtain biopsy specimens and to insert implants. The prosthetic rehabilitation was allowed 4 months after the placement of the dental implants. Follow-up of the bone augmentations and implants that were inserted at these sites, included periodic clinical evaluation and periapical radiographs. All the surgical procedures and postoperative evaluations were performed by the author.

2.1 Technique

Illustration case; 55 years old female was referred to the pre-prosthetic unit at our department for bone augmentation of her posterior mandible bilaterally and placement of dental implants. On examination; a healthy patient presented with bilateral posterior mandibular edentulism (Kennedy class-1).

Both of the residual ridges had more than 20 degrees of bone angulation toward the lingual side (**Figure 1a**). CBCT showed moderate to severe atrophy of both posterior mandibular ridges (**Figure 1b–d**). Short implants were not an option due to the severe lingual angulation, and inadequate bone width of the residual ridges. Guided implant placement was not a treatment option as well due to the central location of the inferior alveolar nerve. This case necessitated bone augmentation and was treated with the WT.

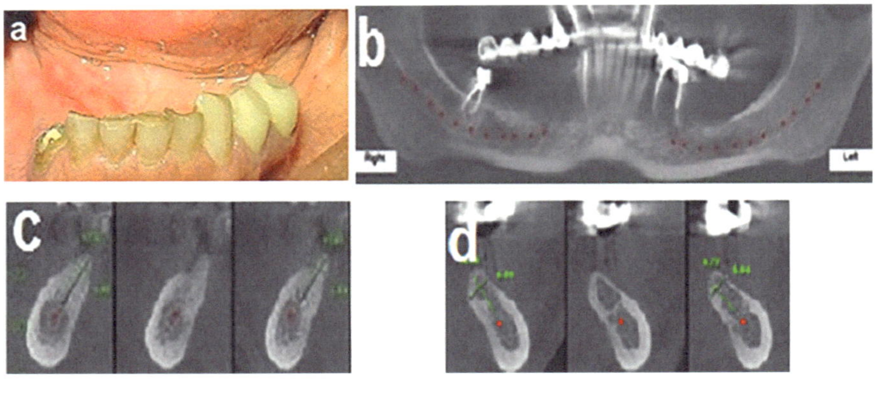

Figure 1.
Bilateral edentulous posterior mandibular ridges. (a) Clinical view. (b–d) Computed tomography shows inadequate bone in height, width, and angulation.

2.2 The donor site

Retromolar/ramus region is the gold standard of this technique. It can provide cortical bone blocks of 3-4 mm thickness, 2–3 cm length, 8-12 mm width (height). In the present case, the left retromolar area was the donor site. Under general anesthesia, administration of IV Augmentin 1 gr, Iv Dexamethasone 20 mg, and local anesthesia with a vasoconstrictor. A full-thickness mucoperiosteal flap was reflected with mid-crestal incision distal to the second premolar. The incision was extended through the retromolar region and the external oblique ridge to the ramus. An anterior release incision was performed at the first premolar and extended to the vestibular depth. This flap exposed the left augmented site (teeth 36 and 37 region), and the donor site of the bone block. In addition, it allowed visualization of the lateral and inferior border of the mandible, the buccal shelf, and the mental neurovascular bundle. The length (posterior–anterior) of the bone block, the width (superior–inferior) were determined and done by three complete osteotomies; posterior, anterior, and inferior (**Figure 2a**), using a micro-Saw (Dentsply Friadent, Mannheim, Germany). The superior (crestal) edge was perforated with small holes by small round bur in a straight hand-piece, those holes determined the thickness of the bone block. The block harvest was completed by a straight osteotome that was tapped along the superior holes. The block was carefully released and removed to avoid injury to inferior alveolar neurovascular bundles, and the donor site was left for spontaneous regeneration.

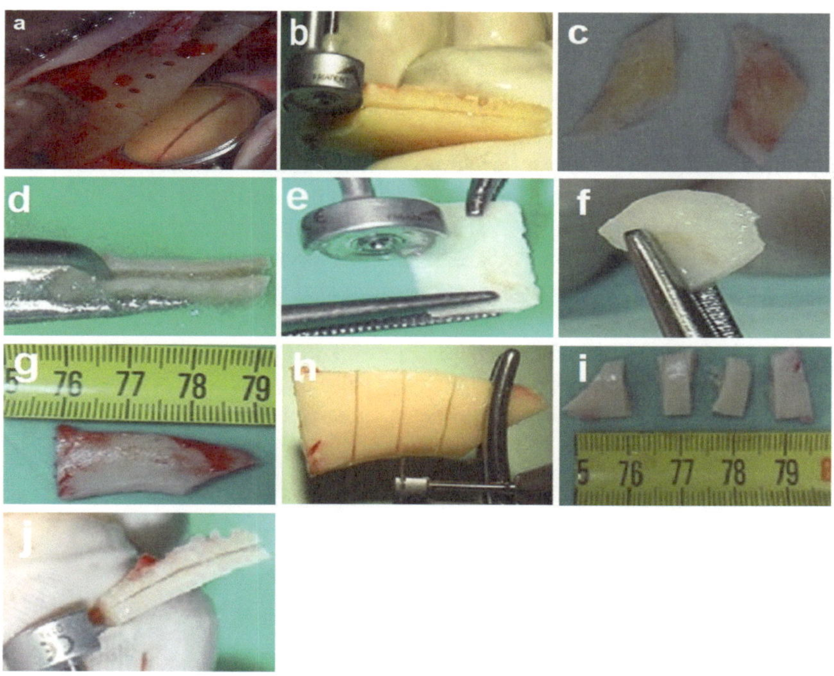

Figure 2.
The donor site and the Wedge preparation. (a) The bone block harvesting from the left retromolar area. (b–f) Multiple splitting of the bone blocks results in multiple small bone wedges. (g–j) Transverse splitting of the harvested bone block, as an additional option to create the bone wedges.

2.3 The wedge preparation

The wedge preparation was made by multiple splittings of the harvested bone block. In the present case, the bone block splitting was performed in the direction of the longitudinal axis, the first split yielded two thinner bone blocks, and further splitting at the same axis gave 4 thin bone blocks from the original bone block (**Figure 2b–d**). Further transverse splitting of the four thin bone blocks provided 8–10 thin bone blocks and each one is called "bone wedge" (**Figure 2e** and **f**). However, the splitting of the harvested block can be also made at the transverse axis of the block to obtain four thick bone blocks. Further splitting of those blocks at their long axis can give 8–10 thin bone wedges (**Figure 2g–j**).

2.4 Recipient site

The left recipient site was already exposed for bone block harvesting. The augmented bed was prepared by making grooves (slots, fissures) with either high speed straight thin bur, low speed small straight bur, or by the saw-shaped piezosurgery device, therefore, at the recipient site, three buccolingual grooves were made (**Figure 3a** and **b**). The number of the grooves is determined by the length of the augmented ridge, on the other hand, the depth of the grooves is limited by its distance from the inferior alveolar nerve which is measured on the dental CT scan. In general, the groove should be extended all the way from the buccal cortices to the lingual cortices, and as deep as possible in the recipient site residual bone. The main role of the groove in the WT is to give biological and mechanical retention of the bone wedge.

2.5 The augmentation procedure

Try-in of the bone wedges into the grooves at the recipient bed was performed in order to adapt one bone wedge to each groove. Thereafter, one wedge was inserted and taped into one groove using a flat edge cylindrical instrument and hummer (**Figure 4a**). It was extremely important to check the stability of each wedge by trying to extract it out from its groove; an unstable wedge should be removed and replaced by a stable one. This procedure is the fixation method of the bone wedge to the recipient site. The next step was the trimming and rounding of the sharp edges of each wedge in order to prevent trauma to the soft tissue overlying the augmentation (**Figure 4b** and **c**), consequently, multiple bone compartments were achieved (**Figure 4d**). The next step was packing those compartments with allograft particulate bone substitutes (**Figure 4e** and **f**), the desired bone volume was achieved

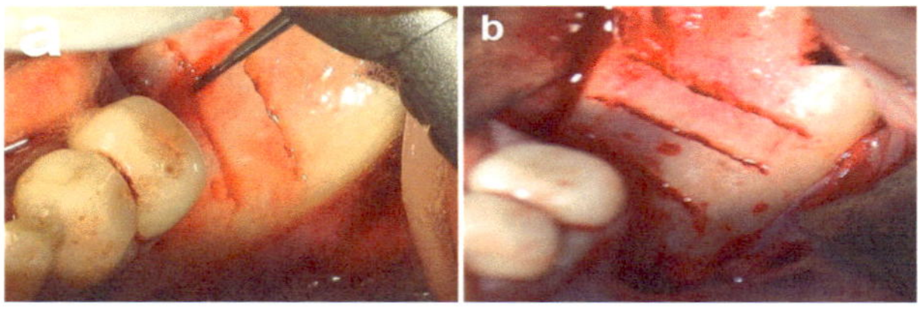

Figure 3.
The recipient site. (a) Grooves are created by height speed, low speed or piezoelectric. (b) Three grooves were created at the recipient site.

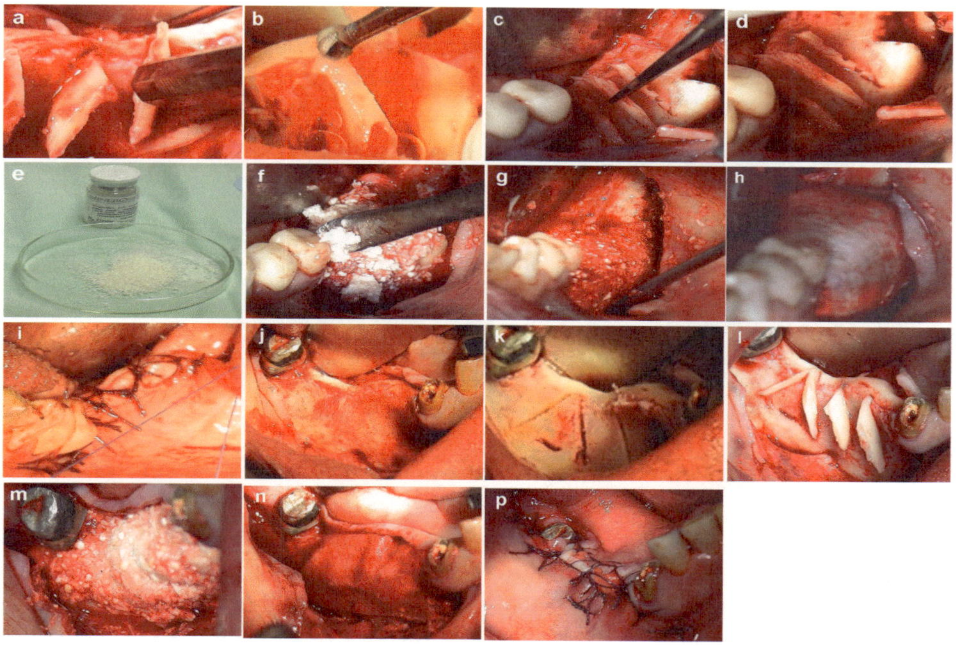

Figure 4.
The bone augmentation procedure. (a) Insertion and tapping of the bone wedges inside the grooves. (b) Trimming of the sharp edges of bone wedge. (c) Stability checking of the bone wedge inside the groove. (d) Bone compartments at the recipient site. (e) The bone filler, allograft particulate bone. (f) The filling of the bone compartments with the allograft particles. (g) The obtained final bone volume. (h) The resorbable membrane covering the bone graft. (i) Tension free closure of the augmented site. (j–o) Bone grafting of the patient's right side with the WT.

(**Figure 4g**), subsequently the bone graft was covered with a resorbable membrane (**Figure 4h**). A tension-free closure of the flap was performed (**Figure 4i**), utilizing a free buccal fat pad graft was used to enhance flap closure. The right side of the mandible was augmented using 4 bone wedges, with the same sequence that was performed to augment the left side (**Figure 4j–o**).

The follow-up was performed every two weeks for the first six weeks, and once a month later on (**Figure 5a**). After 4 months the patient underwent a dental CT scan (CBCT) to evaluate the amount of bone gain that was achieved from the augmentation procedure (**Figure 5b–d**), then dental implants were inserted under local anesthesia (**Figure 6**). Three to four months later the patient was referred for prosthetic rehabilitation (**Figure 7a** and **b**). This case has been followed up for 120 months (**Figure 7c–e**).

2.6 Case presentations

2.6.1 Case 1

A 45-year-old woman was referred to our department to augment atrophic ridges at the anterior and left posterior mandible. On examination, partial edentulism of the mandible with missing anterior and left posterior teeth (43–33 and 35, 36), moreover, the left and right first premolar were with poor prognosis (**Figure 8a–c**). Computed

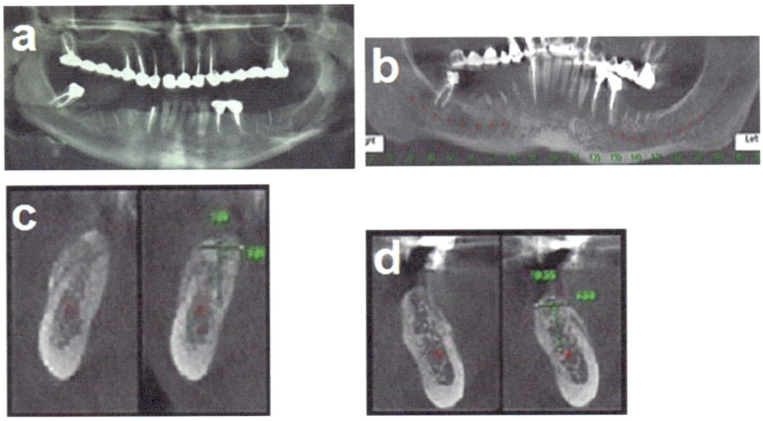

Figure 5.
Follow-up after two weeks. (a) The post-op panoramic view demonstrates one donor site and two recipient sites. (b–d) Computed tomographic views demonstrate the new bone that was obtained.

tomography was performed and demonstrated the bone deficit at the anterior and left mandible (**Figure 8d** and **e**). The patient had been treated in two stages; at the first stage, WT was performed to augment the anterior and left mandibular regions. Under general anesthesia the bone block was harvested from the left retromolar area (the same surgical site), then was split to obtain the bone wedges (**Figure 8f–i**). The recipient sites were prepared by creating grooves, consequently, 7 bone wedges were inserted into the grooves in a stable position and several bone compartments were achieved (**Figure 8j–l**). Then, the compartments were filled with particulate allograft bone substitute, obtaining the desired bone volume (**Figure 8m**), which was covered with a resorbable membrane (**Figure 8n**), and tension free closure of the recipient site was performed

(**Figure 8o**). A temporary bridge based on left and right first premolars was placed. The healing process was uneventful during the follow-up period, after 4 months a Computed dental tomography was performed and demonstrated the bone gain which was 4–6 mm horizontally and vertically (**Figure 8p–r**). At the second stage, the reentry to the augmented sites revealed new bone volume, and integration of the bone wedges into the new bone mass (**Figure 8s**), thereafter, 6 implants were inserted with immediate loading (**Figure 8t–v**). All implants were successfully osseointegrated (**Figure 8w** and **x**) and the final rehabilitation was performed after 3 months (**Figure 8y**). This case is followed for 72 months (**Figure 8y**).

2.6.2 Case 2

A 28-year-old woman was referred complaining of severe atrophy of the anterior maxillary region; after a failed bone augmentation procedure which was done by her surgeon. Clinical and radiographic examinations revealed severe atrophy of the anterior maxillary ridge and pneumatization of the right maxillary sinus (**Figure 9a–e**). She was treated in three stages; bone augmentation of the anterior maxilla with the wedge technique, extraction and socket augmentation of the right second premolar, and right maxillary sinus augmentation. The right mandibular retromolar area was the donor site for the bone block, after splitting the bone block, 7 bone wedges were

DOI: http://dx.doi.org/10.5772/intechopen.100099

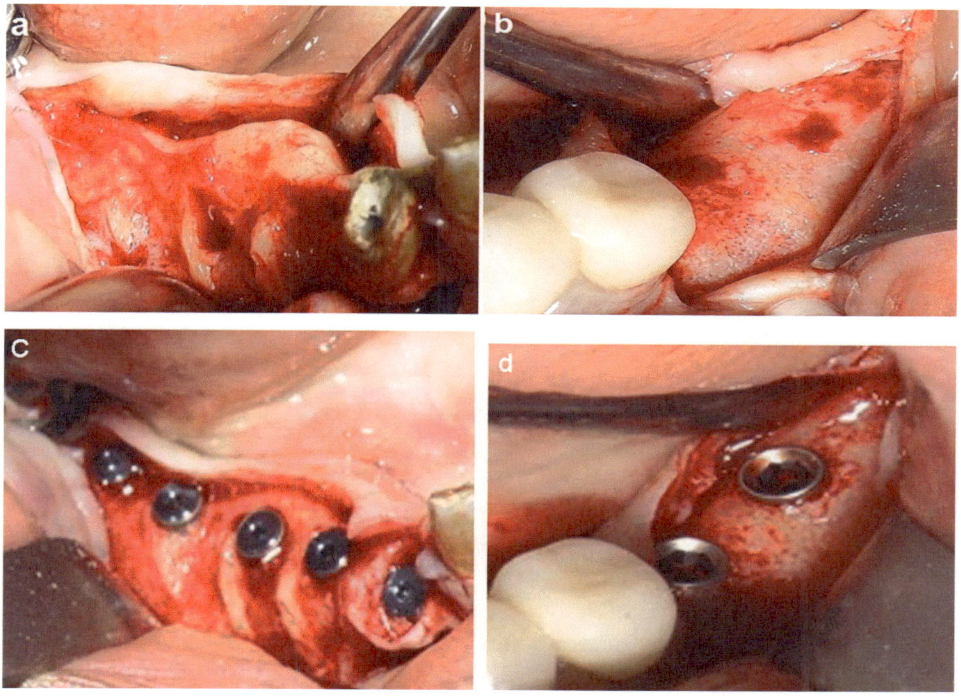

Figure 6.
Reentry after 4 months and implant placement. (a) Shows good bone regeneration after 4 months at the right side. (b) Shows good new bone volume at the left side. (c and d) Implants placement.

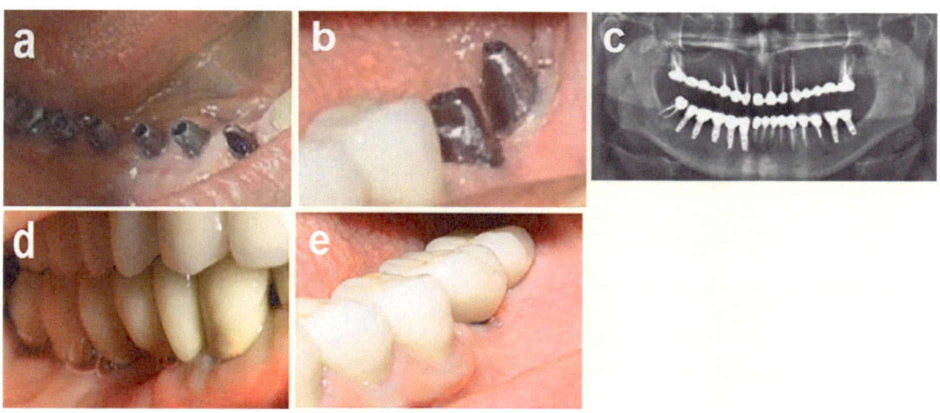

Figure 7.
Rehabilitation and follow up. (a and b) Implant abutments. (c–e) Panoramic radiograph and clinical view 60 months after the surgery.

obtained. Four cortical bone wedges were inserted at the grooves that were prepared at the recipient site (**Figure 9f**). Then, particulate allograft bone substitute was used as the bone filler between the bone wedges (**Figure 9g**). The right maxillary first premolar, and the left maxillary canine were temporarily preserved to hold an acrylic bridge during the healing phase. Follow-up examinations at months showed excellent

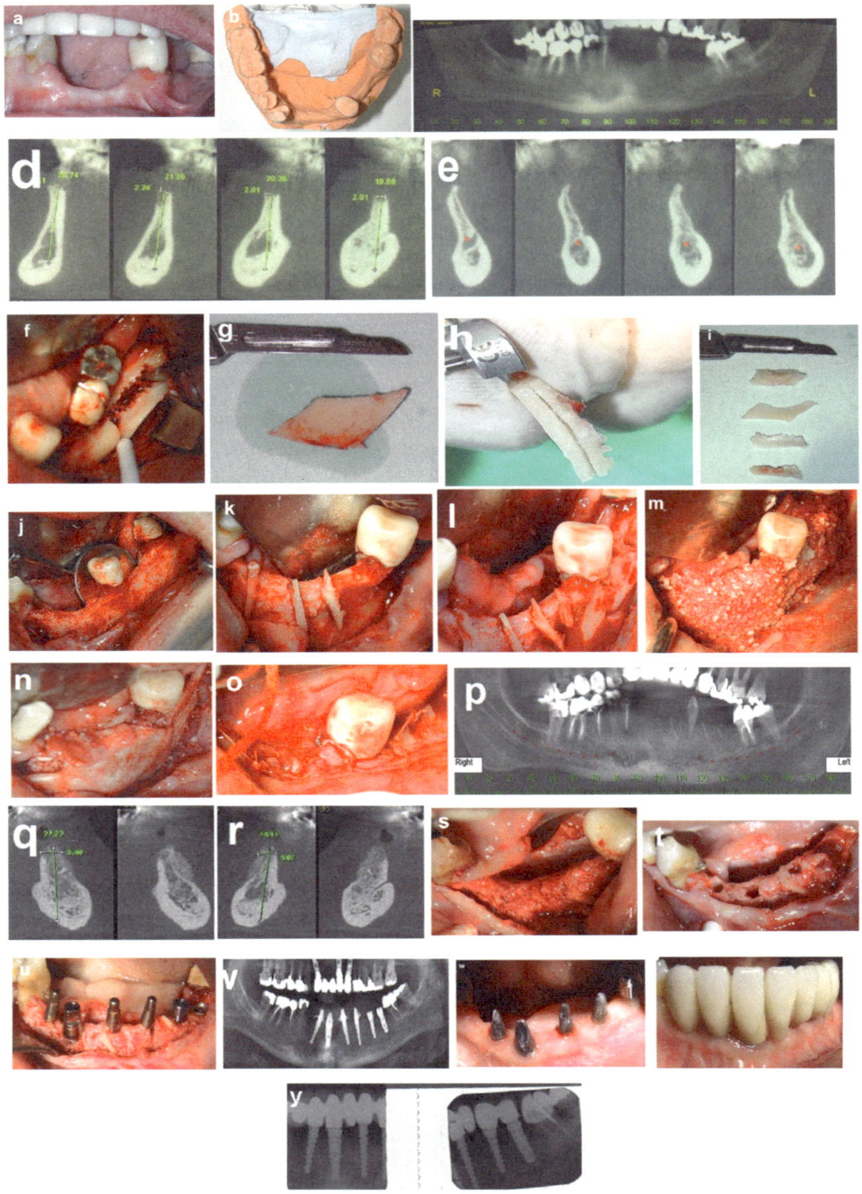

Figure 8.

Case 2. (a–e) Clinical and radiographic view of the mandible. (f–i) Bone block harvest and the preparation of the bone wedges. (j–o) WT bone augmentation at the anterior and the left mandibular ridges. (p–r) Computed tomography 4 months after bone grafting. (s–u) Reentry and implant insertions 4 months after the augmentation surgery. (v) Radiographic view-follow up of the implants. (w and x) Crowns rehabilitation. (y) 72 months follow-up.

recovery (**Figure 9h**) and CBCT showed the new bone gain and the available bone (width; 6 to 10 mm) for implant insertion (**Figure 9i–k**). At the stage-two surgery, the intraoperative views showed a good regeneration, and the bone wedges had excellent integration in the new bone volume (**Figure 9l**). **Figure 9(m)** and **(n)** demonstrate the drilling through those wedges indicating their stability and viability.

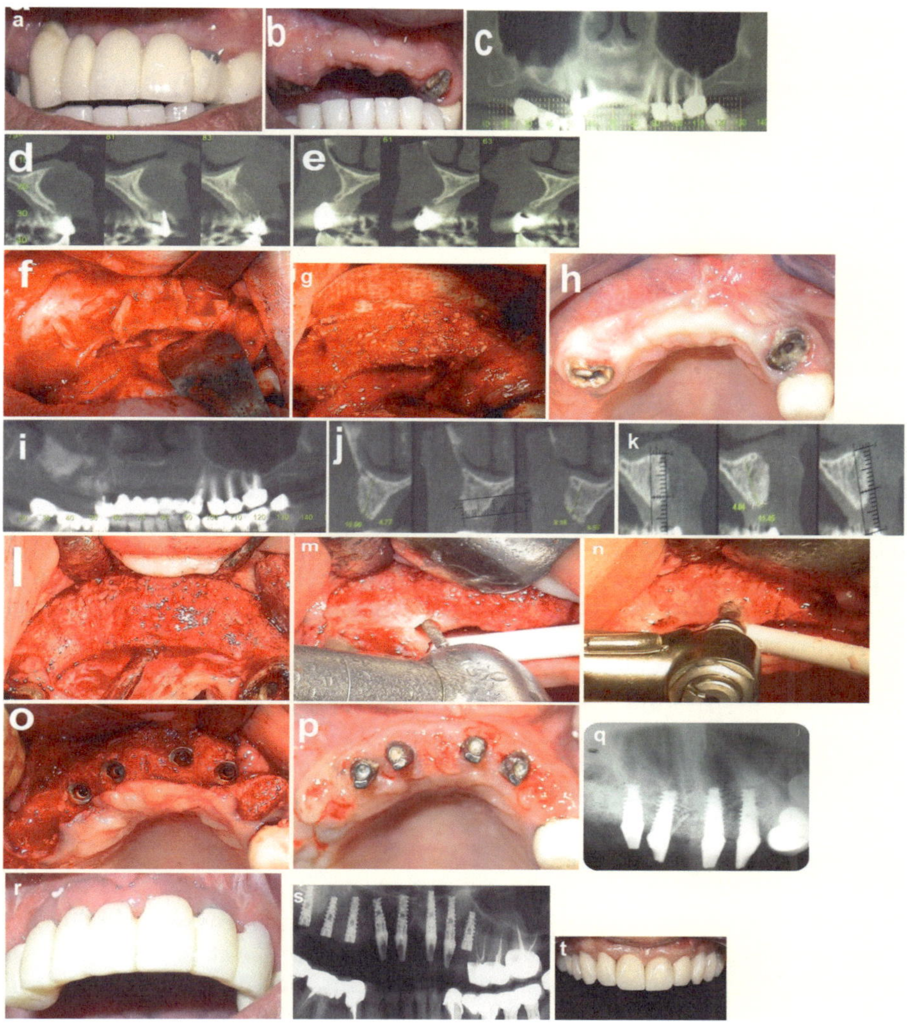

Figure 9.
Case 2. (a and b) Clinical view-anterior maxilla. (c–e) Computed tomography of the anterior maxilla demonstrates the severe atrophy of the residual ridge. (f–g) The WT bone augmentation, intraoperative views. (h–k) Clinical and radiographic views at four months after the surgery. (l) Reentry 4 months after the surgery demonstrates nice bone regeneration. (m and n) Show the drilling for the implants that was performed through the bone wedges. (o) 4 implants were placed at the recipient site. (p and q) Clinical and radiographic view at 4 months after implant placement. (r and s) Temporary rehabilitation follow up 5 months after implants insertion. (t) 60 months follow-up after the surgery, fixed prosthesis supported by dental implants with excellent outcomes.

At the same stage, the right maxillary first premolar, and the left maxillary canine were extracted with socket augmentation. In addition, 4 implants were placed at the anterior augmented region (**Figure 9o**) with immediate loading. **Figure 9(p)** and **(q)** show clinical and radiographic view one month after implant placement. At stage-three surgery, additional 4 implants were placed; 3 at the right maxilla and one implant at the left maxillary canine. Four months later the patient was referred to her dentist for a fixed prosthesis over the implants (**Figure 9r** and **s**). This patient had been followed for 60 months (**Figure 9t**).

3. Results

3.1 Clinical outcomes

Bone augmentation with cortical bone wedges was performed in adult patients, mean age 47 years; ranging from 19 to 67 years. Different sites at the maxilla and the mandible had been treated with the WT, and the majority of the augmented sites were at the posterior mandible (**Figure 10**). The majority of the treated patients had more than one site to augment. The healing process was uneventful. The donor site for the bone block (the retromolar area) healed very well without complications and spontaneous regeneration of the site was observed during the follow-up period, with full regeneration after twelve months. The recipient sites healed very well, and the bone augmentations were maintained without wound dehiscence among almost all the treated patients. However, one patient experienced a partial breakdown of the wound, and the majority of the augmented bone was lost; this patient had completed treatment with nerve transposition for implant placement. Four months after the augmentation surgery, clinical evaluation of the recipient sites revealed new hard tissue volume and good ridge contour. CBCT evaluation showed a good bone volume with 4 to 8 mm bone gain horizontally and 3–6 mm bone gain vertically. The second surgery that was performed for dental implant placement revealed a new and good bone volume, with excellent integration of the bone wedges at the recipient site. The excellent integration of the bone wedges was obvious with no dislodgement during the implant site preparation. Dental implants were inserted of adequate lengths (10-16 mm) and diameters (2.8–4.2 mm). Further follow-up of the augmentation sites and the implants in both the mandible and the maxilla revealed stable long-term outcomes after the implants rehabilitation.

3.2 Histologic findings

At the reentry stage for implant insertion, hard tissue specimens were obtained from the wedge area for histologic evaluation (**Figure 11a** and **b**). The obtained specimen of the bone wedge was stained with hematoxylin and eosin (H&E) after overnight decalcification using Rapid Decalcification Solution containing Hydrochloric Acid, revealed

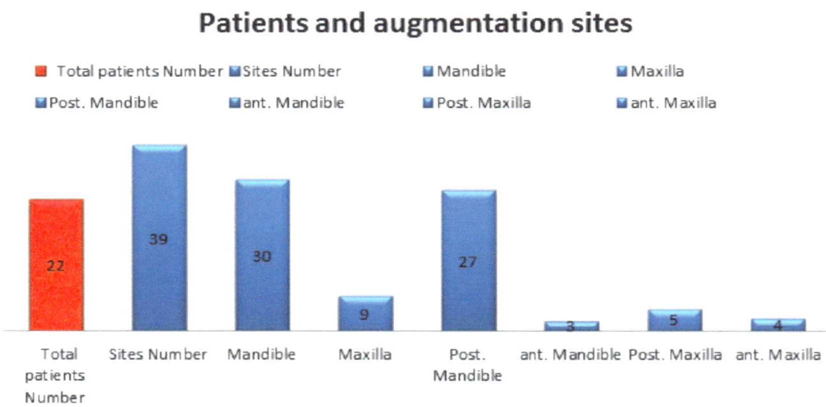

Figure 10.
Patients and augmented sites.

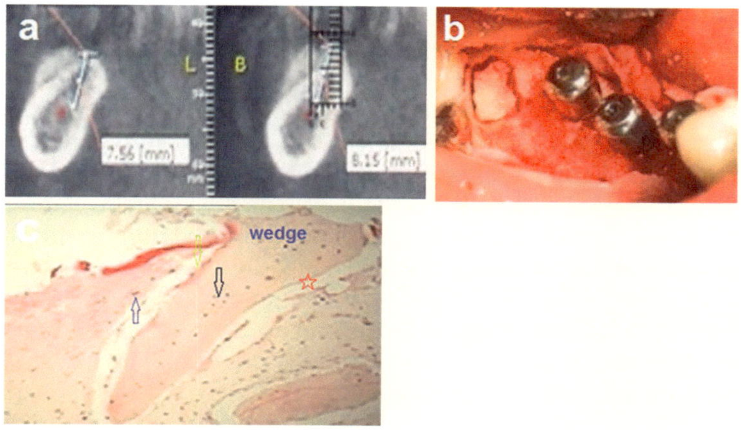

Figure 11.
Histologic examination. (a and b) The site of the wedge biopsy. (c) The bone wedge is obvious at the center of the figure (hematoxylin–eosin). Black arrow, vital osteoclasts; blue arrow, osteoblasts; green arrow, osteoclasts. The red star, the artificial split of the specimens.

vital osteocytes within the entire bone wedge, osteoblasts, and osteoclast in its periphery (**Figure 11c**), with no evidence of necrotic areas inside the bone wedges. Those findings may indicate the vitality and remodeling activities of the graft. More specific histological examinations and stains should be performed to enhance the understanding of the healing process. This could be performed on an animal model.

4. Discussion

Autogenous bone grafts have been used for many years for the reconstruction of alveolar defects and are still considered the gold standard for bone augmentation. The mandibular symphysis and ramus are widely used as intraoral donor sites. Extraoral donor sites are used as well, however, they have some major disadvantages including concomitant morbidities of the donor site, high treatment costs, and high resorption rates [11–17]. The donor site for the WT is the mandibular retromolar/ramus area, therefore, the majority of the bone block consists mainly of cortical bone. Pikos in 2005 stated that one ramus donor site can provide bone volume for a three-tooth segment, and can provide 3–4 mm as horizontal or vertical bone regeneration [41]. If an extensive bone graft is required for one or more sites in the same patient, it may necessitate simultaneous harvest of bone blocks bilaterally from the ramus area and from the symphysis area as well in order to obtain enough bone quantities. Moreover, these cases may necessitate multiple augmentation surgeries to achieve the desired reconstruction of the same site as the report of Schwarts using the Multitier techniques for such cases. In addition, some surgeons may use extraoral donor sites for multiple-site ridge augmentation [42]. Among the concerns of the recipient sites reconstruction with bone blocks, two of them are extremely significant for the final outcome; the First one is bone block dislodgement during the insertion of the implants [43], and the second one is the presence of a connective tissue layer between the block graft and the recipient bed [44]. In addition, micromovements of the bone block graft, loosening the fixation screws, and infection may compromise the desired augmentation outcomes.

The present chapter describes the wedge technique as a novel bone augmentation method that can be useful for multiple site augmentations as horizontal or vertical bone augmentation or both (3-dimensional). The multiple splitting of one harvested block could give 8 to 12 thin cortical bone wedges (0.5 to 1 mm thickness for each wedge), and 3 to 4 wedges that are used in the recipient site can augment at least a three-tooth segment. A simple calculation manifests that one harvested bone block can augment 3 to 4 sites of a three-tooth segment. The fundamental concept of this technique is the use of cortical bone wedges that are inserted into the grooves at the recipient site to create bone compartments that are filled with allograft bone particles.

The grooves at the recipient site have several functions including; mechanical retention of the cortical bone wedge so there is no need for fixation materials like screws, reducing the hazards of hardware infection and eliminating their expenses. Moreover, the grooves act as biological retention of the cortical bone wedge, and may be considered as decortication for the recipient site. The blood vessels injury during the groove preparation can enhance angiogenesis and revascularization of the thin bone wedge in one hand, and it can accelerate the regional acceleratory phenomenon on the other hand which has an important function in the healing of the operated organs. It is well documented in the relevant literature that the success of bone grafting procedures depends mainly on the amount of revascularization (quality and intensity). De Marco et al. in 2005 reported that several vascular sprouts from the recipient bed proliferated toward the graft by the third day, and were demonstrated at the graft periphery. Moreover, revascularization was more intense in the area near the perforation of the recipient bed [38].

According to the author's opinion, the previously mentioned findings regarding the revascularization of a bone graft at the recipient site may explain the integration of the thin bone wedges in the retention grooves. In addition, the use of particulate bone to fill the compartments in the WT plays a significant role in the fast incorporation of the bone graft at the recipient site [4]. The regeneration process can be approved by the histologic finding of specimens obtained from the bone wedges examinations 4 months after the augmentation. Vital Osteocytes were visible inside the bone wedge which indicates the wedge vitality. Moreover, the presence of osteoclasts and osteoblasts at the periphery of the wedge indicate bone graft remodeling.

The cortical bone wedge, in the WT, has several functions; the thin nature of the wedge (0,5-1 mm) may enhance the ingrowth of the vascular sprouts that emerge from the grooves at the recipient bed at two contact surface areas at each wedge, therefore, the revascularization of the wedge graft maybe earlier and faster than that of the standard thick block. Moreover, the bone wedge acts as a space maintainer for the augmented bone, which is achieved by the multiple bone compartments that are created between the bone wedges. In addition, while inserting the bone wedges in the grooves, they tent the membrane that covers the graft. As a result, the bone wedges support the particulate bone filler, and inhibit its deformation at the recipient site. According to the author's point of view, the insertion of several bone wedges at the recipient site creates a site with an increased number of autogenous bone walls that may accelerate the regeneration of the treated sites similar to the reconstruction concept of the periodontal defects. Moreover, the wedge–groove unit increases bone to bone contact surface areas that lead to a faster wedge to groove integration. Successful grafting depends mainly on the close contact between the graft and vascularization tissue, and on its fixation to the recipient bed [35, 39]. Those two principles are fundamental in the wedge-groove unit concept. Moreover, comparing the wedge-groove unit with the standard thick cortical bone graft, the latter has higher failure rates due to the risk of early exposure, slower rates of revascularization with areas of necrosis that may persist for a long time within the graf, and incomplete bone graft replacement [45, 46].

The cortical bone wedge technique has several advantages:

1. One harvested bone block from the ramus can augment two to three recipient sites.

2. Two harvested ramus bone blocks bilaterally can augment multisite in both jaws.

3. There is no need for fixation materials (Screws, mini-plates, or titanium mesh).

4. Decrease the need for extra-oral donor sites. Therefore, reducing the complications and expenses of the standard bone block graft.

An additional key factor for successful bone augmentation relies crucially on adequate volume, quality, and tension-free closure of the soft tissue at the recipient site. The buccal-free fat graft was simultaneously used along with the wedge technique as soft tissue grafting to enhance a double layer tension-free closure of the recipient site. The role of the buccal free fat graft during bone augmentation procedures was proved by Kablan and Laster at their publication [47].

The Resorption of different bone augmentation materials is well documented in the relevant literature in dentistry. Haggery et al. in 2015 stated that the resorption rates of cortical grafts are (0–50%), with the most resorption occurring at the periphery of the graft [4]. In addition, according to the dental implant literature, bone resorption around implants is expected during the first year of function to be approximately 1.2 mm in height, and 0.1 mm additional resorption for every subsequent year [48, 49]. The clinical and radiographic follow-up results among the patients that had been treated with the WT and followed for an average time of 56 months; ranging from 30 to 120 months showed excellent survival and success rates with minimal bone resorption around the implants. According to the author, the long-term stability of the outcomes utilizing the WT results from the use of thin cortical bone wedges that completely revascularized during the healing period, and from the combined use of particulate bone as well; that is readily incorporated at the recipient site.

5. Conclusions

The cortical bone wedge technique's biological rationale is to create multiple autogenic bone compartments that are filled with allogeneic bone particles. This combination can augment multiple sites with intraoral autogenous bone blocks and reduces the need for extraoral donor sites. The wedge-groove unit may enhance revascularization of the bone graft and improve its survival. The long-term follow-up results of the wedge technique indicate the predictability of this treatment modality.

Acknowledgements

Thanks to Dr. Abir Abu Subeh for her technical support.

Conflict of interest

The author declares no conflict of interest.

Abbreviations

WT	wedge technique

Author details

Fares Kablan
Department of Oral and Maxillofacial Surgery, The Galilee Medical Center, Nahariya, Israel

*Address all correspondence to: kablanp1@gmail.com

References

[1] Cross J. Bone augmentation procedures in implant dentistry. Int J Oral Maxillofac Implants [Internet]. 2009;24 Suppl:237-259. Available from: https://pubmed.ncbi.nlm.nih.gov/19885448/.

[2] Esposito M. The efficacy of various bone augmentation procedures for dental implants: A Cochrane systematic review of randomized controlled clinical trials. Int J Oral Maxillofac Implants [Internet]. 2006 [cited 14 August 2021];21(5):696-710. Available from: https://pubmed.ncbi.nlm.nih.gov/17066630/.

[3] Davi Rabelo G. Retrospective study of bone grafting procedures before implant placement. Implant Dent [Internet]. 2010 [cited 14 August 2021];19(4). Available from: https://pubmed.ncbi.nlm.nih.gov/20683291/.

[4] CJ H. Simple bone augmentation for alveolar ridge defects. Oral Maxillofac Surg Clin North Am [Internet]. 2015 [cited 14 August 2021];27(2):203-226. Available from: https://pubmed.ncbi.nlm.nih.gov/25951957/

[5] PJ B. An algorithm for reconstruction of alveolar defects before implant placement. Oral Maxillofac Surg Clin North Am. 2001;13:533-541.

[6] Jensen S. Bone augmentation procedures in localized defects in the alveolar ridge: Clinical results with different bone grafts and bone-substitute materials. Int J Oral Maxillofac Implants [Internet]. 2009 [cited 14 August 2021];24:218-36. Available from: https://pubmed.ncbi.nlm.nih.gov/19885447/

[7] PJW S. A: Interpositional bone graft augmentation of atrophic mandible. J Oral Surg. 1978;36:30-32.

[8] Jensen OT. Anterior maxillary alveolar distraction osteogenesis: A prospective 5-year clinical study. Int J Oral Maxillofac Implants. 2002;17:52-68.

[9] Jensen OT. Alveolar segmental "sandwich" osteotomies for posterior edentulous mandibular sites for dental implants. J Oral Maxillofac Surg. 2006;64:471-475.

[10] Urbani G. Distraction osteogenesis to achieve mandibular vertical bone regeneration: A case report. Int J Oral Maxillofac Implants. 1996;11: 387-394.

[11] Beirne OR. Comparison of complications after bone removal from lateral and medial plates of the anterior ilium for mandibular augmentation. Int J Oral Maxillofac Surg. 1986; 15:269.

[12] Cricchio G. Donor site morbidity in two different approaches to anterior iliac crest bone harvesting. Clin Implant Dent Relat Res. 2003;5(3):161-169.

[13] Kline Jr RM. Complications associated with the harvesting of cranial bone grafts. Plast Reconstr Surg. 1995;95(1):5-13.

[14] Frodel Jr JL. Calvarial bone graft harvest. Techniques, considerations, and morbidity. Arch Otolaryngol Head Neck Surg. 1993 Jan;119(1):17-23.

[15] Restoy-Lozano A. Calvarial bone grafting for three-dimensional reconstruction of severe maxillary defects: A case series. Int J Oral Maxillofac Implants. 2015;30(4):880-890.

[16] Chen YC. Donor site morbidity after harvesting of proximal tibia bone. Head Neck. 2006 Jun;28(6):496-500.

[17] Nkenke E. Morbidity of harvesting of bone grafts from the iliac crest for preprosthetic augmentation procedures: A prospective study. Int J Oral Maxillofac Surg. 2004 Mar;33(2):157-163.

[18] Khoury F. Augmentation of the sinus floor with mandibular bone blocks and simultaneous implantation. A 6-year clinical investigation. Int J Oral Maxillofac Implants. Jul-Aug 1999;14(4):557-564.

[19] Misch CM. Ridge augmentation using mandibular ramus bone grafts for the placement of dental implants: Presentation of a technique. Pract Periodontics Aesthet Dent. 1996 Mar;8(2):127-135; quiz 138.

[20] Mish CM. Comparison of intraoral donor sites for onlay grafting prior to implant placement. Int J Oral Maxillofac Implants. Nov-Dec 1997;12(6):767-776.

[21] Schwartz-Arad D. Surgical success of intraoral autogenous block onlay bone grafting for alveolar ridge augmentation. Implant Dent. 2005 Jun;14(2):131-138.

[22] Garg AK. Autogenous mandibular bone grafts in the treatment of the resorbed maxillary anterior alveolar ridge rationale and approach. Implant Dent. 1998;7(3):169-176.

[23] Silva FM. Complications of intraoral donor site for bone grafting prior to implant placement. Implant Dent. 2006 Dec;15(4):420-426.

[24] Joshi A. An investigation of post-operative morbidity following chin graft surgery. Br Dent J. 2004 Feb 28;196(4):215-218.

[25] Clavero J. Ramus or chin grafts for maxillary sinus inlay and local onlay augmentation: Comparison of donor site morbidity and complications. Clin Implant Dent Relat Res. 2003;5(3):154-160.

[26] Nkenke E. Morbidity of harvesting of retromolar bone grafts: A prospective study. Clin Oral Implants Res. 2002 Oct;13(5):514-521.

[27] Nkenke E. Morbidity of harvesting of chin grafts: A prospective study. Clin Oral Implants Res. 2001 Oct;12(5):495-502.

[28] Widmark G. Rehabilitation of patients with severely resorbed maxillae by means of implants with or without bone grafts. A one year follow up study. Int J Oral Maxillofac Implants. Jul-Aug 1998;13(4):474-482.

[29] Cammack GV 2nd. Histologic evaluation of mineralized and demineralized freeze-dried bone allograft for ridge and sinus augmentations. Int J Periodontics Restorative Dent. 2005 Jun;25(3): 231-237.

[30] Simon M. Vertical ridge augmentation by expanded-polytetrafluoroethylene membrane and a combination of intraoral autogenous bone graft and deproteinized anorganic bovine bone (Bio Oss). Clin Oral Implants Res. 2007 Oct;18(5):620-629.

[31] Koll A. Current trends and future perspectives of bone substitute materials – From space holders to innovative biomaterials. J Craniomaxillofac Surg. 2012 Dec;40(8):706-718.

[32] Gomes KU. Use of allogenic bone graft in maxillary reconstruction for installation of dental implants. J Oral Maxillofac Surg. 2008 Nov;66(11):2335-2338.

[33] Le B. Cortical tenting grafting technique in severely atrophic alveolar

ridge for implant site preparation. Implant Dent. 2008 Mar;17(1):40-50.

[34] Khojasteh A. Localized bone augmentation with cortical bone blocks tended over different particulate bone substitutes: A retrospective study. Int J Oral Maxillofac Implants. Nov-Dec 2012;27(6):1481-1493.

[35] Burchardt H. Transplantation of bone. Surg Clin North Am. 1978 Apr;58(2):403-427.

[36] Nathanson A. The early vascularization of an autogenous bone inlay into an artificial defect in the rabbit mandibular. Acta Otolaryngol. Jan-Feb 1978;85(1-2):135-148.

[37] Hammack BL. Comparative vascularization of autogenous and homogenous-bone transplants. J Bone Joint Surg Am. 1960 Jul;42-A:811-817.

[38] De Marco AC. Revascularization of autogenous block grafts with or without an e-PTFE membrane. Int J Oral Maxillofac Implants. Nov-Dec 2005;20(6):867-874.

[39] Scardina GA. Microcirculation in the healing of surgical wounds in the oral cavity. Int J Oral Maxillofac Surg. 2013 Jan;42(1):31-35.

[40] LaTenta GS. The role of rigid fixation in bone graft augmentation of the craniofacial skeleton. Plast Reconstr Surg. 1989 Oct;84(4):578-588.

[41] Pikos MA. Mandibular block autografts for alveolar ridge augmentation. Atlas Oral Maxillofac Surg Clin North Am. 2005 Sep;13(2):91-107.

[42] Schwarts AD. Multitier of harvesting technique for bone augmentation using intraoral autogenous bone blocks. Implant Den. 2007 Mar;16(1):5-12.

[43] Proussaefs P. The use of intraorally harvested autogenous block grafts for vertical alveolar ridge augmentation: A human study. Int J Periodontics Restorative Dent. 2005 Aug;25(4):351-363.

[44] De Carvalho PS. Influence of bed preparation on the incorporation of autogenous bone grafts: A study in dogs. Int J Oral Maxillofac Implants. Jul-Aug 2000;15(4):565-570.

[45] Andrade MG. Pattern of osteogenesis during onlay bone graft healing. Oral Surg Oral Med Oral Pathol Oral Radiol Endod. 2010 Dec;110(6):713-719.

[46] Oppenheimer AJ. Craniofacial bone grafting: Wolff's law revisited. Craniomaxillofac Trauma Reconstr. 2008 Nov;1(1):49-61.

[47] Kablan F. The use of free fat tissue transfer from the buccal fat pad to obtain and maintain primary closure and to improve soft tissue thickness at bone-augmented sites: Technique presentation and report of case series. Int J Oral Maxillofac Implants. Mar-Apr 2014;29(2):e220-e231.

[48] Adell R. A 15-year study of osseointegrated implants in the treatment of the edentulous jaw. Int J Oral Surg. 1981 Dec;10(6):387-416.

[49] Albrektsson T. The long-term efficacy of currently used dental implants: A review and proposed criteria of success. Int J Oral Maxillofac Implants. Summer 1986;1(1):11-25.

Section 3

Advanced Clinical Techniques and Peri-Implantitis

Chapter 11

Peri-Implant Soft Tissue Augmentation

Marko Blašković and Dorotea Blašković

Abstract

The peri-implant soft tissue (PIS) augmentation procedure has become an integral part of implant-prosthetic rehabilitation. Minimal width of keratinized mucosa (KM) of 2 mm is deemed necessary to facilitate oral hygiene maintenance around the implant and provide hard and soft peri-implant tissue stability. PIS thickness of at least 2 mm is recommended to achieve the esthetic appearance and prevent recessions around implant prosthetic rehabilitation. The autogenous soft tissue grafts can be divided into two groups based on their histological composition—free gingival graft (FGG) and connective tissue graft (CTG). FGG graft is used mainly to increase the width of keratinized mucosa while CTG augment the thickness of PIS. Both grafts are harvested from the same anatomical region—the palate. Alternatively, they can be harvested from the maxillary tuberosity. Soft tissue grafts can be also harvested as pedicle grafts, in case when the soft tissue graft remains attached to the donor site by one side preserving the blood supply from the donor region. Clinically this will result in less shrinkage of the graft postoperatively, improving the outcome of the augmentation procedure. To bypass the drawback connected with FGG or CTG harvesting, substitutional soft tissue grafts have been developed.

Keywords: connective tissue graft, CTG, free gingival graft, FGG, apically positioned flap, APF, peri-implant soft tissue augmentation, subepithelial connective tissue graft, de-epithelized free gingival graft, keratinized mucosa

1. Introduction

Peri-implant soft tissue (PST) thickness and width of keratinized mucosa (KM) have a major impact on the esthetic appearance, stability, and health of implant/prosthetic reconstruction. Dental implants were introduced 50 years ago as a treatment modality for edentulous patients and, later on, for partially edentulous patients with shortened arches and single-tooth gaps [1]. Until lately, the success of implant treatment was based on implant survival rates, prosthetic stability, radiographic bone loss, and absence of infection [2, 3]. Today, patients' implant treatment expectations have changed. They have shifted from healthy and functional to healthy, functional, esthetic, and natural-looking tooth replacement [4]. Consequently, the PST augmentation procedure became a fundamental part of implant treatment algorithms.

There are two main objectives of soft tissue augmentation around implants—(1) to restore an adequate width of KM and (2) to increase the volume of peri-implant soft tissue [5].

1.1 KM width around implants

The displacement and loss of the KM can be a consequence of—(1) flap mobilization in order to achieve primary flap closure during horizontal or vertical bone augmentation procedures and (2) vertical bone resorption and reduction of distance between the bone crest and mucogingival line [6].

Today, the vast majority of published evidence supports the necessity of at least 2 mm of keratinized mucosa width around the implant.

The presence of an adequate amount of KM around implants (>2 mm) will facilitate maintenance of oral hygiene, which can lead to less plaque accumulation and lower incidence of peri-implant mucositis. Furthermore, KM can be associated with soft and hard tissue stability, resulting in decreased incidence in the recession of peri-implant mucosa, marginal bone resorption, and attachment loss (**Figure 1**) [5, 7–13].

KM is fundamental in maintaining health around implants in erratic maintenance compliers patients. Less than 2 mm of KM around implants is erratic compliers seems to be associated with a higher incidence of peri-implantitis [12, 14].

1.2 PIS volume

In literature, the suggested PIS thickness is at least 2 mm. PIS thickness has a major influence on two factors—(1) esthetic appearance of the implant/prosthetic rehabilitation and (2) marginal bone stability [13, 15].

1.2.1 Esthetic appearance

The color, texture, volume, level of mucosal margin of the PIS, and presence of papilla has a major influence on the overall esthetical outcome. The aforementioned elements must be in line with those of soft tissue around adjacent teeth in order to obtain a harmonious and natural-looking restoration. These parameters are influenced

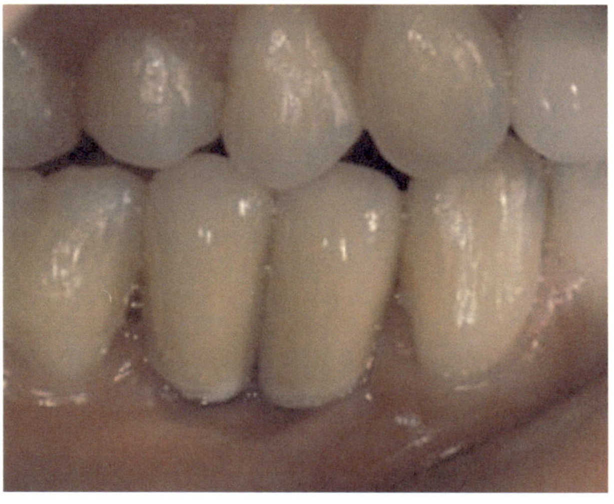

Figure 1.
Recession of the marginal mucosa caused by inadequate width of KM.

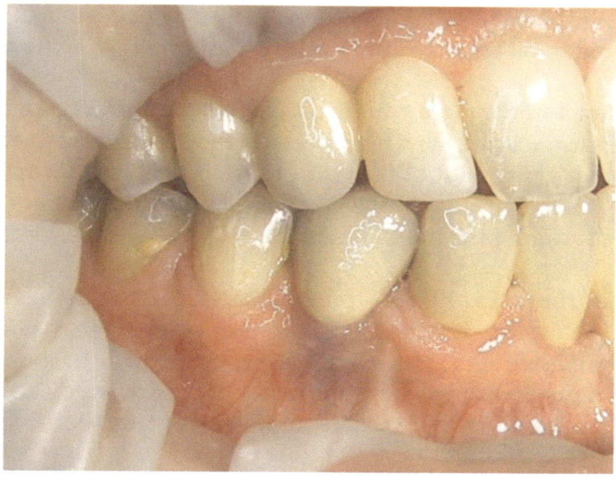

Figure 2.
Visible discoloration of the thin marginal mucosa caused by titanium abutment in the region of the lower right canine.

mainly by soft tissue thickness. Several indexes were developed to objectively evaluate the esthetical appearance of the implant/prosthetic restoration [16].

In literature, the suggested PIS thickness is at least 2 mm [15].

Inadequate PIS volume can be improved with soft tissue augmentation techniques. Furthermore, thick soft tissue can even mask and hide alveolar bone loss on the buccal side of implants [12, 13, 15]. Therefore, soft tissue augmentation is recommended in esthetical regions where a certain amount of buccal bone remodeling is expected, like immediate implant placement in situations with thin biotype or thin buccal bone plate [17, 18].

PIS thickness is essential for concealing the color of the prosthetic restoration and preventing PIS discoloration caused by prosthetic material. In cases with thin PIS (< 2 mm) titanium abutments will cause a visible color change of the buccal PIS (**Figure 2**) [12, 19–21].

1.2.2 Peri-implant marginal bone stability

PIS has a predetermined thickness of 2.5–4 mm, termed biologic width [22]. PIS is formed after healing abutment installation. In case when soft tissue is thinner than 2 mm, peri-implant marginal bone resorption will be initiated in order to establish sufficient space for the biological width [22, 23]. Augmentation of PIS volume with soft tissue grafts can prevent marginal bone resorption in the case of thin PIS [5, 14, 24].

2. General principles of PIS grafting

After transplantation to the recipient region, the soft tissue graft depends on plasmatic imbibition in order to receive sufficient nourishment. In the later stages, after 3–4 days, the soft tissue graft will be transvascularized with newly formed blood vessels. Blood vessel anastomoses will be formed between vessels of the recipient site and vessels already present in the graft [21, 25–29]. In order to achieve plasmatic imbibition and transvascularization certain factors must be met:

1. Rigid immobilization of the graft-excessive movement can hamper plasmatic imbibition and transvascularization of the flap

2. Intimate contact of the graft with the recipient site—decreased distance for the plasmatic diffusion or for new blood vessels to reach the graft will result in faster and complete nourishment of the graft. Furthermore, the formation of a blood clot or active hemorrhage between the vascular surface of the recipient site and graft can compromise the nourishment of the graft

3. Vascularity of the recipient site—the root surface of the tooth and the surface of the implant are avascular surfaces. In those situations, the survival of the graft will be accomplished either by using a larger graft than the avascular surface in order to obtain nourishment from the adjacent vascularized surfaces, preparing a split-thickness flap in order to assure nourishment from both sides of the flap, or by using a pedicle graft.

4. The PIS grafting procedure should begin with the preparation of the recipient site in order to decrease the time between graft harvest and graft transfer into recipient bed [21, 25, 26].

Most of the aforementioned conditions are met when the periosteum is used as a recipient site. The periosteum is well irrigated and it is immobile (**Figure 3**) [25, 30].

Likewise, to achieve those factors care must be taken while harvesting the soft tissue graft. The graft should be of uniform thickness to ensure even intimate contact of the inner surface of the graft and the recipient site [25, 26].

The composition of the graft can influence the nourishment of the graft—adipose and glandular tissue may hinder the nourishment of the rest of the graft so they should be dissected from the graft [26, 31].

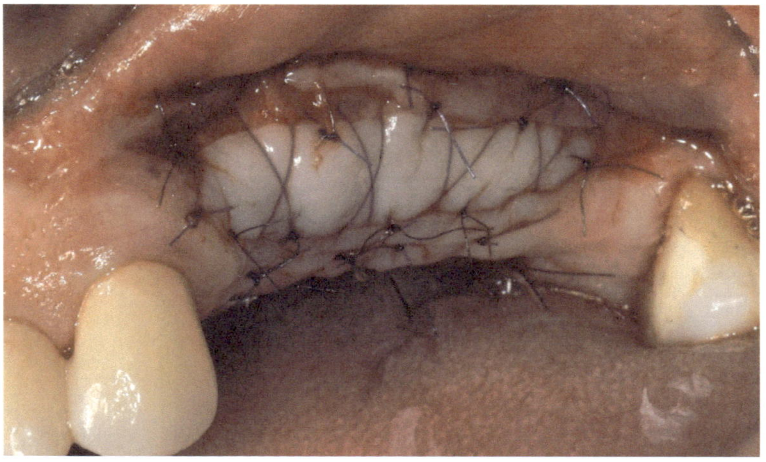

Figure 3.
Stabilization and intimate contact of the autologous soft tissue graft (free gingival graft) in the recipient site achieved with simple interrupted and cross mattress sutures. After the dissection and apical displacement of the mucosal flap, only the exposed periosteal surface is present in the recipient site. The periosteum is well irrigated and immobile surface, suitable for graft nutrition and stabilization.

3. Connective tissue graft (CTG)

The first description in literature of the use of connective tissue graft was by Alan Edel in 1974 for increasing the width of gingiva [32]. Since than the indications and the use of CTG graft increased significantly. Today, CTG is still regarded as the gold standard for most soft tissue augmentation treatments. It is indicated for:

1. Increasing the width of the keratinized gingiva [33]

2. Treatment of single and multiple gingival recession around teeth [34]

3. Treatment of mucosal recession around implants [35]

4. Furcation treatment [36]

5. Regeneration of infrabony defects [37]

6. Augmentation of edentulous alveolar ridge defects [38]

7. Augmentation of PIS [39]

Some of the aforementioned indications are overlapping with those of the FGG. The main advantage of the CTG over FGG is the superior esthetic outcome in terms of color and texture of the augmented area (**Figure 4**) [25, 26, 40–42].

3.1 Connective tissue graft harvesting (CTG)

The harvesting technique of the CTG has a direct influence on the graft dimension, histological composition, harvesting complications, morbidity, healing dynamics of

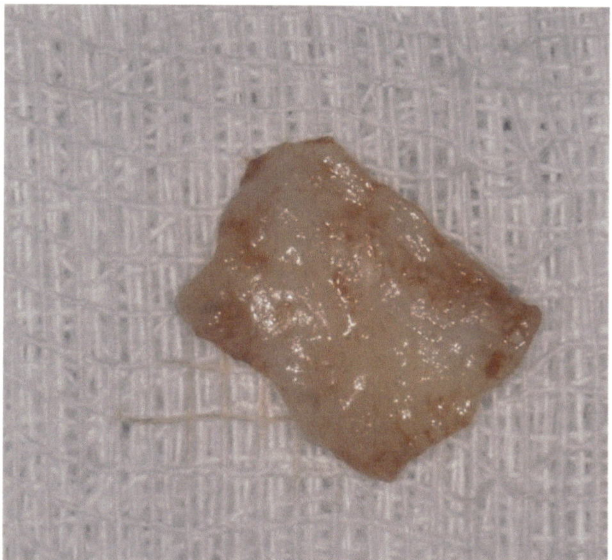

Figure 4.
Connective tissue graft.

the donor site, healing dynamics of the recipient site, and outcome of the grafting procedure. The ideal technique should enable the maximum volume and quality of the graft to be harvested, while concurrently limiting trauma, postoperative morbidity, and possible complications connected with CTG harvesting [43]. A variety number of techniques have been described in the literature for connective tissue graft harvesting. All the techniques can be divided into two groups—(1) connective tissue harvesting with the preparation of the primary flap (offend referred to as subepithelial connective tissue graft, sCTG) and (2) free gingival graft harvesting with extraoral de-epithelization. The first group can be further subdivided into free CTG or pedicle CTG depending if the CTG is completely dissected or remains attached by one side of the palatal soft tissue [26, 40, 42–45].

The palate is the most frequent site donor site for CTG or FGG harvesting [40]. Histologically, it is composed of different layers—the most superficial epithelial layer, covering a dense connective tissue layer (lamina propria). The submucosal layer is located below the lamina propria and above the periosteum, containing fatty and glandular tissue. Preferably, the CTG should consist only or mostly of the lamina propria layer, with little or no submucosa [26, 46]. Fatty and glandular tissue can hinder or slow the revascularization of the graft after its transplantation [31]. Furthermore, they can be responsible for the increased shrinkage rate of the CTG during healing, influencing the outcome of the grafting procedure [40, 47, 48].

Palatal soft tissue thickness differs greatly among the various areas of the palate and among individuals [49–51].

Limited data in the literature suggest that patients with thick palatal soft tissue have increased thickness mainly of the submucosal layer while the dimensions of lamina propria remain unchanged [49]. It could be hypothesized that CTG harvesting with the primary flap techniques in thick palatal soft tissue would always result in a graft composed of a lower percentage of lamina propria. The only layer that would have increased share in graft thickness would be the submucosal layer [49].

In the case of thin palatal soft tissue, there is not enough connective tissue thickness to prepare the primary flap and the CTG. The result of CTG harvesting with the primary flap in those situations can lead either to (1) primary flap necrosis if the primary flap is prepared to thin in order to increase the composition of the lamina propria inside CTG, or (2) CTG with a decreased thickness and composition of lamina propria which can result in the improper outcome of the harvesting procedure [48].

To overcome the aforementioned drawbacks, a new harvesting procedure was described—harvesting of an FGG and afterward, intra- or extra-oral de-epithelization of the FGG. As a consequence of the de-epithelization, the epitel layer is removed and the FGG graft is converted into CTG. With this harvesting procedure, the most valuable tissue (lamina propria) is almost completely inside the graft regardless of the initial thickness of the palatal soft tissue. In contrast, when the primary flap is used, a varying percentage of the lamina propria remains unutilized, attached to the inner side of the primary flap [40, 49, 52]. Furthermore, CTG obtained with the new harvesting procedure (de-epithelized FGG) is firmer and easier to manage during the grafting procedure with less variations in compositions among different CTG [48, 49].

The main disadvantage of the de-epithelized FGG procedure is the secondary intention healing of the donor site resulting in a slower healing process related to a higher percentage of complications linked to the donor site (pain and bleeding). Patients who underwent CTG graft harvesting experienced a lower incidence of donor site pain in the early postoperative period compared to FGG graft harvesting patients (**Table 1**) [49, 52–55].

Harvesting techniques of free CTG		
	CTG with primary flap (subepithelial connective tissue graft)	de-epithelized FGG
Advantages	Primary healing of the donor site	Larger graft dimensions
	Faster healing with less complications (pain, bleeding)	Higher quality of graft composition
	Better patient acceptance	Easier management of the graft
		Lower percentage of graft contraction during healing
Disadvantages	Reduced graft dimensions	Secondary healing of the donor site
	Lower quality of graft composition	Slower healing with more complication
	Higher percentage of contraction during healing	Lower patient acceptance
	Poor handling properties	

Table 1.
Advantages and disadvantages of CTG harvesting techniques: CTG with the primary flap and de-epithelized CTG.

3.1.1 Connective tissue harvesting with the preparation of primary flap- subepithelial connective tissue graft (sCTG)

3.1.1.1 The role of the primary flap

The main purpose of the primary flap is the protection of the donor wound region. At the end of the surgical procedure, the primary flap is repositioned and sutured in its original position, completely covering the wound area beneath it. Thus, thanks to the primary flap, the wound area is healing with primary intention. This will result in a reduced time of haling and postoperative morbidity. In case when the primary flap has reduced vascularity as a consequence of a surgical error during flap preparation (flap thinner than 1 mm, perforation of the flap) it will necrotize, leaving the donor area unprotected and left to heal with secondary intention 26, 25, 40, 42, 43, 47, 52 (**Figure** 5).

3.1.1.2 Donor area

The donor area for CTG graft harvesting is located in the palatal masticatory mucosa extending:

1. Mesiodistally: the donor iste is extending from the distal line angle of the canine to the mesial line angle of the platal root of the first molar. In this region, the soft tissue thickness is suitable for the CTG harvesting procedure.

2. Apically the donor area is limited with a zone containing blood vessels. The average distance between blood vessels and CEJ of adjacent teeth is 12 mm. The recommended apical limit of the donor area is set at 10 mm from CEJ, leaving 2 additional millimeters of the safety zone between the apical border of the CTG and the blood vessels.

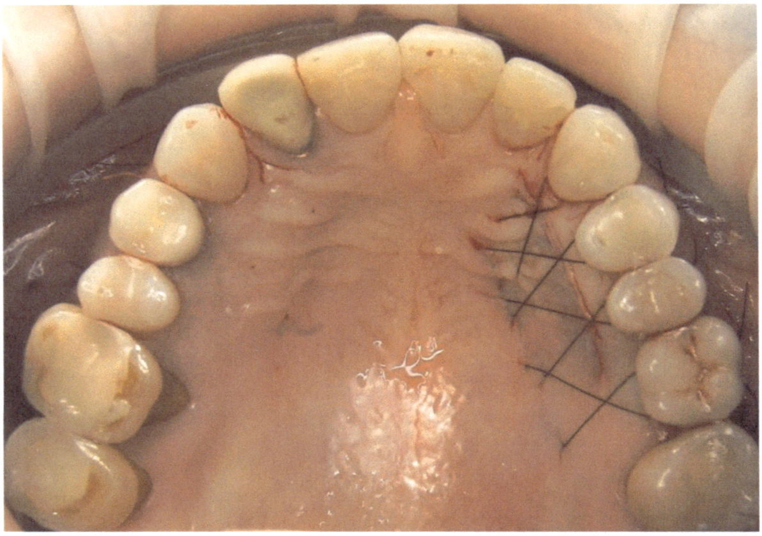

Figure 5.
sCTG harvesting. After the harvesting procedure of the sCTG the primary flap is repositioned in its original position. The primary flap protects the wound beneath it, enabling primary healing of the donor area.

3. The coronal incision is displaced 2 mm from the CEJ to prevent soft tissue recession on the palatal side of the adjacent teeth.

In patients with a flat palate, the palatine artery is closer to the CEJ, located 7 mm apically of the CEJ of adjacent teeth resulting in a limited height of the CTG [25, 26, 56–59].

Another limiting factor for CTG harvesting with the preparation of the primary flap is the palatal soft tissue thickness. The palatal soft tissue should be at least 3 mm thick, to allow the preparation of primary flap thick 1.0–1.5 mm and harvesting of 1.5–2.0 mm thick CTG. Therefore, before starting the grafting procedure, it is advisable to examine the thickness of the donor area [42, 60–63].

In case when inadequate palatal soft tissue thickness is present, three different solutions are available—(1) two-step procedures: Augmentation of the palatal soft tissue with the collagen sponge and after 8 weeks harvesting of the sCTG from the thickened donor site [60–62], (2) different grafting techniques of the CTG (de-epithelized CTG) [42, 48, 64], and (3) use of a substitutional soft tissue graft (allogenic or xenogenic soft tissue substitute graft) [65–68].

3.1.1.3 Surgical technique

The first part of the harvesting procedure consists of the preparation of the primary flap. The dissection of the primary flap starts with a horizontal incision 1.0–1.5 mm deep, 2 mm apical from the cementoenamel junction, and perpendicular to the mucosal surface. The blade angulation is changed to approximately 135° and a split-thickness flap is prepared in the apical direction. With the progression of the flap preparation, the angle of the blade is flattened until it becomes parallel with the gingival surface. The dissection is controlled from the external aspect of the flap in order to prevent flap perforation. The partial-thickness flap preparations end after reaching 8 mm from the first horizontal incision, this is 10 mm apically from the cementoenamel junction, leaving a safe zone with 2 mm of distance from the possible location of blood vessels. This will result in the maximal apico-coronal graft dimension of 8 mm.

The primary flap is prepared with the sharp dissection, in a split-thickness manner. During the partial-thickness preparation, the blade is oriented parallel with the mucosal surface to prevent perforations or overthinning of the primary flap. Care must be taken to leave the minimum residual thickness of the primary flap at least 1.5 mm, otherwise it could be necrotized.

After finishing its dissection, the primary flap is partially reflected and the connective tissue graft is dissected just beneath it. It is suggested to place the coronal dissection line 1.0–1.5 mm apical from the coronal incision line of the primary flap. This will result in a 1.0–1.5 mm connective tissue band along the coronal incision line, improving the healing of the primary flap, but at the same reducing the apico-coronal dimension of the connective tissue graft from the maximal 8 to 7 or 6.5 mm [26, 44, 69–71].

The connective tissue graft can be harvested with or without the periosteum layer depending on if it is inner surface is prepared with sharp or blunt dissection. The CTG with the periosteum has better mechanical stability and better clinical handling. On the other hand, leaving a periosteal surface on the bone in the donor area will improve the healing of the primary flap. In clinical situations where the primary flap was prepared with reduced thickness (equal or less than the lower value of the recommended thickness) or perforated during dissection, it could be advisable to leave the periosteum covering the bone surface [26, 44, 69–71].

After the completion of the harvesting procedure, the primary flap is repositioned and sutured in its original position. Although, cross matters or a combination of parallel and cross sutures were recommended [26, 69, 70], it seems that the suturing technique does not have an influence on early wound healing in the donor area [72].

Once the CTG is harvested it must be kept in a moist environment, usually draped in wet gauze, until is transferred to the recipient site [26, 69–71].

3.2 Connective tissue pedicle flaps

Connective tissue can be harvested from the palatal donor site as a free graft or pedicle graft. Free grafts are completely dissected from the donor site while pedicle flaps remain attached by one part to the donor site. In that way, they retain the vascularization of the donor site which will influence positively the graft volume stability reducing the shrinkage of the graft postoperatively and improving the outcome of the augmentation procedure [44, 45, 73].

Pedicle palatal connective tissue was first described in 1980 [74].

The preparation of the primary flap is equal to the primary flap for the free connective tissue graft. The only difference is the length of the primary flap which can be elongated if the defect is located in the frontal region [45]. The main variation to conventional free connective tissue graft is the harvesting of the CTG. During the preparation of the pedicle, the connective tissue graft below the primary flap is freed from the rest of the palatal tissue on three sides, while one side remains attached to it [45, 73, 75–77].

Different modifications of this technique have been described, which can be divided into two groups—roll techniques and vascularized interpositional periosteal connective tissue flap. In the first group, the pedicle is attached by its coronal part to the buccal flap and rolled under the buccal flap. This flap is used mostly for minor augmentation of the buccal PIS during the single implant uncovering procedure

[78–80]. Other indications include soft tissue augmentation for pontic site development [81, 82] and multiple implants PIS augmentation and pontic site development at implant uncover procedure (**Figures 6–11**) [83].

The vascularized interpositional periosteal connective tissue flap (VIP-CTG) consists of a connective tissue pedicle that remains attached to the palatal tissue on the

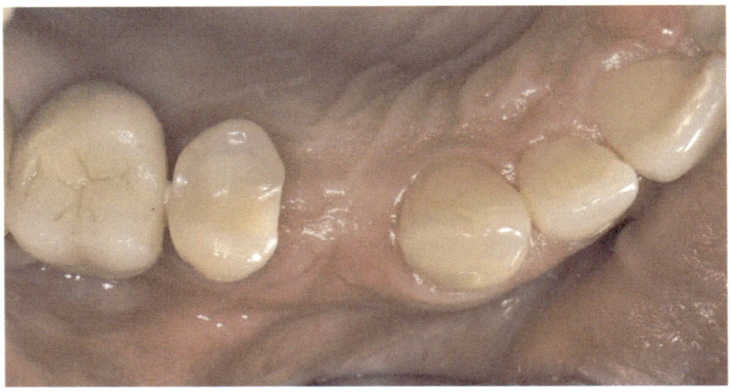

Figure 6.
Palatal roll technique for PIS augmentation around the single implant at uncovering procedure. Initial situation.

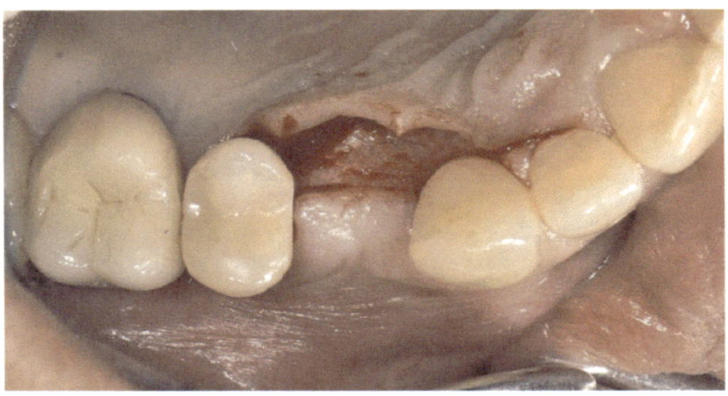

Figure 7.
The primary flap has been prepared.

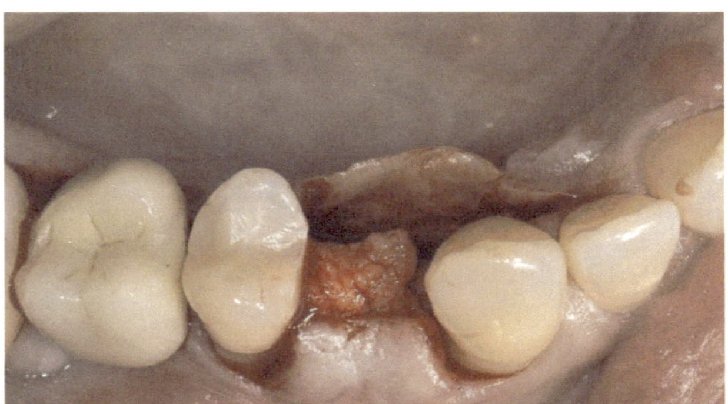

Figure 8.
The CTG remains attached to the buccal flap, while it is dissected from the adjacent palatal soft tissue on the apical, mesial, and distal side.

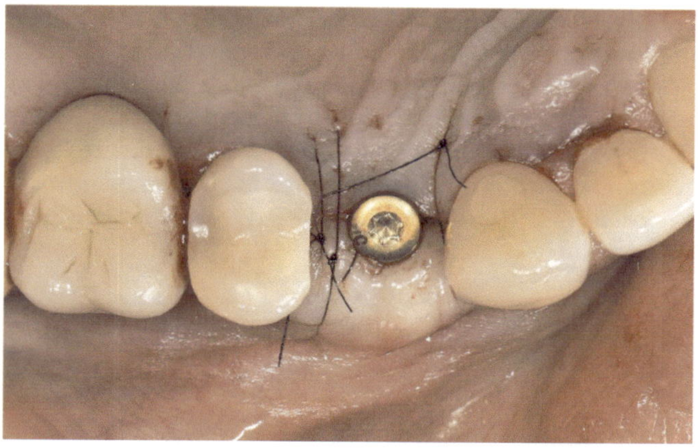

Figure 9.
The CTG pedicle graft has been rotated beneath the buccal flap and sutured in this position. The thickness of the buccal PIS has been visibly augmented.

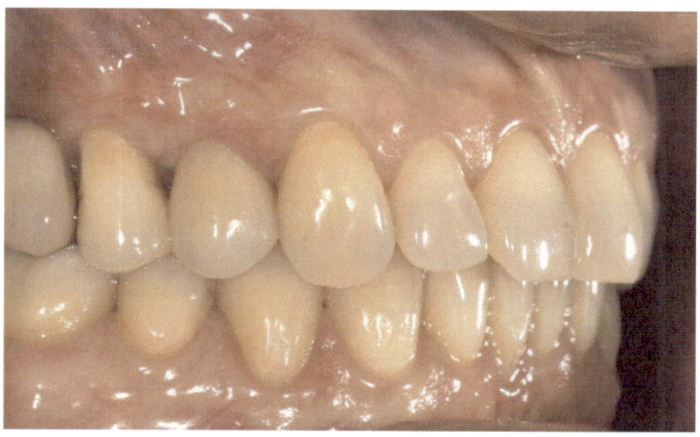

Figure 10.
Definitive zircon-ceramic screw-retained crown 14.

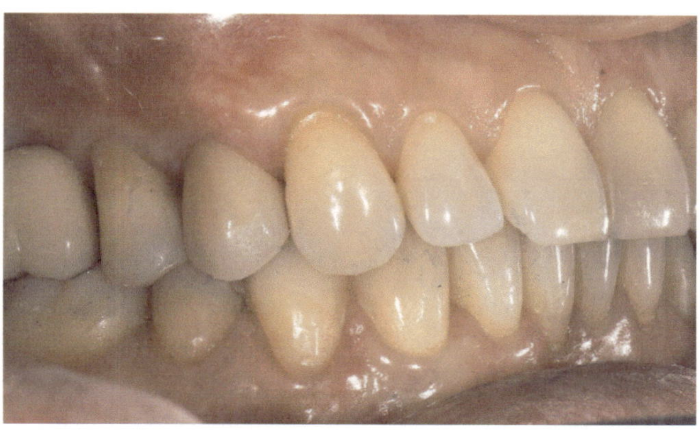

Figure 11.
Two years follow up.

distal or mesial side, depending on the defect location. It can be used for more pronounced soft-tissue defect augmentation (horizontal and vertical), allowing grafting of large soft tissue defects with only one procedure. Furthermore, VIP-CTG can be used for simultaneous soft and hard tissue augmentation procedures, reducing patient treatment time and morbidity. This procedure is indicated before implant placement, concomitant with implant placement, or during the implant osseointegration period [45, 75, 76] or pontic site development (**Figures 12–18**) [44, 73, 74, 84].

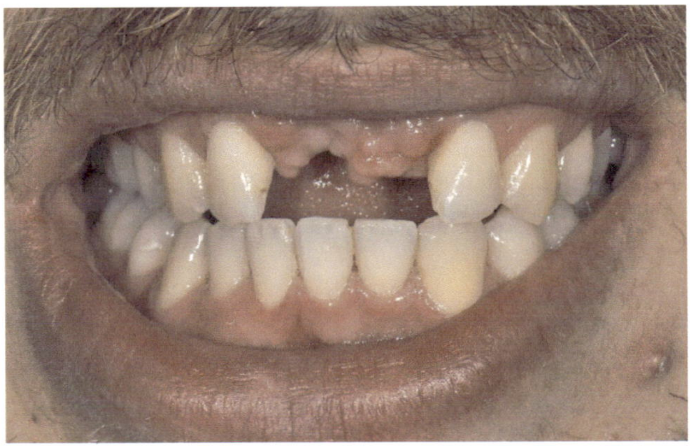

Figure 12.
VIP-CTG for the treatment of the vertical soft-tissue defect in an esthetical demanding situation. Initial situation.

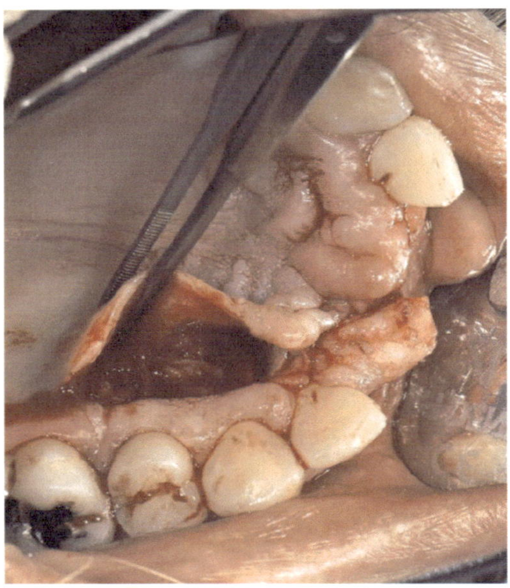

Figure 13.
The incision line of the primary flap is extending mesially until the defect site is located in the region of the central incisor. The VIP-CTG is dissected from the rest of the palatal soft tissue on three sides (distal, coronal, apical) and rolled over the buccal soft tissue in order to determine the size of the buccal pouch that will be prepared. The mesial side of the VIP-CTG will remain attached to the adjacent palatal soft tissue.

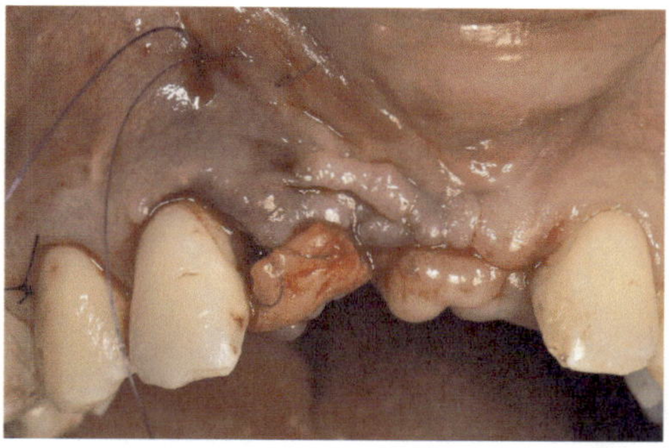

Figure 14.
With the help of two horizontal mattress sutures the VIP-CTG will be positioned and stabilized inside the pouch.

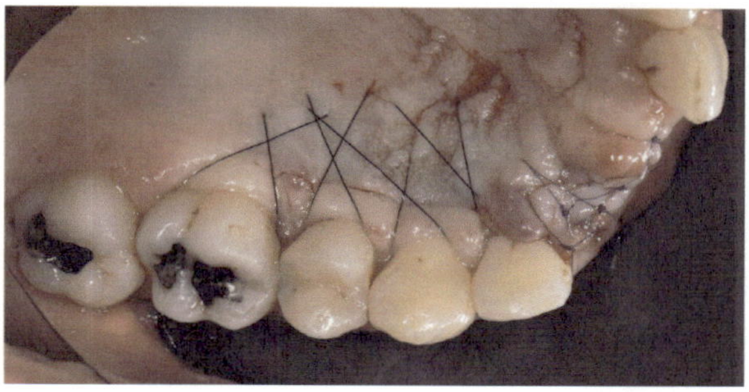

Figure 15.
Suturing of the donor and defect area. The donor and the defect sites will heal by primary intention.

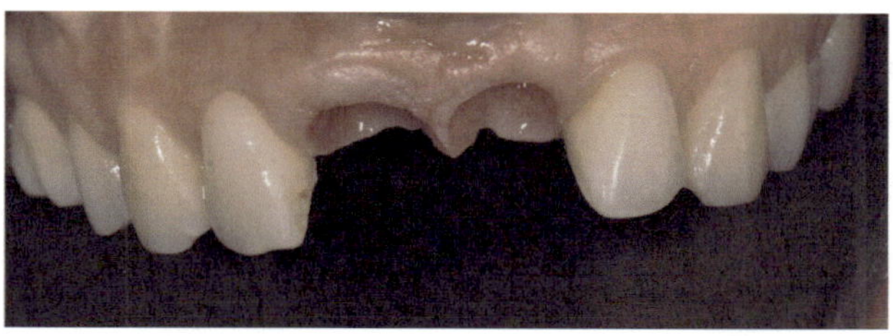

Figure 16.
Final appearance of the PIS after soft tissue conditioning with provisional crowns-frontal view.

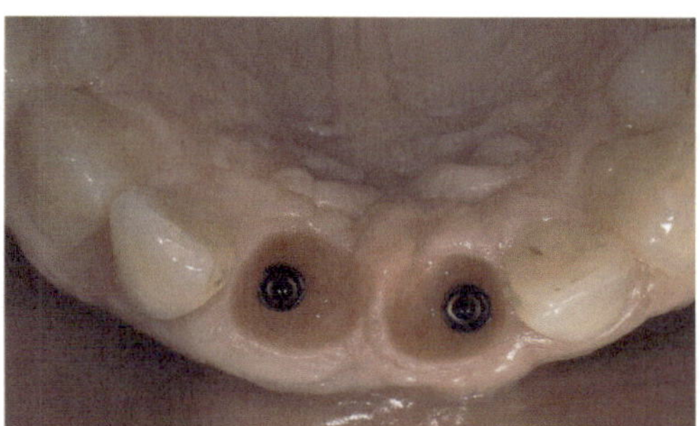

Figure 17.
Final appearance of the PIS after soft tissue conditioning with provisional crowns-occlusal view

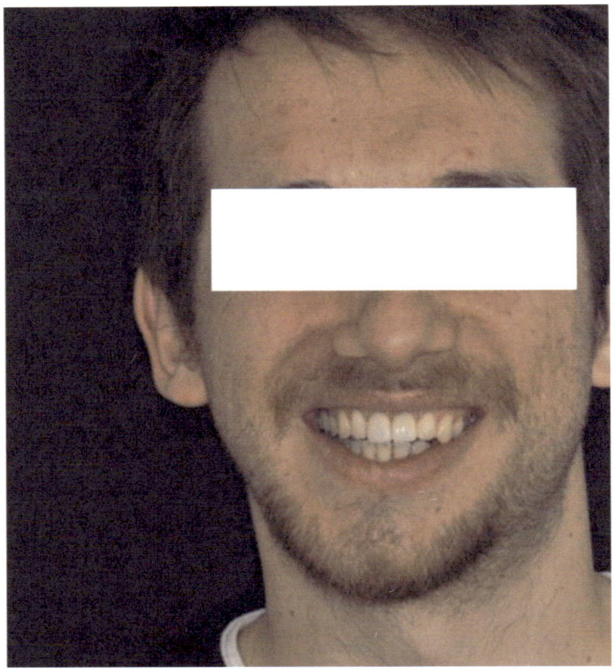

Figure 18.
Final screw-retained zirconia-ceramic crowns 21, 11.

3.3 Preparation of recipient site for CTG

The recipient site can be prepared with different surgical techniques. The techniques can be categorized in three groups:

1. Tunnel technique: The recipient site is prepared without vertical incisions and papilla incisions [21].

2. Coronally advanced flap without vertical incisions [85]

3. Single or double vertical incisions [86]

The vertical incision can compromise the vascular supply of the flap and cause an esthetical appearance. Incision through the papilla can cause papilla height reduction after healing, a likewise vertical incision can cause scare formation. On the other hand, the vertical incisions will facilitate the coronal advancement of the flap or the correct positioning and the stabilization of the graft [25].

4. Free gingival graft (FGG)

Soft tissue graft consisting of epithelial and connective tissue layer which is completely detached from the rest of the palatal soft tissue is defined as a free gingival graft (FGG) [40].

The FGG was introduced in 1966 [87]. Historically, FGG was used to expand the band of keratinized gingiva around teeth [32], cover exposed root surfaces [88], soft tissue augmentation of edentulous ridges [89, 90], and expand the band of keratinized tissue around implants [91]. Since the esthetic appearance of the augmented tissue is poor due to inadequate color blending with the adjacent soft tissue and a "patch" like appearance, today FGG grafts are used mostly to increase the band of keratinized mucosa around implants in nonesthetic areas. Other indications for FGG are seldom performed only in nonesthetic areas 38, 40. The combination of apically positioned flap and autogenous graft is considered the gold standard technique for increasing the width of keratinized mucosa around implants [15].

4.1 Recipient site preparation

The recipient site is prepared with the apically positioned flap technique.

A split-thickness flap is prepared along the mucogingival border. Usually, the flap design consists of a horizontal incision and two vertical incisions that are elongated to or apically to the mucogingival border depending on the amount of the apical displacement of the partial-thickness flap. The split-thickness flap is prepared with sharp dissection in the apical direction taking care to leave intact periosteal surface covering the bone; a 15C or 12D blade is used. In order to prevent perforations of the flap, the blade is oriented parallel with the mucosal surface during the dissection. Additionally, the progression of the flap dissection is monitored from the external flap surface. Muscle attachment, loose connective tissue fibers are removed from the periosteal surface. Care is taken to prepare an even surface that will allow an intimate contact of the graft with the vascularized surface. After the partial-thickness flap has been prepared, the flap is sutured in a new apical position. Sutures must engage the flap and the rigid periosteal surface in order to stabilize the flap [59]. The FGG is stabilized on the exposed periosteal surface with sutures or cyanoacrylate [40, 92]. After stabilization, the graft must be completely immobile, intimately adapted to the periosteal surface with no dead space remaining between the inner surface of the graft and the periosteal surface otherwise plasmatic imbibition and neovascularization bill be hindered. Furthermore, care must be taken to harvest an FGG with an even thickness to allow even precise adaptation to the recipient site throughout the inner surface of the graft. If present, fat tissue should be cut out from the FGG as it can slow down or prevent revascularization of the flap [25, 31, 40, 64].

4.2 Donor site preparation

The palatal masticatory mucosa is the most used donor site for FGG harvesting. Usually, the donor site is located inside the premolar and molar areas. The anterior palatal region where rugae are present is usually avoided since the rugae will remain present inside the FGG and will be transplanted to the recipient site, further deteriorating the appearance of the grafted site. The presence of the rugae can render the harvesting of the FGG challenging, especially in situations where the thin (1.0–1.5 mm) FGG grafts are harvested.

The harvesting procedure can be done freehand or with the help of a template.

The design of the flap consists of four incisions outlining the graft—coronal horizontal incision, mesial and distal vertical incision, and apical horizontal incision. Usually, the goal is to harvest an FGG which thickness is not exceeding 1.5 mm. For depth orientation during the performance of the outlining incision of the future graft, only the beveled part of the blade can be used which dimensions are approximately 1 mm [25, 44].

During healing, FGG undergoes contraction of around 30% of initially gain keratinized tissue band [7, 40, 93]. This fact should be taken into consideration while determining the dimension of the graft, which should be 30% larger than the site needing augmentation (**Figures 19–22**) [40].

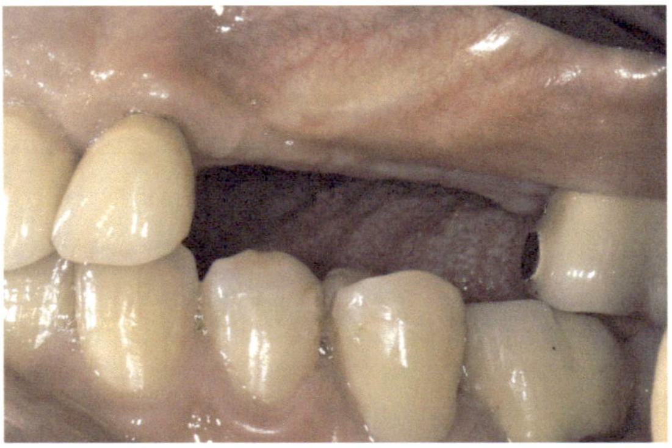

Figure 19.
Figure loss of vestibular depth and coronal and palatal displacement of keratinized mucosa after guided bone regeneration.

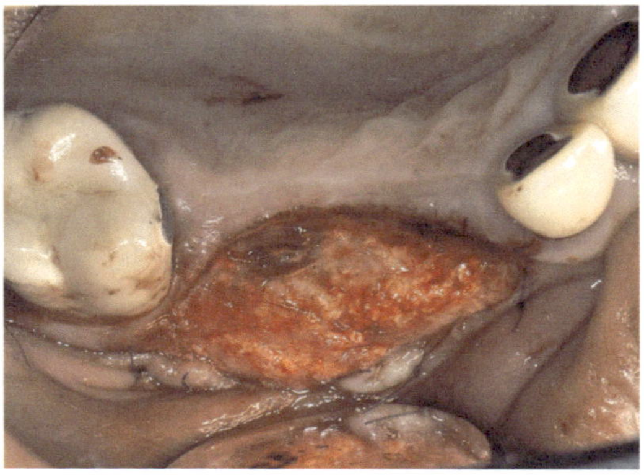

Figure 20.
Apically positioned flap-the recipient site has been prepared with the apical displacement of a split-thickness buccal flap. The exposed periosteal surface is present in the recipient site.

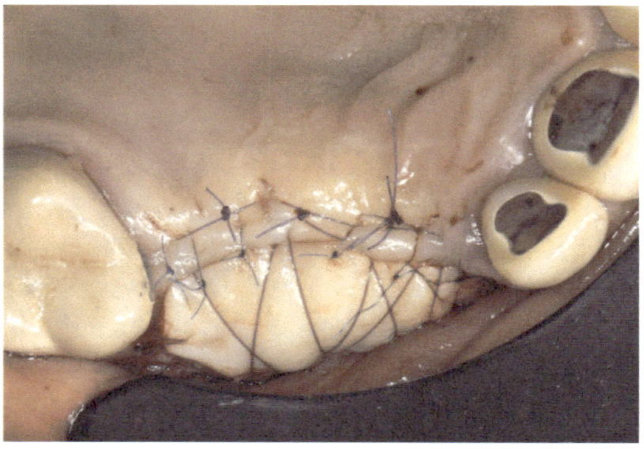

Figure 21.
Free gingival graft stabilized in the recipient site, on the exposed periosteal surface, with the help of sutures.

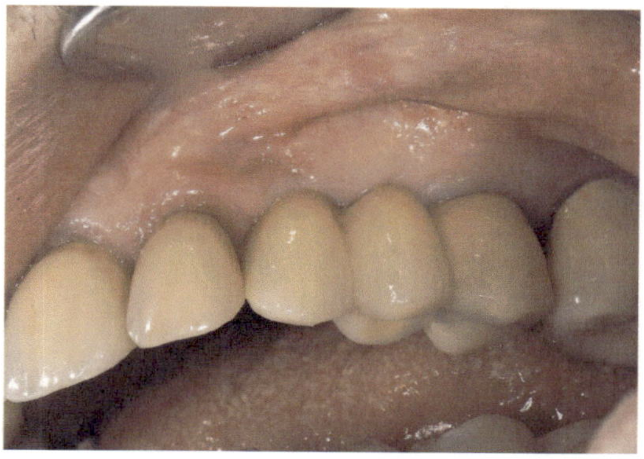

Figure 22.
Final three-unit screw-retained bridge. On the buccal side a wide zone of KM and deepen vestibule is present.

After completion of graft dissection, the wound in the donor site is protected. Different techniques have been proposed—sutures, absorbable gelatin sponge, cyanoacrylate bioadhesive, periodontal dressing, palatal stents, platelet-rich fibrin, or a combination of some of the aforementioned techniques (**Figures 23–34**) [25, 26, 48, 53, 94, 95].

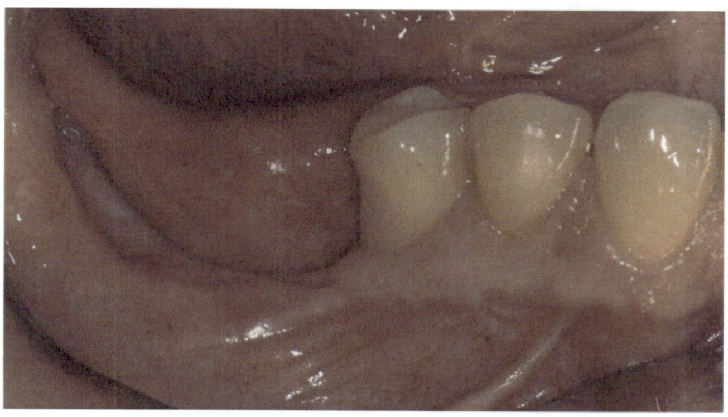

Figure 23.
Two months after implant insertion in the region 36. Visible loss of keratinized mucosa-lateral view.

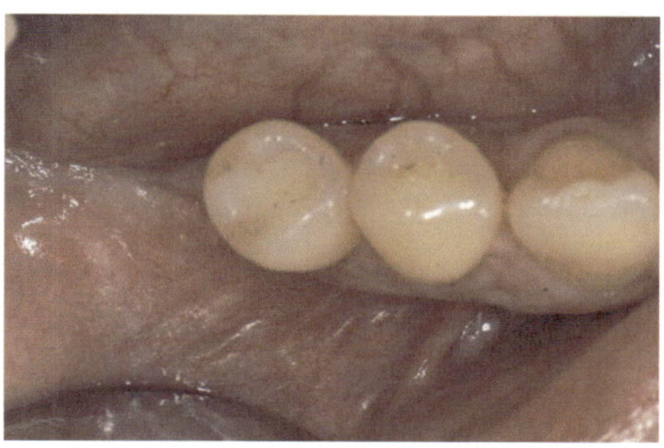

Figure 24.
Two months after implant insertion in the region 36. Visible loss of keratinized mucosa-occlusal view.

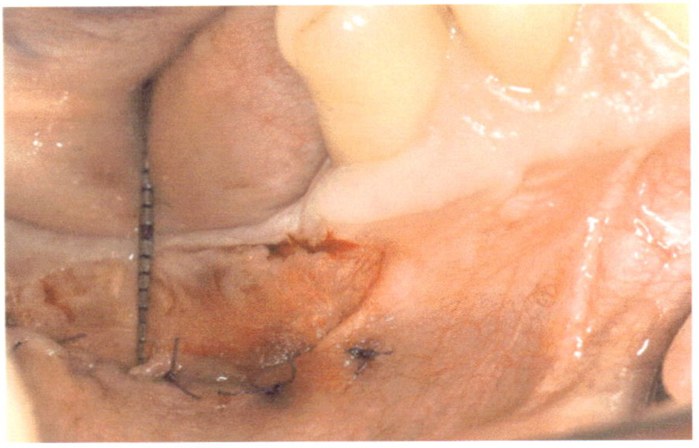

Figure 25.
Recipient site preparation—Apically positioned flap was prepared in the recipient region. The partial-thickness flap was stabilized in the new apical position using resorbable sutures. The height of the recipient site was measured.

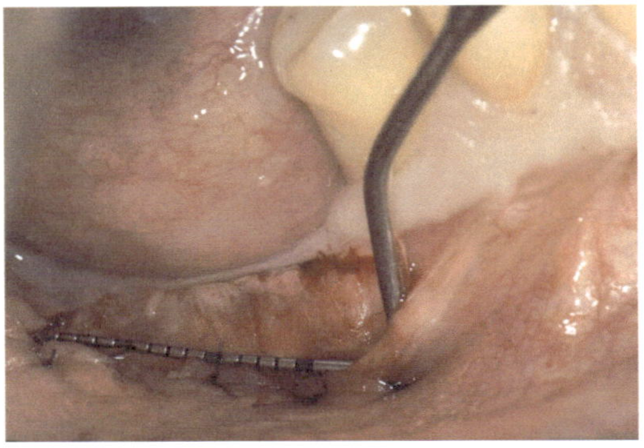

Figure 26.
Recipient site preparation—Apically positioned flap was prepared in the recipient region. The partial-thickness flap was stabilized in the new apical position using resorbable sutures. The width of the recipient site was measured.

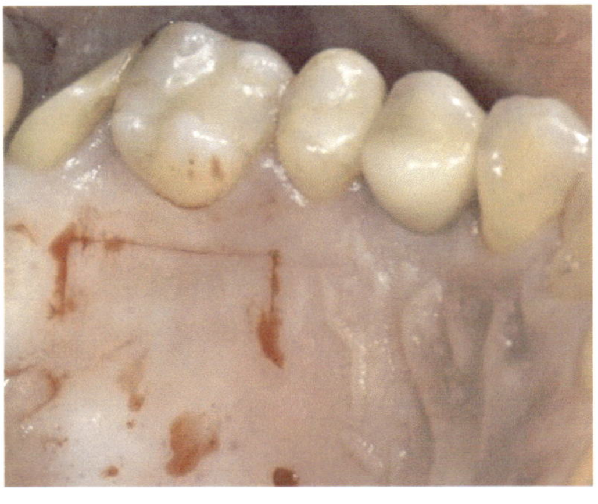

Figure 27.
Initial incisions outlining the future FGG—The dimensions of the graft were determined based on the measurements of the recipient site. The donor site was located in the region of the first molar, posterior to the rugae area. To avoid exercise bleeding during FGG preparation, the last outlining incision (horizontal apical incision) was done at the end of the procedure.

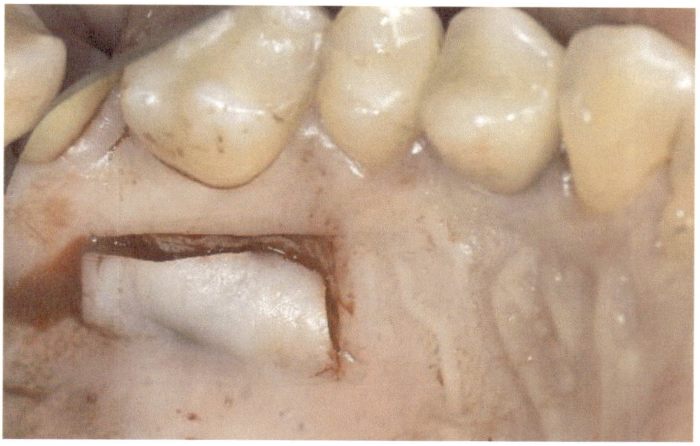

Figure 28.
1–1.5 mm thick flap was prepared, starting from the coronal horizontal incision extending apically until reaching the imaginary line connecting the apical end of the two vertical incisions. The preparation of the FGG was terminated with the horizontal apical incision which completely dissected the FGG from the rest of the palatal soft tissue.

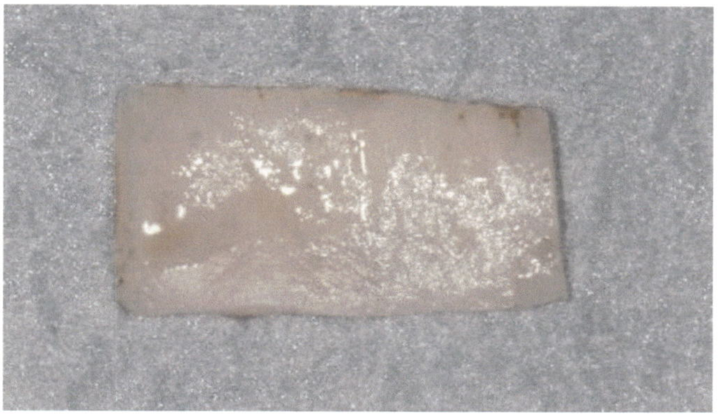

Figure 29.
FGG after harvesting.

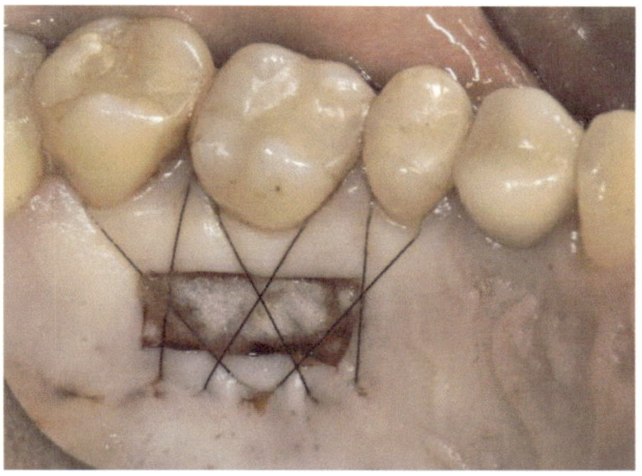

Figure 30.
Donor site protection—Absorbable gelatin sponge and compressive crossed mattress sutures.

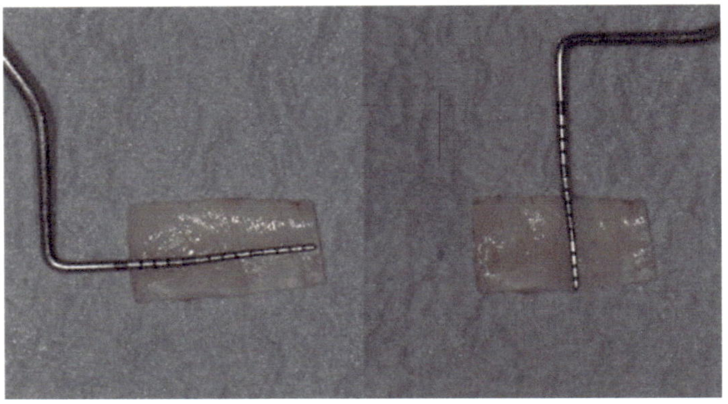

Figure 31.
Dimensions of the harvested FGG.

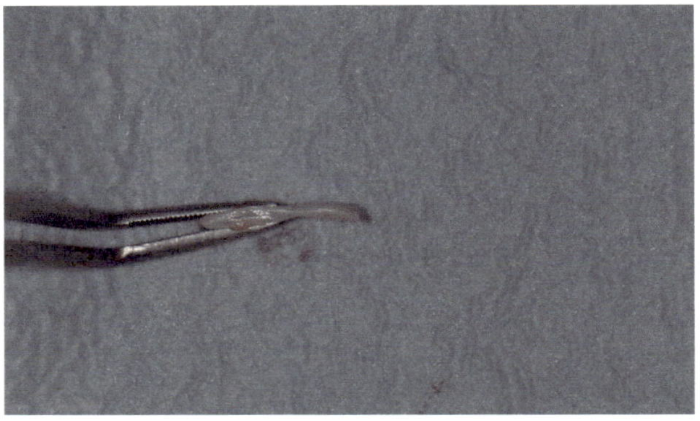

Figure 32.
Thickness of the harvested FGG—The thickness of the graft should not exceed 1.5 mm in order to reduce the postoperative morbidity associated with the donor site.

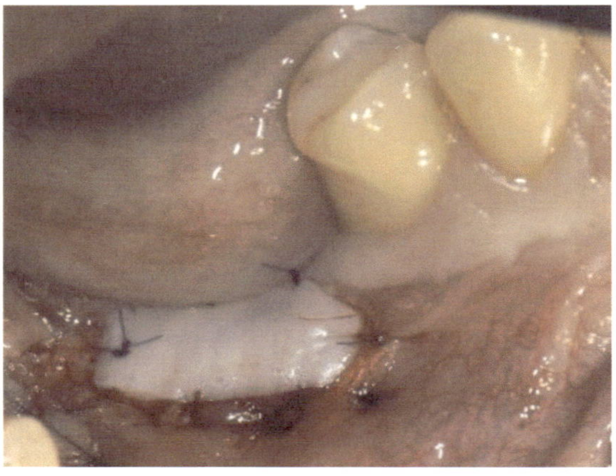

Figure 33.
Initial stabilization of the FGG in the recipient site—The stabilization of the graft is initiated by applying simple interrupted sutures on the coronal part of the graft. Afterward, one to two additional simple interrupted sutures are applied on the mesial and distal vertical border of the flap- stretching the flap over the exposed periosteal surface in the donor area. In order to stabilize the graft, the needle must engage the graft and the periosteal surface.

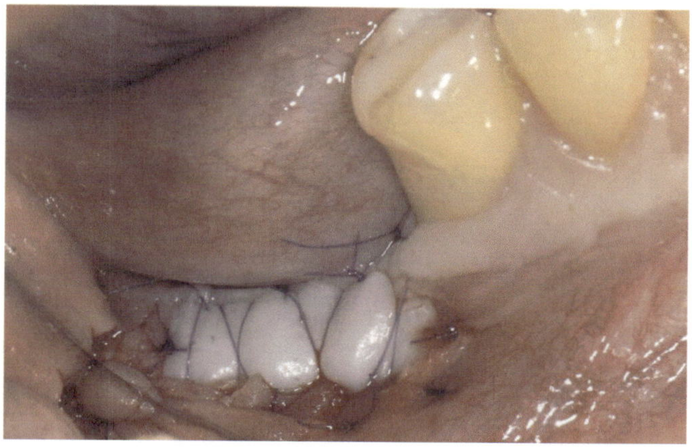

Figure 34.
Final graft stabilization—Mattress crossed sutures extending from the coronal to the apical part of the recipient site are used to secure even contact throughout the inner surface of the graft and the periosteal surface.

5. Alternative sites for free autogenous graft harvesting-maxillary tuberosity

Harvesting autogenous free grafts from the tuberosity are linked to different advantages compared to the classical palatal donor sites—the presence of a lower percentage of fatty/glandular tissue within the graft, higher percentage of collagen fibers within the graft, increased thickness of soft tissue in the donor area, and reduced patient morbidity and a lower percentage of other postoperative complications [26, 47, 96].

Soft tissue grafts from the tuberosity undergo minimal shrinkage during healing as a result of a higher quality of harvested soft tissue [47, 97]. A lower level of pain after tuber soft tissue graft harvesting may be explained by the faster rate of donor site healing compared to palatal donor sites. Additionally, the tuberosity donor site is less prone to masticatory friction [47, 96–98].

The presence of the fully erupted or semi-impacted third molar can prevent soft tissue grafting from the tuber region. In seldom clinical cases, hyperplastic response during haling of tuberosity CTG was observed, leading to an esthetic results (**Figures 35–38**) [47, 96].

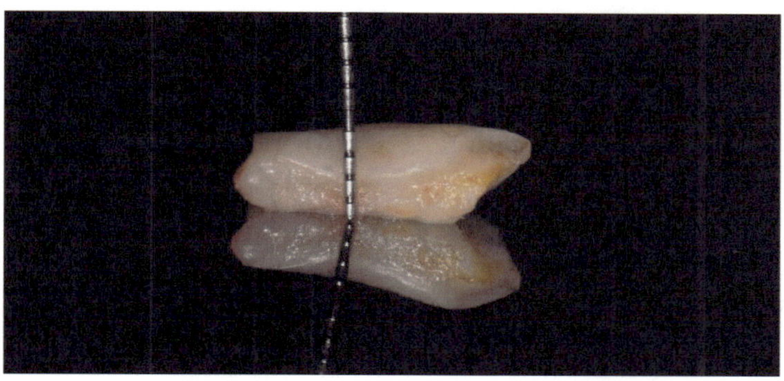

Figure 35.
CTG harvesting from the tuberosity. Autologous graft has been harvested as a free gingival graft. Note the increased thickness and the absence of the fatty tissue inside the CTG.

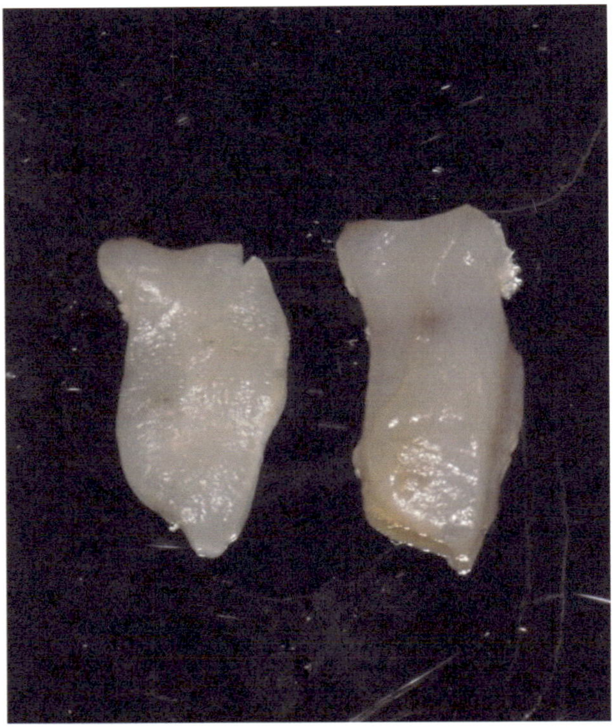

Figure 36.
After extraoral de-epithelization: Epithelial layer (left part of the picture) removed from the rest of CTG (right part of the picture).

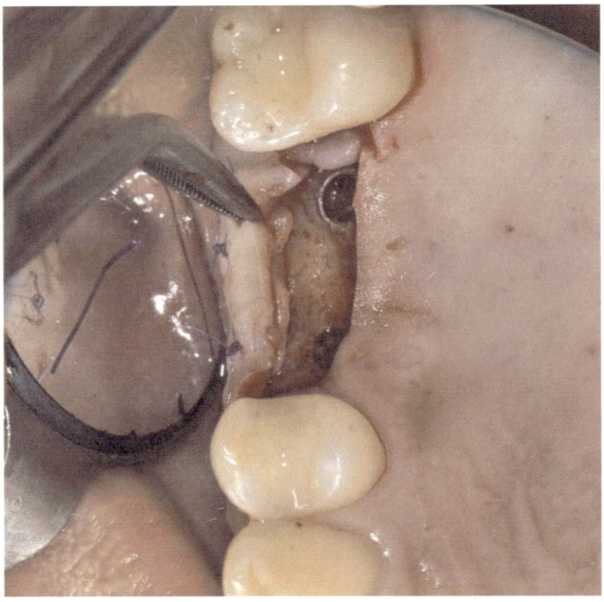

Figure 37.
The CTG from the tuberosity is stabilized beneath the buccal flap with horizontal matrasses suture.

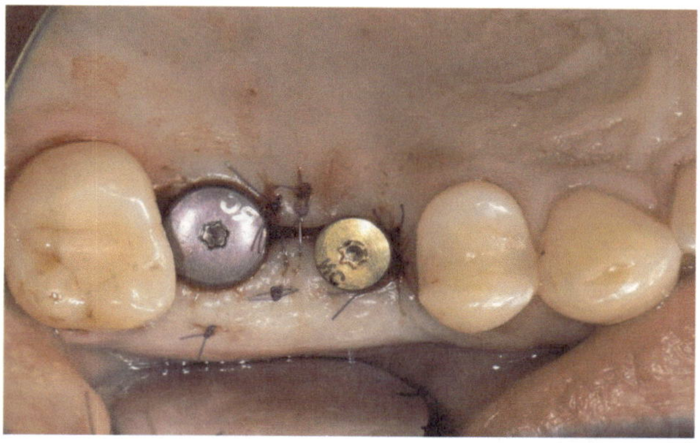

Figure 38.
Flap adaptation around healing abutments.

6. Substitutional soft tissue grafts

Although the results of PIS grafting with substitutional grafts, at the present are inferior to the results obtained after autogenous soft tissue grafting [5, 8, 65, 66, 93, 99], the absence of the donor site makes this treatment modality appealing to the patient and practitioners, as well [26, 42, 100].

The elimination of the harvesting procedure [25, 65] will lead to the reduction of surgical time [65], simplify the surgical procedure [42, 100], decrease the patient morbidity [26, 42, 65, 93], allow the unlimited supply of the soft tissue graft [26, 101, 102], and increase patient acceptance for the procedure [42, 65, 100, 103].

The augmentation procedure with substitutional soft tissue grafts will result in PIS with perfect color and texture blending to the adjacent soft tissue [65, 101].

Two types of substitutional grafts are available—xenogenic and allogeneic soft tissue grafts. Both of the grafts can be used for augmenting the volume and the width of keratinized mucosal band [25, 26, 65, 93, 99, 104].

The substitutional grafts are deprived of vital cells. During the manufacturing procedure, cells and antigenic components are removed, preserving only the extracellular matrix consisting mainly of collagen and elastin fibers. The three-dimensional structures of the aforementioned scaffold will promote fibroblast and keratinocyte migration and vascular ingrowth from the surrounding tissue [105–107]. This will result in an excellent color match since the keratinocytes are derived from the surrounding tissue. Nevertheless, compared to autogenous soft tissue grafts, they do not possess the ability to promote keratinization, limiting their application for increasing the width of KM [105, 106]. To overcome this drawback, a combination of an FGG graft with reduced apico-coronal dimensions to 2 mm and an XCM was proposed [6].

When used to augment PIS thickness, substitutional grafts are less resistant to compression of the overlaying flap compared to CTG. Loss of the initial volume of the substitutional graft can lead to the compromised outcome of the grafting procedure. To overcome this drawback, a volume stable collagen matrix was developed [105]. As a result of the cross-linking process of the collagen fibers, the collagen matrix becomes more volume stable and prone to withstand soft-tissue pressure [108, 109]. At the moment there is a lack of literature on the long-term stability of augmented PIS with the substitutional grafts (**Figures 39–66**) [105].

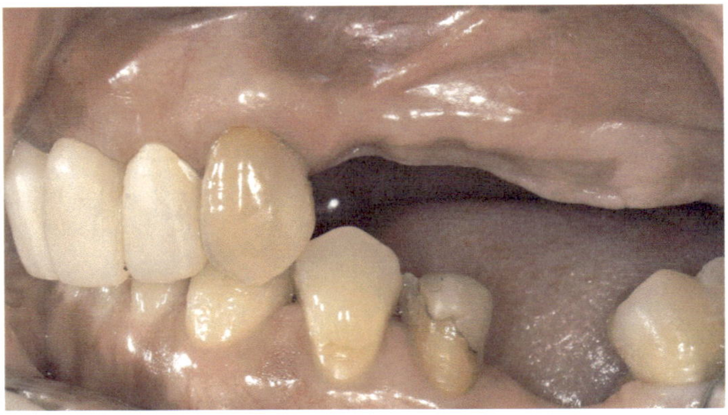

Figure 39.
Initial situation—Lateral view.

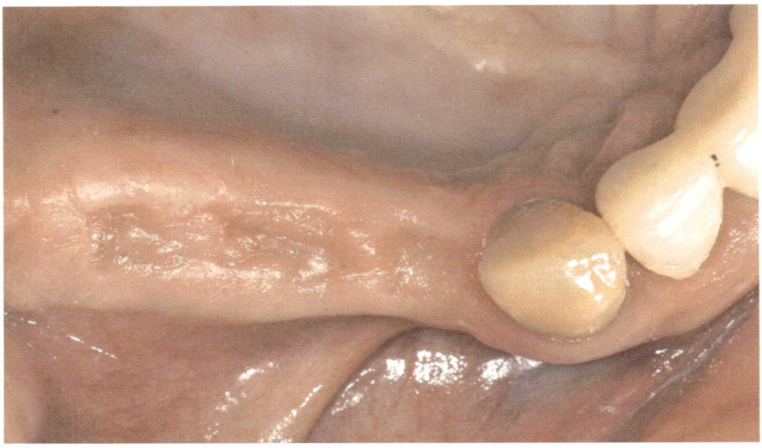

Figure 40.
Initial situation.

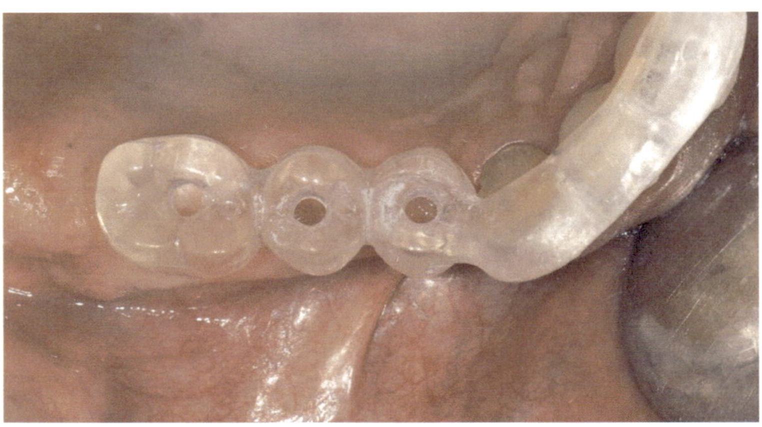

Figure 41.
Surgical stent.

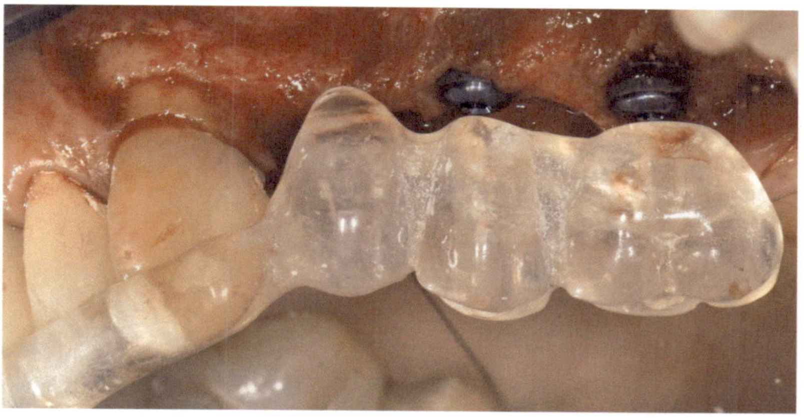

Figure 42.
Dehiscence bone defects around implant 16 and 15.

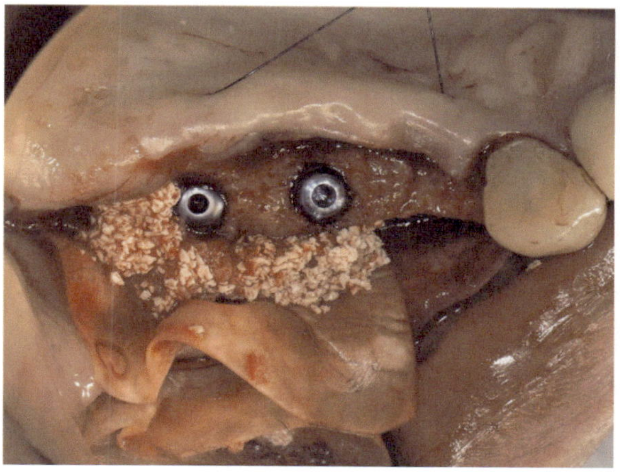

Figure 43.
GBR: A composite bone graft was used consisting of 50% autogenous and 50% xenogenic graft. The bone graft was applied in two layers—The internal layer which is covering the exposed implant surface, is made out of autogenous bone and the external layer is consisting of a xenogenic bone graft.

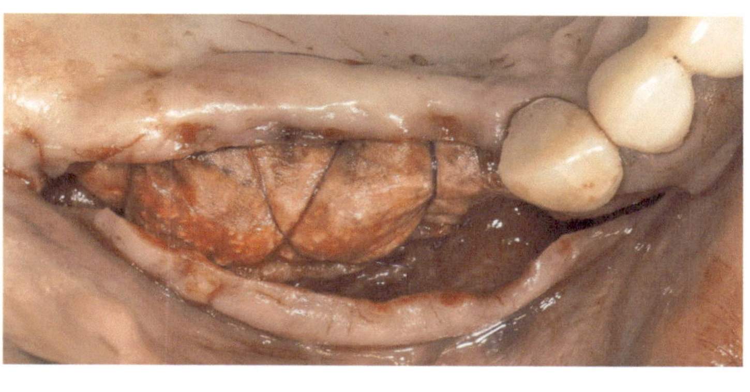

Figure 44.
GBR: Native collagen membrane stabilized with resorbable sutures.

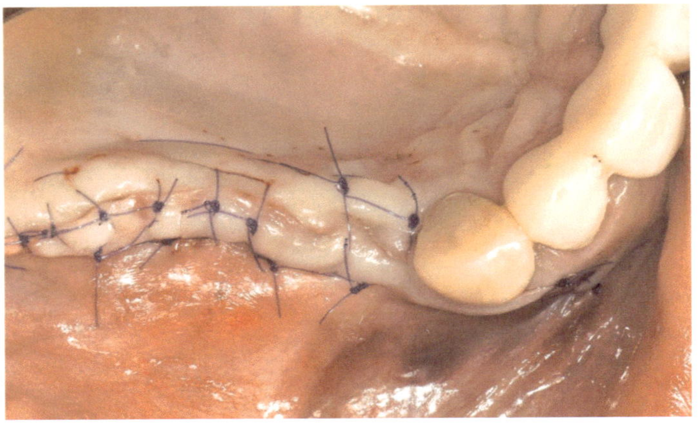

Figure 45.
Suturing in three layers;(1) palatal-apical position—Mattress sutures for membrane stabilization, (2) buccal-apical—Mattress sutures for initial closing of the flap, and (3) bucco-coronal—Simple interrupted suture for the final closure of the flap.

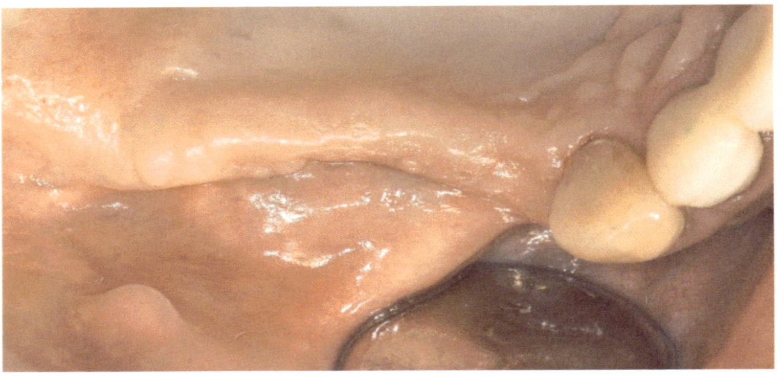

Figure 46.
Four months after the GBR, the palatal displacement of the mucogingival line is evident. Occlusal view.

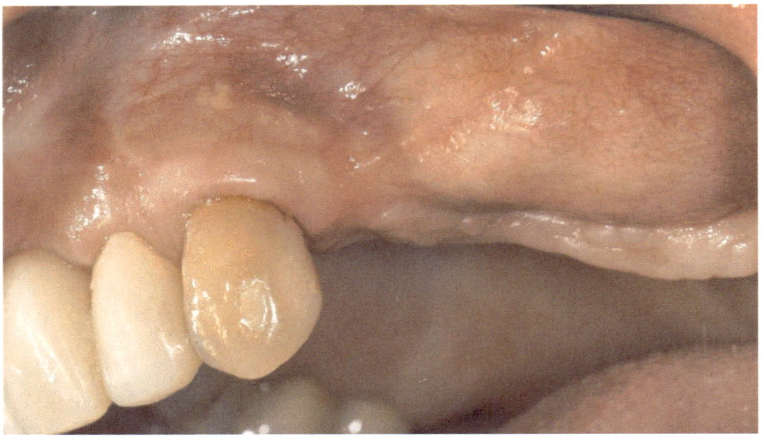

Figure 47.
Four months after the GBR, the palatal displacement of the mucogingival line is evident. Lateral view.

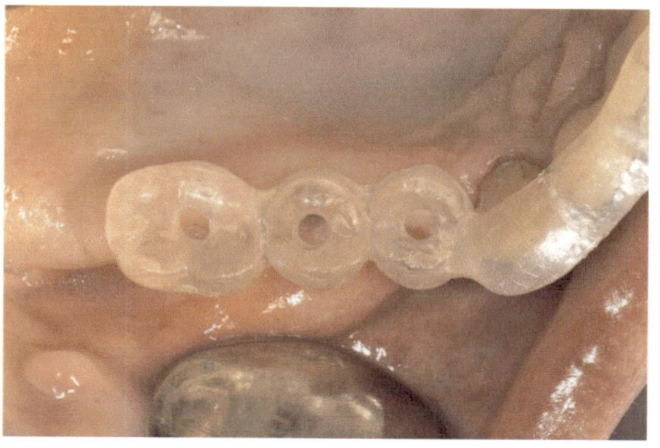

Figure 48.
The surgical stent was used to determine the dimensions of the flap.

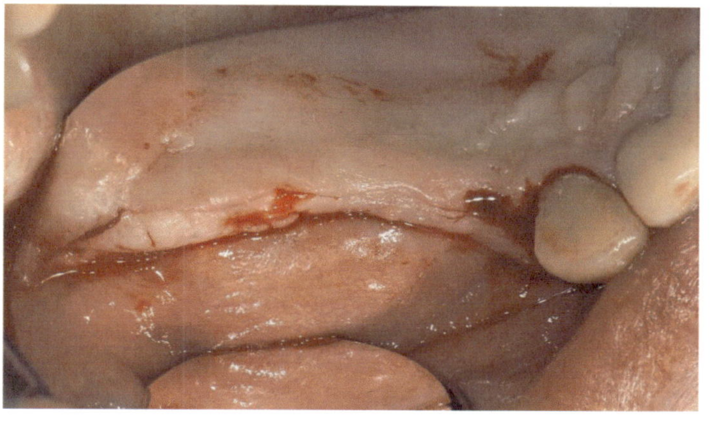

Figure 49.
The flap incision is made not at the mucogingival junction but 4 mm within the keratinized mucosa, therefore the buccal split-thickness flap will include a band of keratinized mucosa which is 4 mm wide.

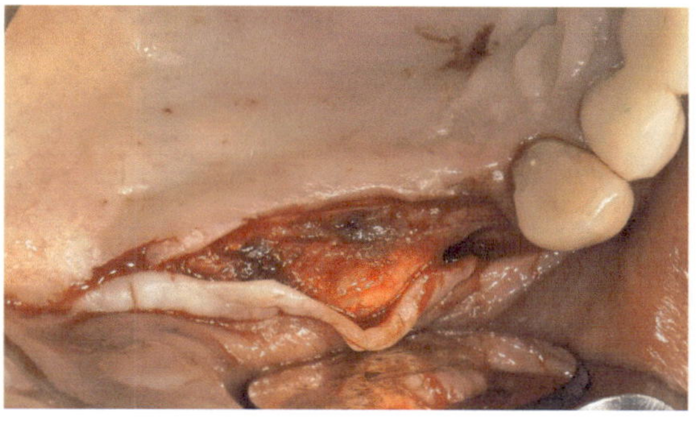

Figure 50.
Finalized preparation of the buccal split-thickness flap. The most coronal part of the partial-thickness flap consists of keratinized mucosa.

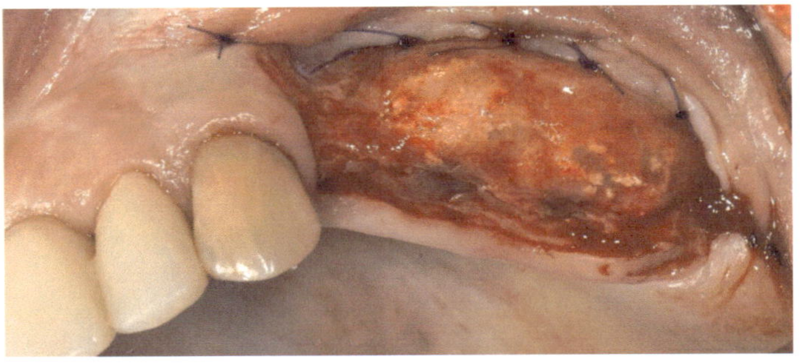

Figure 51.
Apically positioned flap—Stabilization of the buccal partial-thickness flap in the new apical position. The exposed periosteal surface is completely surrounded by keratinized mucosa.

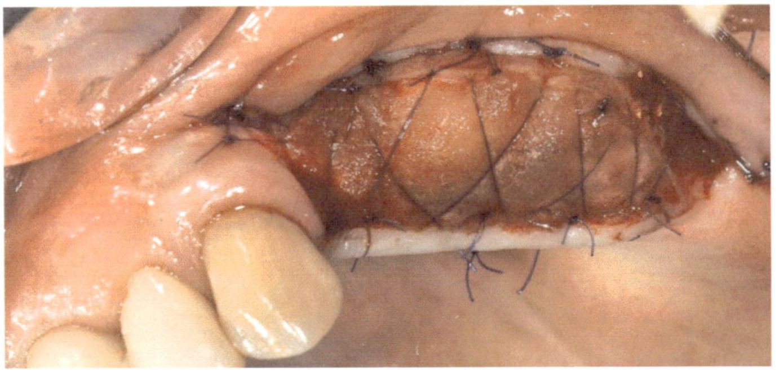

Figure 52.
The exposed periosteal surface is covered with xenogenic collagen matrix (Mucoderm, Botiss gmbh, Berlin).

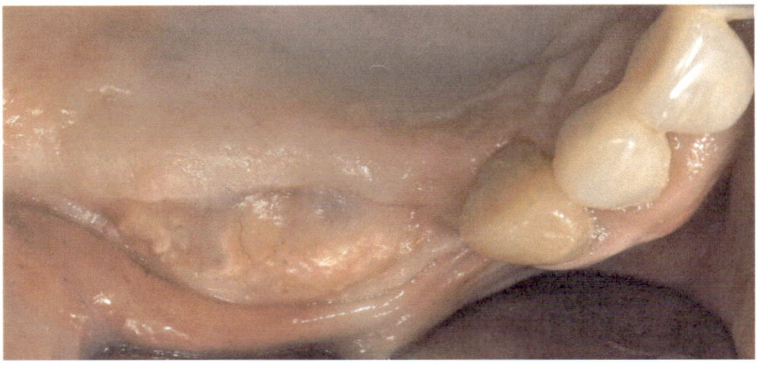

Figure 53.
Healing two months after the keratinized mucosa widening procedure. The gain of the keratinized mucosa is evident but the thickness of the gained tissue is unsatisfactory. Occlusal view.

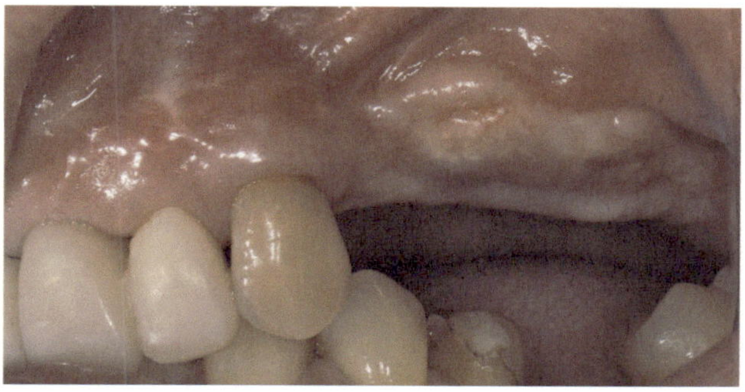

Figure 54.
Healing two months after the keratinized mucosa widening procedure. The gain of the keratinized mucosa is evident but the thickness of the gained tissue is unsatisfactory. Lateral view.

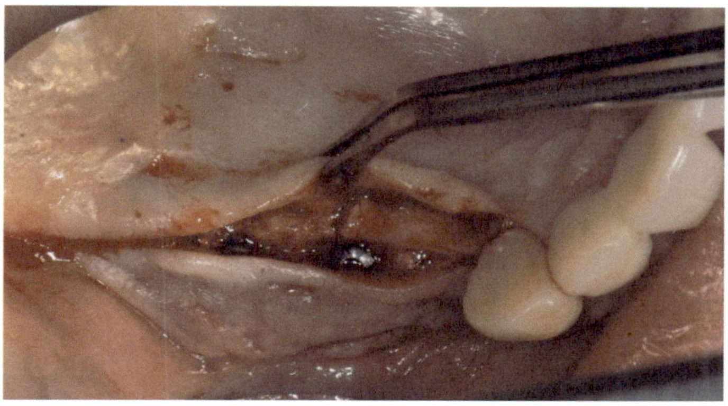

Figure 55.
During the implant uncovering procedure, a primary flap was prepared on the palatal side. The minimal thickness of 1.5 mm of the primary flap was respected, and the connective tissue was exposed.

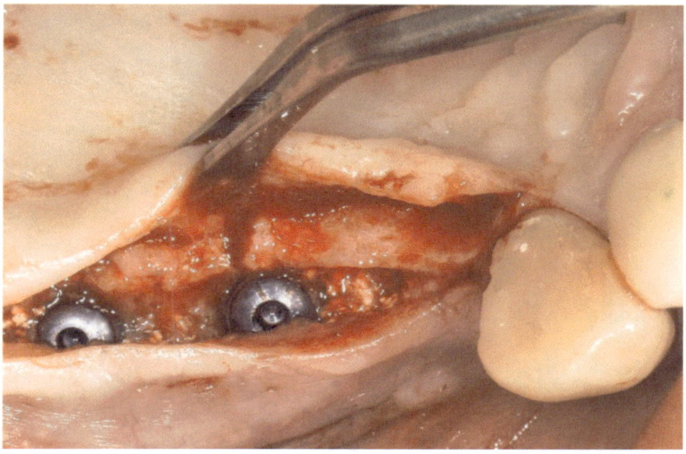

Figure 56.
Mesial, distal and apical incisions were made inside the connective tissue graft in order to completely dissect the CTG from the rest of the adjacent soft tissue.

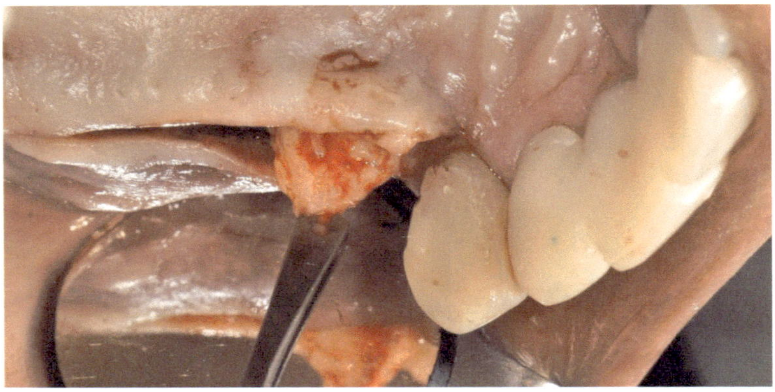

Figure 57.
The CTG is completely dissected from the rest of the adjacent soft tissue.

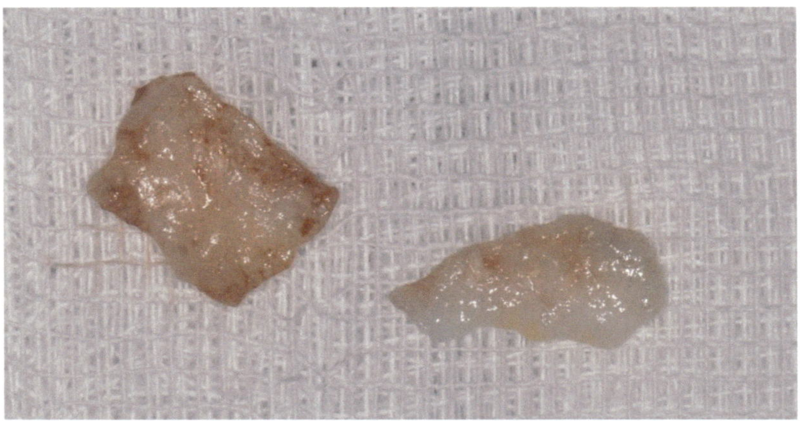

Figure 58.
On the left: CTG harvested from the palate (the harvesting procedure was displayed on the previous pictures), on the right additional CTG harvested from the tuberosity on the same side.

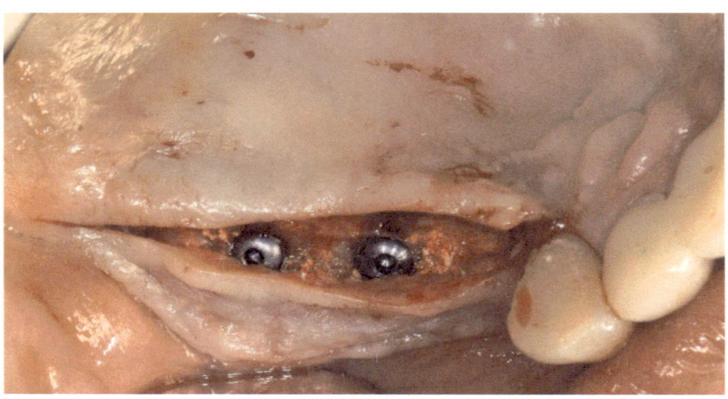

Figure 59.
Appearance of the palatal and tuber donor site after CTG harvesting.

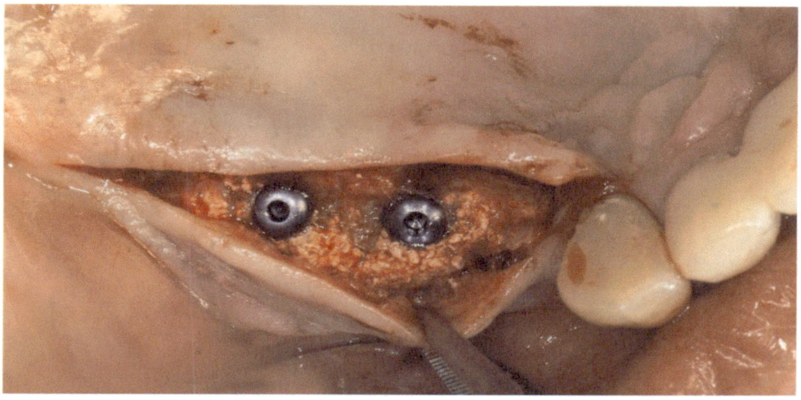

Figure 60.
Appearance of the regenerated bone on the buccal side of the implants.

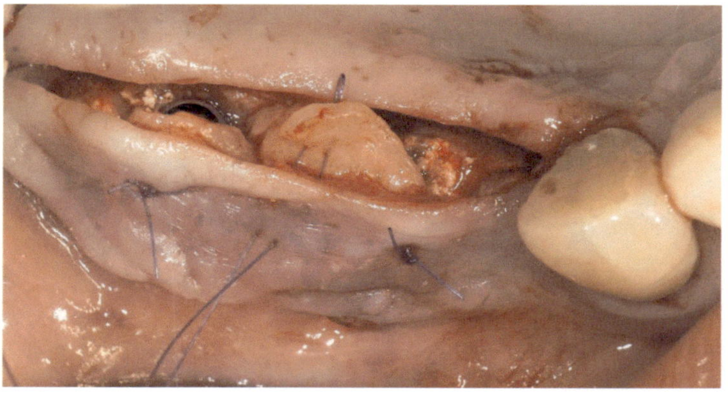

Figure 61.
Both of the CTG grafts were stabilized with sutures to the buccal flap.

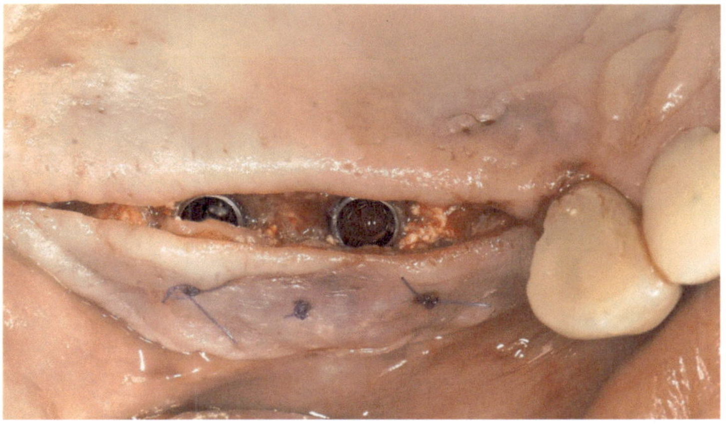

Figure 62.
Final stabilization of the CTG grafts to the inner aspect of the buccal flap.

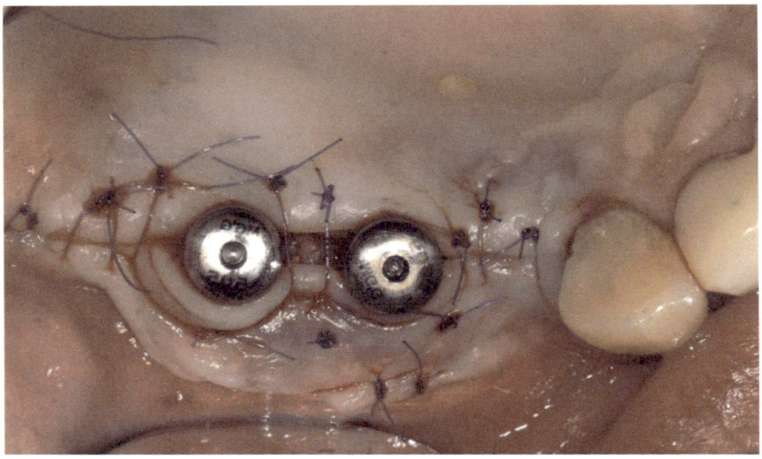

Figure 63.
Final suturing of the flap.

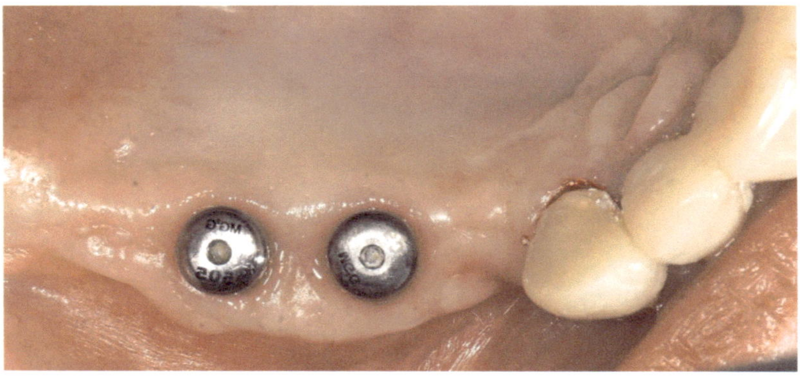

Figure 64.
After 2 months of healing adequate quantity (soft tissue thickness) and quality (width of keratinized mucosa) of soft tissue surrounding the healing abutments.

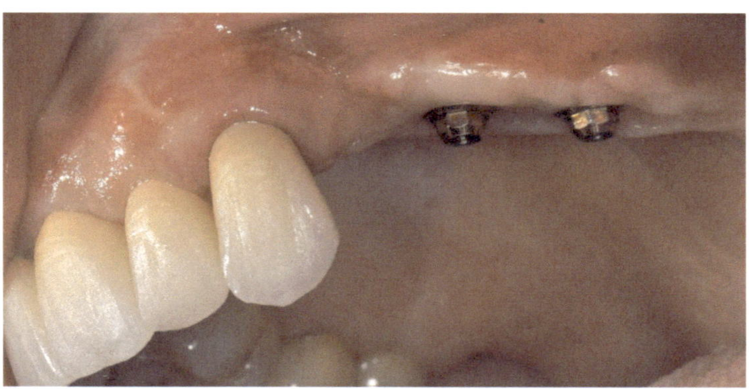

Figure 65.
Screw retained abutments.

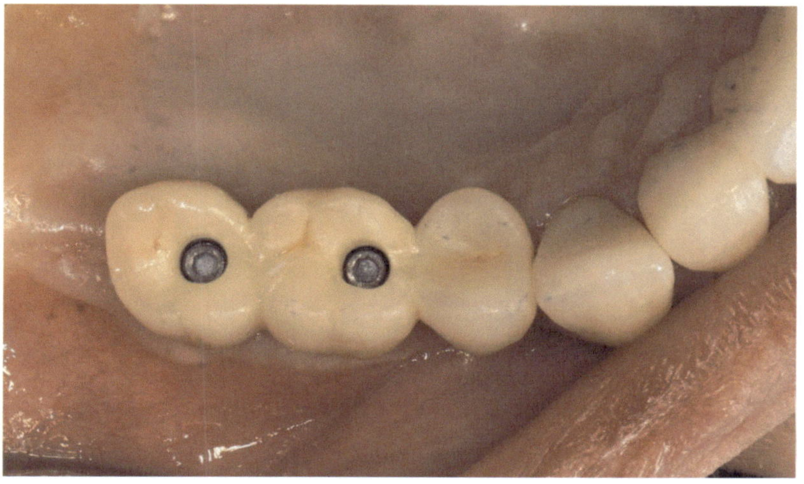

Figure 66.
Three units screw-retained bridge.

7. Conclusion

PIS augmentation procedure has become an integral part of implant-prosthetic rehabilitation. The aim of PIS augmentation is adequate quality and quantity of PIS—at least 2 mm of the width of peri-implant KM and 2 mm or more, of the thickness of PIS. These dimensions of PIS will result in stable peri-implant hard and soft tissue, better esthetical outcome and facilitate oral hygiene maintenance around the implant.

The use of autogenous soft tissue graft for PIS augmentation is considered the gold standard. FGG is primarily used for increasing the KM width and CTG for increasing the thickness of PIS. Different techniques have been developed for the harvesting of the CTG graft. The grafting technique and the choice of the donor site can influence different aspects of the procedure, from patient discomfort in the postoperative period to the quality and dimension of the graft. The choice of the grafting technique should be addressed individually based on the parameters of the specific clinical case (patient desire for decreased morbidity, anatomical limitations of the donor site, dimensions, and quality of the required graft).

The use of substitutional soft tissue grafts has different advantages—reduced length, the complexity of the procedure and patient morbidity, availability of the unlimited amount of the graft, and better patient acceptance. At the moment, the results of the use of substitutional grafts are inferior compared to soft tissue autografts. There is a lack of published long-term results of PIS augmentation with substitutional soft tissue grafts. Therefore, they should be used in cases where patient denial for soft tissue autografts would lead to rejection of the PIS augmentation procedure. In all other cases, priority should be given to soft tissue autografts.

Author details

Marko Blašković[1,2]* and Dorotea Blašković[2]

1 Faculty of Dental Medicine, University of Rijeka, Rijeka, Croatia

2 Private Practice, Stomatološka poliklinika dr. Blašković, Rijeka, Croatia

*Address all correspondence to: marko_blaskovic@yahoo.com

References

[1] Buser D, Sennerby L, De Bruyn H. Modern implant dentistry based on osseointegration: 50 years of progress, current trends and open questions. Periodontology 2000. 2017;**73**(1):7-21

[2] Albrektsson T, Zarb G, Worthington P, Eriksson AR. The long-term efficacy of currently used dental implants: A review and proposed criteria of success. The International Journal of Oral & Maxillofacial Implants. 1986;**1**(1): 11-25

[3] Smith DE, Zarb GA. Criteria for success of osseointegrated endosseous implants. The Journal of Prosthetic Dentistry. 1989;**62**(5):567-572

[4] Papaspyridakos P, Chen CJ, Singh M, Weber HP, Gallucci GO. Success criteria in implant dentistry: A systematic review. Journal of Dental Research. 2012; **91**(3):242-248

[5] Tavelli L, Barootchi S, Avila-Ortiz G, Urban IA, Giannobile WV, Wang HL. Peri-implant soft tissue phenotype modification and its impact on peri-implant health: A systematic review and network meta-analysis. Journal of Periodontology. 2021;**92**(1):21-44

[6] Urban IA, Lozada JL, Nagy K, Sanz M. Treatment of severe mucogingival defects with a combination of strip gingival grafts and a xenogeneic collagen matrix: a prospective case series study. The International Journal of Periodontics & Restorative Dentistry. 2015;**35**(3): 345-353

[7] Chackartchi T, Romanos GE, Sculean A. Soft tissue-related complications and management around dental implants. Periodontology 2000. 2019;**81**(1):124-138

[8] Thoma DS, Naenni N, Figuero E, Hämmerle CHF, Schwarz F, Jung RE, et al. Effects of soft tissue augmentation procedures on peri-implant health or disease: A systematic review and meta-analysis. Clinical Oral Implants Research. 2018;**29**(15):32-49

[9] Lin GH, Chan HL, Wang HL. The significance of keratinized mucosa on implant health: A systematic review. Journal of Periodontology. 2013;**84**(12): 1755-1767

[10] Longoni S, Tinto M, Pacifico C, Sartori M, Andreano A. Effect of peri-implant keratinized tissue width on tissue health and stability: Systematic review and meta-analysis. The International Journal of Oral & Maxillofacial Implants. 2019; **34**(6):1307-1317

[11] Iorio-Siciliano V, Blasi A, Sammartino G, Salvi GE, Sculean A. Soft tissue stability related to mucosal recession at dental implants: A systematic review. Quintessence International. 2020;**51**(1):28-36

[12] Avila-Ortiz G, Gonzalez-Martin O, Couso-Queiruga E, Wang HL. The peri-implant phenotype. Journal of Periodontology. 2020;**91**(3):283-288

[13] Giannobile WV, Jung RE, Schwarz F. Groups of the 2nd osteology foundation consensus meeting. Evidence-based knowledge on the aesthetics and maintenance of peri-implant soft tissues: Osteology foundation consensus report part 1. Effects of soft tissue augmentation procedures on the maintenance of peri-implant soft tissue health. Clinical Oral Implants Research. 2018;**29**(15):7-10

[14] Monje A, Blasi G. Significance of keratinized mucosa/gingiva on peri-implant and adjacent periodontal

conditions in erratic maintenance compliers. Journal of Periodontology. 2019;**90**(5):445-453

[15] Thoma DS, Mühlemann S, Jung RE. Critical soft-tissue dimensions with dental implants and treatment concepts. Periodontology 2000. 2014;**66**(1):106-118

[16] Arunyanak SP, Pollini A, Ntounis A, Morton D. Clinician assessments and patient perspectives of single-tooth implant restorations in the esthetic zone of the maxilla: A systematic review. The Journal of Prosthetic Dentistry. 2017; **118**(1):10-17

[17] Seyssens L, De Lat L, Cosyn J. Immediate implant placement with or without connective tissue graft: A systematic review and meta-analysis. Journal of Clinical Periodontology. 2021; **48**(2):284-301

[18] Atieh MA, Alsabeeha NHM. Soft tissue changes after connective tissue grafts around immediately placed and restored dental implants in the esthetic zone: A systematic review and meta-analysis. Journal of Esthetic and Restorative Dentistry. 2020;**3**:280-290

[19] Martínez-Rus F, Prieto M, Salido MP, Madrigal C, Özcan M, Pradíes G. A clinical study assessing the influence of anodized titanium and zirconium dioxide abutments and peri-implant soft tissue thickness on the optical outcome of implant-supported lithium disilicate single crowns. The International Journal of Oral & Maxillofacial Implants. 2017;**32**(1): 156-163

[20] Jung RE, Sailer I, Hämmerle CH, Attin T, Schmidlin P. In vitro color changes of soft tissues caused by restorative materials. The International Journal of Periodontics & Restorative Dentistry. 2007;**27**(3):251-257

[21] Zuhr O, Rebele SF, Cheung SL, Hürzeler MB. Research group on oral soft tissue biology and wound healing. Surgery without papilla incision: Tunneling flap procedures in plastic periodontal and implant surgery. Periodontology 2000. 2018;**77**(1): 123-149

[22] Abrahamsson I, Berglundh T, Wennström J, Lindhe J. The peri-implant hard and soft tissues at different implant systems. A comparative study in the dog. Clinical Oral Implants Research. 1996; **7**(3):212-219

[23] Linkevicius T, Apse P, Grybauskas S, Puisys A. The influence of soft tissue thickness on crestal bone changes around implants: A 1-year prospective controlled clinical trial. The International Journal of Oral & Maxillofacial Implants. 2009;**24**(4):712-719

[24] Puisys A, Linkevicius T. The influence of mucosal tissue thickening on crestal bone stability around bone-level implants. A prospective controlled clinical trial. Clinical Oral Implants Research. 2015;**26**(2):123-129

[25] Luo RM, Chvartszaid D, Kim SW, Portnof JE. Soft-tissue grafting solutions. Dental Clinics of North America. 2020; **64**(2):435-451

[26] Zuhr O, Bäumer D, Hürzeler M. The addition of soft tissue replacement grafts in plastic periodontal and implant surgery: Critical elements in design and execution. Journal of Clinical Periodontology. 2014;**41**(15):S123-S142

[27] Mörmann W, Bernimoulin JP, Schmid MO. Fluorescein angiography of free gingival autografts. Journal of Clinical Periodontology. 1975;**2**(4):177-189

[28] Nobuto T, Imai H, Yamaoka A. Microvascularization of the free gingival

autograft. Journal of Periodontology. 1988;**59**(10):639-646

[29] Oliver RC, Löe H, Karring T. Microscopic evaluation of the healing and revascularization of free gingival grafts. Journal of Periodontal Research. 1968;**3**(2):84-95

[30] Sculean A, Gruber R, Bosshardt DD. Soft tissue wound healing around teeth and dental implants. Journal of Clinical Periodontology. 2014;**41**(15):S6-S22

[31] Sullivan HC, Atkins JH. Free autogenous gingival grafts. I. Principles of successful grafting. Periodontics. 1968;**6**(3):121-129

[32] Edel A. Clinical evaluation of free connective tissue grafts used to increase the width of keratinised gingiva. Journal of Clinical Periodontology. 1974;**1**(4): 185-196

[33] Baltacıoğlu E, Bağış B, Korkmaz FM, Aydın G, Yuva P, Korkmaz YT. Peri-implant plastic surgical approaches to increasing keratinized mucosa width. The Journal of Oral Implantology. 2015; **41**(3):e73-e81

[34] Cairo F. Periodontal plastic surgery of gingival recessions at single and multiple teeth. Periodontology 2000. 2017;**75**(1):296-316

[35] Mazzotti C, Stefanini M, Felice P, Bentivogli V, Mounssif I, Zucchelli G. Soft-tissue dehiscence coverage at peri-implant sites. Periodontology 2000. 2018;**77**(1):256-272

[36] Bouchard P, Ouhayoun JP, Nilvéus RE. Expanded polytetrafluoroethylene membranes and connective tissue grafts support bone regeneration for closing mandibular Class II furcations. Journal of Periodontology. 1993;**64**(12):1193-1198

[37] Santoro G, Zucchelli G, Gherlone E. Combined regenerative and mucogingival treatment of deep intrabony defects associated with buccal gingival recession: Two case reports. The International Journal of Periodontics & Restorative Dentistry. 2016;**36**(6):849-857

[38] Langer B, Calagna LJ. The subepithelial connective tissue graft. A new approach to the enhancement of anterior cosmetics. The International Journal of Periodontics & Restorative Dentistry. 1982;**2**:22-33

[39] Tunkel J, de Stavola L, Khoury F. Changes in soft tissue dimensions following three different techniques of stage-two surgery: A case series report. The International Journal of Periodontics & Restorative Dentistry. 2013;**33**(4): 411-418

[40] Zucchelli G, Tavelli L, McGuire MK, Rasperini G, Feinberg SE, Wang HL, et al. Autogenous soft tissue grafting for periodontal and peri-implant plastic surgical reconstruction. Journal of Periodontology. 2020;**91**(1):9-16

[41] Marzadori M, Stefanini M, Mazzotti C, Ganz S, Sharma P, Zucchelli G. Soft-tissue augmentation procedures in edentulous esthetic areas. Periodontology 2000. 2018;**77**(1):111-122

[42] Zucchelli G, Mounssif I. Periodontal plastic surgery. Periodontology 2000. 2015;**68**(1):333-368

[43] Puri K, Kumar A, Khatri M, Bansal M, Rehan M, Siddeshappa ST. 44-year journey of palatal connective tissue graft harvest: A narrative review. Journal of Indian Society of Periodontology. 2019;**23**(5):395-408

[44] Sclar AG. Soft Tissue and Esthetic Considerations in Implant Therapy. Carol Stream, IL: Quintessence; 2003

[45] Tseng ES, Tavelli L, Wang HL. Palatal pedicle flaps for soft tissue augmentation. The International Journal of Periodontics & Restorative Dentistry. 2020;**40**(4):581-588

[46] Harris RJ. Histologic evaluation of connective tissue grafts in humans. The International Journal of Periodontics & Restorative Dentistry. 2003;**23**(6):575-583

[47] Tavelli L, Barootchi S, Greenwell H, Wang HL. Is a soft tissue graft harvested from the maxillary tuberosity the approach of choice in an isolated site? Journal of Periodontology. 2019;**90**(8): 821-825

[48] Zucchelli G, Mele M, Stefanini M, Mazzotti C, Marzadori M, Montebugnoli L, et al. Patient morbidity and root coverage outcome after subepithelial connective tissue and de-epithelialized grafts: A comparative randomized-controlled clinical trial. Journal of Clinical Periodontology. 2010; **37**(8):728-738

[49] Bertl K, Pifl M, Hirtler L, Rendl B, Nürnberger S, Stavropoulos A, et al. Relative composition of fibrous connective and fatty/glandular tissue in connective tissue grafts depends on the harvesting technique but not the donor site of the hard palate. Journal of Periodontology. 2015;**86**(12):1331-1339

[50] Studer SP, Allen EP, Rees TC, Kouba A. The thickness of masticatory mucosa in the human hard palate and tuberosity as potential donor sites for ridge augmentation procedures. Journal of Periodontology. 1997;**68**(2):145-151

[51] Stipetić J, Hrala Z, Celebić A. Thickness of masticatory mucosa in the human hard palate and tuberosity dependent on gender and body mass index. Collegium Antropologicum. 2005; **29**(1):243-247

[52] Wessel JR, Tatakis DN. Patient outcomes following subepithelial connective tissue graft and free gingival graft procedures. Journal of Periodontology. 2008;**79**(3):425-430

[53] Tavelli L, Asa'ad F, Acunzo R, Pagni G, Consonni D, Rasperini G. Minimizing patient morbidity following palatal gingival harvesting: A randomized controlled clinical study. The International Journal of Periodontics & Restorative Dentistry. 2018;**38**(6): e127-e134

[54] Griffin TJ, Cheung WS, Zavras AI, Damoulis PD. Postoperative complications following gingival augmentation procedures. Journal of Periodontology. 2006;**77**(12):2070-2079

[55] Del Pizzo M, Modica F, Bethaz N, Priotto P, Romagnoli R. The connective tissue graft: A comparative clinical evaluation of wound healing at the palatal donor site. A preliminary study. Journal of Clinical Periodontology. 2002; **29**(9):848-854

[56] Reiser GM, Bruno JF, Mahan PE, Larkin LH. The subepithelial connective tissue graft palatal donor site: Anatomic considerations for surgeons. The International Journal of Periodontics & Restorative Dentistry. 1996;**16**(2): 130-137

[57] Monnet-Corti V, Santini A, Glise JM, Fouque-Deruelle C, Dillier FL, Liébart MF, et al. Connective tissue graft for gingival recession treatment: Assessment of the maximum graft dimensions at the palatal vault as a donor site. Journal of Periodontology. 2006; **77**(5):899-902

[58] Tavelli L, Barootchi S, Ravidà A, Oh TJ, Wang HL. What is the safety zone for palatal soft tissue graft harvesting based on the locations of the

greater palatine artery and foramen? A systematic review. Journal of Oral and Maxillofacial Surgery. 2019;**77**(2):271.e1-271.e9

[59] Deeb JG, Deeb GR. Oral soft tissue grafting. Oral and Maxillofacial Surgery Clinics of North America. 2020;**32**(4):611-630

[60] Carnio J, Koutouzis T. Palatal augmentation technique: A predictable method to increase the palatal connective tissue at donor sites—A consecutive case series. The International Journal of Periodontics & Restorative Dentistry. 2015;**35**(5):707-713

[61] Carnio J, Hallmon WW. A technique for augmenting the palatal connective tissue donor site: Clinical case report and histologic evaluation. The International Journal of Periodontics & Restorative Dentistry. 2005;**25**(3):257-263

[62] Rocha AL, Shirasu BK, Hayacibara RM, Magro-Filho O, Zanoni JN, Araújo MG. Clinical and histological evaluation of subepithelial connective tissue after collagen sponge implantation in the human palate. Journal of Periodontal Research. 2012;**47**(6):758-765

[63] Jahnke PV, Sandifer JB, Gher ME, Gray JL, Richardson AC. Thick free gingival and connective tissue autografts for root coverage. Journal of Periodontology. 1993;**64**(4):315-322

[64] Tavelli L, Ravidà A, Lin GH, Del Amo FS, Tattan M, Wang HL. Comparison between subepithelial connective tissue graft and de-epithelialized gingival graft: A systematic review and a meta-analysis. Journal of the International Academy of Periodontology. 2019;**21**(2):82-96

[65] Moraschini V, Guimarães HB, Cavalcante IC, Calasans-Maia MD. Clinical efficacy of xenogeneic collagen matrix in augmenting keratinized mucosa round dental implants: A systematic review and meta-analysis. Clinical Oral Investigations. 2020;**24**(7):2163-2174

[66] Cairo F, Barbato L, Tonelli P, Batalocco G, Pagavino G, Nieri M. Xenogeneic collagen matrix versus connective tissue graft for buccal soft tissue augmentation at implant site. A randomized, controlled clinical trial. Journal of Clinical Periodontology. 2017;**44**(7):769-776

[67] Basegmez C, Karabuda ZC, Demirel K, Yalcin S. The comparison of acellular dermal matrix allografts with free gingival grafts in the augmentation of peri-implant attached mucosa: a randomised controlled trial. European Journal of Oral Implantology. 2013;**6**(2):145-152

[68] de Resende DRB, Greghi SLA, Siqueira AF, Benfatti CAM, Damante CA, Ragghianti Zangrando MS. Acellular dermal matrix allograft versus free gingival graft: A histological evaluation and split-mouth randomized clinical trial. Clinical Oral Investigations. 2019;**23**(2):539-550

[69] Zuhr O, Hürzeler M. Plastic-esthetic periodontal and implant surgery—A microsurgical approach. Batavia, IL: Quintessence Publishing Co. 2011

[70] Hürzeler MB, Weng D. A single-incision technique to harvest subepithelial connective tissue grafts from the palate. The International Journal of Periodontics & Restorative Dentistry. 1999;**19**(3):279-287

[71] Lorenzana ER, Allen EP. The single-incision palatal harvest technique: A

strategy for esthetics and patient comfort. The International Journal of Periodontics & Restorative Dentistry. 2000;**20**(3):297-305

[72] Maino GNE, Valles C, Santos A, Pascual A, Esquinas C, Nart J. Influence of suturing technique on wound healing and patient morbidity after connective tissue harvesting. A randomized clinical trial. Journal of Clinical Periodontology. 2018;**45**(8):977-985

[73] Akcalı A, Schneider D, Ünlü F, Bıcakcı N, Köse T, Hämmerle CH. Soft tissue augmentation of ridge defects in the maxillary anterior area using two different methods: A randomized controlled clinical trial. Clinical Oral Implants Research. 2015;**26**(6):688-695

[74] Abrams L. Augmentation of the deformed residual edentulous ridge for fixed prosthesis. The Compendium on Continuing Education in General Dentistry. 1980;**1**(3):205-213

[75] El Chaar E, Oshman S, Cicero G, Castano A, Dinoi C, Soltani L, et al. Soft tissue closure of grafted extraction sockets in the anterior maxilla: A modified palatal pedicle connective tissue flap technique. The International Journal of Periodontics & Restorative Dentistry. 2017;**37**(1):99-107

[76] El Chaar ES. Soft tissue closure of grafted extraction sockets in the posterior maxilla: The rotated pedicle palatal connective tissue flap technique. Implant Dentistry. 2010;**19**(5):370-377

[77] Mathews DP. The pediculated connective tissue graft: A technique for improving unaesthetic implant restorations. Practical Procedures & Aesthetic Dentistry. 2002;**14**(9):719-724

[78] Park SH, Wang HL. Pouch roll technique for implant soft tissue augmentation: A variation of the modified roll technique. The International Journal of Periodontics & Restorative Dentistry. 2012;**32**(3):e116-e121

[79] Barone R, Clauser C, Prato GP. Localized soft tissue ridge augmentation at phase 2 implant surgery: A case report. The International Journal of Periodontics & Restorative Dentistry. 1999;**19**(2):141-145

[80] Kulkarni MR, Bakshi PV, Kavlekar AS, Thakur SL. Applications of a modified palatal roll flap in peri-implant soft-tissue augmentation—A case series. Journal of Indian Society of Periodontology. 2017;**21**(4):333-336

[81] Saquib SA, Bhat MYS, Javali MA, Shamsuddin SV, Kader MA. Modified roll technique for soft tissue augmentation in prosthetic rehabilitation: A case report. Clinical Practice. 2019;**9**(1):1110

[82] Scharf DR, Tarnow DP. Modified roll technique for localized alveolar ridge augmentation. The International Journal of Periodontics & Restorative Dentistry. 1992;**12**(5):415-425

[83] Man Y, Wu Q, Wang T, Gong P, Gong T, Qu Y. Split pedicle roll envelope technique around implants and pontics: A prospective case series study. International Journal of Oral and Maxillofacial Surgery. 2015;**44**(10):1295-1301

[84] Khoury F, Happe A. The palatal subepithelial connective tissue flap method for soft tissue management to cover maxillary defects: A clinical report. The International Journal of Oral & Maxillofacial Implants. 2000;**15**(3):415-418

[85] Zucchelli G, Mazzotti C, Mounssif I, Marzadori M, Stefanini M. Esthetic

treatment of peri-implant soft tissue defects: A case report of a modified surgical-prosthetic approach. The International Journal of Periodontics & Restorative Dentistry. 2013;**33**(3): 327-335

[86] Lee CT, Hamalian T, Schulze-Späte U. Minimally invasive treatment of soft tissue deficiency around an implant-supported restoration in the esthetic zone: Modified VISTA technique case report. The Journal of Oral Implantology. 2015;**41**(1):71-76

[87] Nabers JM. Free gingival grafts. Periodontics. 1966;**4**(5):243-245

[88] Miller PD Jr. Root coverage using the free soft tissue autograft following citric acid application. III. A successful and predictable procedure in areas of deep-wide recession. The International Journal of Periodontics & Restorative Dentistry. 1985;**5**(2):14-37

[89] Seibert JS. Reconstruction of deformed, partially edentulous ridges, using full thickness onlay grafts. Part I. Technique and wound healing. The Compendium of Continuing Education in Dentistry. 1983;**4**(5):437-453

[90] Camargo PM, Melnick PR, Kenney EB. The use of free gingival grafts for aesthetic purposes. Periodontology 2000. 2001;**27**(1):72-96

[91] Han Z, Wei Y, Wang C, Yang G, Hu W, Chung KH. Clinical evaluations of free gingival grafting before implant placement to increase keratinized tissue width in molar regions: A retrospective case series. Clinical Oral Implants Research. 2021;**32**(7):799-807

[92] Gümüş P, Buduneli E. Graft stabilization with cyanoacrylate decreases shrinkage of free gingival grafts. Australian Dental Journal. 2014; **59**(1):57-64

[93] Thoma DS, Benić GI, Zwahlen M, Hämmerle CH, Jung RE. A systematic review assessing soft tissue augmentation techniques. Clinical Oral Implants Research. 2009;**20**(4):146-165

[94] Shanmugam M, Kumar TS, Arun KV, Arun R, Karthik SJ. Clinical and histological evaluation of two dressing materials in the healing of palatal wounds. Journal of Indian Society of Periodontology. 2010;**14**(4):241-244

[95] Meza-Mauricio J, Furquim CP, Geldres A, Mendoza-Azpur G, Retamal-Valdes B, Moraschini V, et al. Is the use of platelet-rich fibrin effective in the healing, control of pain, and postoperative bleeding in the palatal area after free gingival graft harvesting? A systematic review of randomized clinical studies. Clinical Oral Investigations. 2021;**25**(7):4239-4249

[96] Dellavia C, Ricci G, Pettinari L, Allievi C, Grizzi F, Gagliano N. Human palatal and tuberosity mucosa as donor sites for ridge augmentation. The International Journal of Periodontics & Restorative Dentistry. 2014;**34**(2): 179-186

[97] Jung UW, Um YJ, Choi SH. Histologic observation of soft tissue acquired from maxillary tuberosity area for root coverage. Journal of Periodontology. 2008;**79**(5):934-940

[98] Amin PN, Bissada NF, Ricchetti PA, APB S, Demko CA. Tuberosity versus palatal donor sites for soft tissue grafting: A split-mouth clinical study. Quintessence International. 2018;**49**(7): 589-598

[99] Bassetti RG, Stähli A, Bassetti MA, Sculean A. Soft tissue augmentation

around osseointegrated and uncovered dental implants: A systematic review. Clinical Oral Investigations. 2017;**21**(1):53-70

[100] Tonetti MS, Cortellini P, Pellegrini G, Nieri M, Bonaccini D, Allegri M, et al. Xenogenic collagen matrix or autologous connective tissue graft as adjunct to coronally advanced flaps for coverage of multiple adjacent gingival recession: Randomized trial assessing non-inferiority in root coverage and superiority in oral health-related quality of life. Journal of Clinical Periodontology. 2018;**45**(1):78-88

[101] Agarwal C, Tarun Kumar AB, Mehta DS. Comparative evaluation of free gingival graft and AlloDerm(®) in enhancing the width of attached gingival: A clinical study. Contemporary Clinical Dentistry. 2015;**6**(4):483-488

[102] McGuire MK, Scheyer ET. Randomized, controlled clinical trial to evaluate a xenogeneic collagen matrix as an alternative to free gingival grafting for oral soft tissue augmentation. Journal of Periodontology. 2014;**85**(10):1333-1341

[103] Tavelli L, Barootchi S, Di Gianfilippo R, Kneifati A, Majzoub J, Stefanini M, et al. Patient experience of autogenous soft tissue grafting has an implication for future treatment: A 10- to 15-year cross-sectional study. Journal of Periodontology. 2021;**92**(5):637-647

[104] Cairo F, Barbato L, Selvaggi F, Baielli MG, Piattelli A, Chambrone L. Surgical procedures for soft tissue augmentation at implant sites. A systematic review and meta-analysis of randomized controlled trials. Clinical Implant Dentistry and Related Research. 2019;**21**(6):1262-1270

[105] Tavelli L, McGuire MK, Zucchelli G, Rasperini G, Feinberg SE, Wang HL, et al. Extracellular matrix-based scaffolding technologies for periodontal and peri-implant soft tissue regeneration. Journal of Periodontology. 2020;**91**(1):17-25

[106] Nocini PF, Castellani R, Zanotti G, Gelpi F, Covani U, Marconcini S, et al. Extensive keratinized tissue augmentation during implant rehabilitation after Le Fort I osteotomy: using a new porcine collagen membrane (Mucoderm). The Journal of Craniofacial Surgery. 2014;**25**(3):799-803

[107] Yu SH, Tseng SC, Wang HL. Classification of soft tissue grafting materials based on biologic principles. The International Journal of Periodontics & Restorative Dentistry. 2018;**38**(6):849-854

[108] Thoma DS, Zeltner M, Hilbe M, Hämmerle CH, Hüsler J, Jung RE. Randomized controlled clinical study evaluating effectiveness and safety of a volume-stable collagen matrix compared to autogenous connective tissue grafts for soft tissue augmentation at implant sites. Journal of Clinical Periodontology. 2016;**43**(10):874-885

[109] Thoma DS, Gasser TJW, Jung RE, Hämmerle CHF. Randomized controlled clinical trial comparing implant sites augmented with a volume-stable collagen matrix or an autogenous connective tissue graft: 3-year data after insertion of reconstructions. Journal of Clinical Periodontology. 2020;**47**(5):630-639

Chapter 12

The Effect of Implant Surface Design and Their Decontamination Methods in Peri-Implantitis Treatment

Dragana Rakašević and Dragana Gabrić

Abstract

Different titanium implant surfaces are prone to microbial colonization and dental plaque accumulation contributing to peri-implantitis pathogens adherence and growth. In conjunction with systemic, local, and implant-based factors such as micro- and macro-designs, implant location, and region, these pathogens can cause a complex inflammatory response resulting in peri-implantitis and deleterious bone loss. Implant surface decontamination plays a crucial and important step in peri-implantitis therapy. The primary goal of implant surface decontamination is to eradicate bacteria and their products outside of implant pits and grooves reducing inflammation and promoting tissue regeneration and/or reparation. Various implant surface decontamination methods such as mechanical, chemical or physical methods have been proposed to prevent bacterial resistance development or/and surface damage. The chapter aimed to assess if implant microdesign could influence the decontamination method choice.

Keywords: peri-implantitis, implant design, implant surface, decontamination methods, peri-implantitis therapy

1. Introduction

Dental implants have become highly predictable routine therapeutic strategy in daily practice for a missing teeth replacement in the partial or total edentulous patients' treatment.

Osseointegration presents close bone-to-implant contact (BIC) and depends on several factors such as implant micro- and macro-design which play crucial roles in long-term implant survival success rate. Implant macro-construction (implant shape, number and shape of implant threads) is designed to improve osseointegration mechanism and obtain implant primary stability resisting detrimental forces occurring during physiological functions [1–4]. Various implant surfaces were developed to enhance osseointegration mechanism accelerating and strengthening bone formation providing better stability [5]. Additional modification of implant surfaces increases surface roughness with aim to improve bone healing especially in the region with poor bone quantity or quality stimulating bone growth, and enabling immediate or early loading protocols [6]. This modification increases surface roughness as well, making it another important parameter for effective osseointegration.

The mechanism of osseointegration could invert unpredictably into a pathological process leading to inflammatory reactions in soft tissue (peri-mucositis) or a subsequent bone loss around an osseointegrated implant. This process could cause peri-implantitis onset, and as consequence implant failure [7–9]. As a disease of the modern era, peri-implantitis is defined as a plaque-associated pathological condition characterized by clinical signs of inflammation such as bleeding on probing (BOP) with or without suppuration, peri-implant probing depths increase (PPD), and clinical attachment loss (CAL) along with radiographic bone loss [10].

Major aetiological factors in the peri-implantitis development are virulent pathogenetic anaerobic bacteria (*Porphyromonas gingivalis, Prevotella intermedia, A. actinomycetemcomitans, Tannerella forsythia, Treponema denticola)* isolated from dental biofilm around the implant triggering the deleterious immunological reaction of the host tissue, and causing progressive surrounding bone loss [11]. Furthermore, some facultative isolated a gram-positive pathogen (*Staphylococcus aureus*) and fungi (*C. albicans*) are considered to contribute to peri-implantitis onset [12, 13].

In addition, a myriad of patient-related factors (genetic, diabetes mellitus, cardiovascular diseases, genetics, smoking), local factors (periodontitis, residual cement, poor oral hygiene, etc.), and implant-based factors are introduced as risks that could induce onset and severity of peri-implantitis [8, 14–18].

1.1 Implant-based and implant-related factors in peri-implantitis

1.1.1 Implant macro-design associated with peri-implantitis

Specific implant topography, i.e., its macro-design such as body shape, threads number, and collar design as well as micro-design aimed to speed the process of osseointegration enabling a rapid implant loading [19]. However, these dental implant components themselves could be addressed as one of the implant-based risk factors associated with peri-implantitis onset.

A variety of commercially available implants with cylindrical or conical body shape, one-, double- or triple-threads number and different thread shapes are constructed not only to accelerate the osseointegration process but also to minimize a hazard shear force acting instantaneously. Moreover, the implant macro-design aimed to prevent additional further marginal bone loss that could jeopardize implant long-term stability after prosthetic rehabilitation. In contrast, cylindric implants and implants with triple-threads demonstrated the production of greater detrimental shear forces [19] resulting in higher bone loss with implant failure, respectively.

To speed up and shorten implant placement by increasing the threads number on the implant body (double- and triple-thread) could, unfortunately, induce more pressure forces [2]. This resulted in increased bone loss, especially at triple-threads compared to single-thread [19]. In a laboratory model, using finite element analysis (FEA), threads shape was used to stimulate and estimate stress distribution between implants and cortical or cancellous bone [20] indicating that "V" shape and a broader-square shape generated less stress in cancellous bone than other examined threads. In contrast, implants with "V" and butter thread shapes generated higher forces that induced bone defect formation [20, 21], and may consequently contribute to peri-implantits. Although these facts arising from *in vitro* and *in vivo* conditions, localisation and bone quality could affect the success of implant therapy associated with implant macro-design. However, a significant incidence of peri-implantitis has been reported in the posterior region of the mandible [22–25] suggesting that the location and region of implant placement might be associated with peri-implantitis development.

Implant macro-design could also cause excess cement retention that could act as rough surface facilitating an adherence of microorganism and inflammation around peri-implant mucosa with subsequent bone loss. Moreover, other implant-based factors such as implant-abutment connection type, prosthetic rehabilitation, and occlusal overload, could also be taken into consideration as risks for peri-implantitis onset [8, 18, 26–28].

Since the current literature are insufficient in providing evidence whether the implant macrodesign parameters such as implant body shape and dimension, and threads number could be the possible risk factors associated with the initiation and progression of peri-implantitis, further studies are required.

1.1.2 Implant micro-design in correlation with peri-implantitis onset

Over the last few decades, implant surfaces topography has been modified to enhance BIC rates, primary implant stability as well as positive host-to-implant response aiming to attain long-term implant treatment success rates. Bone response to implant topography modification has been specifically related to surface roughness, surface free energy and surface chemistry.

The implant's surface could be "smooth" (machined) or rough. Roughness Average (Ra) or Arithmetical Mean Height (Sa) parameters are used to describe the roughness of dental implant surfaces referring to the height of the surface structure in two or three dimensions. Mostly, implant surface roughness could be divided into four groups: smooth implant surface with Sa roughness value less than 0.5 μm, minimally rough surface (Sa value 0.5–1.0 μm), moderately rough surface (Sa value 1.0–2.0 μm), and rough surface (Sa value more than 2.0 μm). Several methods are reported in the literature to create implant roughness including acid etching, sand-blasting, titanium plasma spraying, and hydroxyapatite (HA) coating, contributing to changes in implant physicochemical properties [5, 29, 30]. Currently available dental implant systems could have either moderately rough surfaces such as SLA, TiUnite, OsseoSpeed, and TiOblast implants or a rough surface such as Ankylos, IMZ or TPS implants [29]. Nevertheless, these implant topography features may play a role in peri-implantitis onset [5, 29, 31].

A study by Polizzi and al. demonstrated that peri-implantitis was more commonly detected at implants with a rough TiUnite surface compared with the minimally rough machined surface [32]. Furthermore, the spontaneous and greater bone loss occurred at the implants with a TiUnite surface compared to Turned, SLA or TiOblast surfaces [33–35]. The hazardous effect of TiUnite surface could be explained by its microdesign and the presence of grooves and pits that might encourage bacterial adhesion [35]. Although microbial plaque accumulation had been detected on novel modified anodized surfaces (TiUltra), this surface affected minimal bone loss and inflammation resulting in marginal bone stability [36]. Additionally, zirconium surface promoted plaque reduction *in vitro* conditions compared to Ti-machined, sandblasted and acid-etched surfaces.

Implant roughness and surface free energy influenced the dental plaque accumulation and biofilm formation inducing peri-implantitis [37, 38]. According to a literature review by Teughels et al. [37] increasing surface roughness above 0.2 μm resulted in biofilm formation and bacteria adhesion. Despite differences in surface roughness, another *in vivo* study recorded plaque accumulation on three different titanium disk surfaces (machined, RBM sandblasted and Xpeed) [39]. Additionally, some periodontal bacteria such as *P. gingivalis* could have the ability and greater bacterial viability on titanium compared with zirconium abutments [40]. *S. aureus*, which is introduced as one of the main harmful bacteria in peri-implantitis development, has an immense affinity to colonize on titanium implant surfaces [41, 42]. Even though the role of *C. albicans* in peri-implantitis disease is still being investigated, this species has also been isolated around implants with diagnosed peri-implantitis. In combination with *Streptococcus* species, *C. albicans* has the ability to grow on titanium surfaces forming a robust mixed biofilm that could cause inflammatory tissue reactions with potential tissue damage [43–45].

The development of bioactive titanium surface coatings with antibacterial properties has been considered as an additional strategy for controlling biofilm formation [46]. Different antimicrobials, active molecules, compounds, and ions were incorporated into implant surface to stimulate bactericidal or/and bacteriostatic effect on surrounding tissue decreasing in this way bacterial adhesion on implant surface. Unfortunately, this strategy has a short-term effect since the remains of dead cells on the uncleaned surfaces may act as bridges for bacteria coaggregation and colonization [47] leading to possible peri-implantitis onset.

1.2 Other peri-implantitis risk factors

Other risk factors such as smoking, diabetes, medications used in the treatment of chronic diseases may influence bone metabolism supporting plaque accumulation and adversely impacting the periimplant-tissue response. Despite limited evidence, survival of implants in patients with diabetes could be disturbed by high blood glucose level, that affects the immune system impairing tissue repair and host defenses against dental plaque [48], therefore accelerating peri-implantitis development or progression. Special caution in the peri-implantitis treatment should be advised in patients with chronic disorders/ diseases.

2. Treatment of peri-implantitis

Peri-implantitis is a complex multi-microbial and multifactorial disease, thus, therapy continues to be a challenge. It has been suggested that peri-implantitis surgical therapy is superior to non-surgical one [49]. Implant surface decontamination is an important but at the same time difficult step in peri-implantitis treatment. The goal of implant surface decontamination is to completely remove all causative bacteria from the implant surface preparing the tissue for regeneration and re-osseointegration [12]. Considering the possible role of micro- and micro-design on peri-implantitis initiation, special care should be taken in the process of implant surface decontamination.

The removal of microbes from the implant surface may cause possible implant surface damage. As a result of surface damage, surface chemical oxide layer changes could lead to induced corrosion, acidic pH, changes in surface roughness, plaque accumulation, and osteoclast activation impairing implants biocompatibility [50].

Additionally, different methods of decontamination could generate mechanical or chemical processes on implant surfaces releasing titanium' ions and particles, and promoting the pathogenic biofilm growth on treated surfaces as well [45].

Although there is no standardized protocol for peri-implantitis treatment, many methods of implant surface decontamination have been proposed including mechanical methods, chemical methods, laser, photodynamic therapy, and implantoplasty, usually combined with systemic antibiotics administration [51–60]. Accordingly, this chapter aimed to determine which method of implant surface decontamination could be successfully performed assessing comparably if implant topography could have influenced the decontamination method choice in peri-implantitis treatment.

2.1 Mechanical and chemical methods of implant surface decontamination

The removal of biofilms and calculus is essential for long-term clinical success and bone regeneration [12]. Therefore, mechanical removal of granulation tissue and surface cleaning presents the first steps in peri-implantitis or periodontal therapy. Ideal mechanical methods should be capable of completely removing deposits and bacteria along with their products from the implant surface without altering or damaging implant surface integrity and biocompatibility, or affecting the implant-tissue interface. Due to implant surface macro- and micro-design as well as bacterial characteristics, it is difficult to achieve long-term results using a mechanical method alone. Therefore, this method is usually combined with chemical methods, photodynamic or laser therapy.

Several instruments such as curettes and brushes have been proposed for mechanical implant surface decontamination. Metal (stainless steel) curettes, burs and conventional sonic and ultrasonic scalers, have been shown to damage the smooth or rough (TPS and SLA) implant surface leaving behind the debris by removing the surface coating, threads and edges. Nevertheless, these instruments are only used when smooth surface of implant, implantoplasty, is required [61]. Titanium curettes were also advised to be used with caution due to their tendency to leave marks on the implant surface increasing the depth of the surface roughness and in this way causing an inability to effectively remove biofilm [62]. Plastic curettes did not leave any surface scratches on different implants surfaces. However, their limited flexibility and size resulted in incomplete plaque removal in screw-type implants [63]. Even when combined with chemical methods such as chlorhexidine gluconate (CHX), plastic curette was not effective in biofilm removal from Osseotite® or SLA titanium disks [64] thereby only being recommended for use during maintenance care [65].

Peri-implantitis treatment performing the Vector system improved oral hygiene, yet showing no improvement in clinical parameters compared to carbon curettes after six months of follow-ups [66]. According to systematic reviews, Vector systems with carbon tips efficiently removed biofilms from polished titanium and SLA surfaces. Hence, the potential to produce SLA and TPS surface damage was found to be a drawback, and could be possible explanation for poor clinical outcomes [61, 63, 67].

The market offers a variety of rotating titanium brushes that are successfully used in combination with other chemical agents or physical methods for implant surface decontamination (**Figure 1**). Rotating brushes effectively clean SLA, TiUnite, and OsseoSpeed surfaces without compromising their properties [67]. Contrary to this, *in vitro* study demonstrated that titanium brushes could create titanium surface craters with remaining titanium particles on SLA surface. The significance of this result must be interpreted carefully since this study was conducted under *in vitro* conditions, the coating surfaces

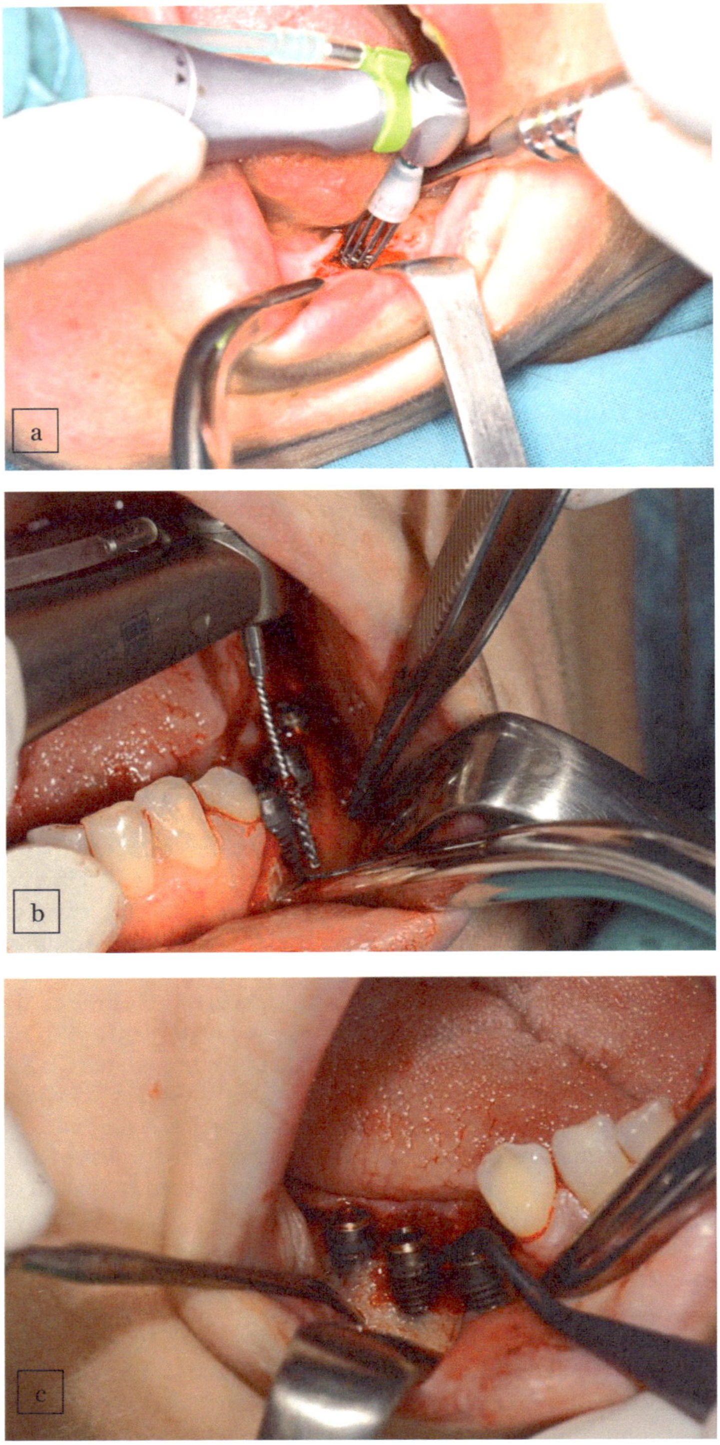

Figure 1.
Mechanical methods of implant surface decontamination by performing two different titanium brushes (a, b,) and graphite curette (c).

were not contaminated, and the treatment was done on "sterile" surfaces [68]. In a recent randomized clinical trial (RCT), rotating titanium brushes combined with 3% H_2O_2 during regenerative surgical procedures of peri-implantitis significantly reduced both PPD and BOP after 12 months from the surgery [69]. The titanium brushes could be proposed for implant surface decontamination during the surgery.

Other mechanical methods of implant surface decontamination, air powder-water sprays, have not shown to be superior in terms of improvement in clinical parameters and possible re-osseointegration compared to other mechanical methods. Recent *in vitro* study revealed that air-power-water spray was not effective in removing biofilms from titanium surfaces, grades 4 and 5, acid-etched, sandblasted, or functionally anodized surfaces compared to electrolytic methods that completely eradicate biofilms from treated surfaces [70]. Furthermore, air-powder system properties such as water flow, powder medium, air pressure, and exposure time seemed to influence biofilm removal and implant surface changes. There was a significant difference in the effectiveness of the medium for hydroxyapatite/tricalcium phosphate and hydroxyapatite, while the cleaning effect was less pronounced on titanium dioxide and phosphoric acid. In addition, amino acid glycine powder effectively removed microbes from implants without altering implant surface as compared to classical sodium bicarbonate powder. It was found that the sodium bicarbonate powder left craters and abrasive residue on the surface. As a result of this, the immune system may be impaired causing an inflammatory response of the tissue [67].

Implantoplasty is another mechanical method of implant surface decontamination that is usually used during surgical peri-implantitis therapy to smoothen the supra-crestal exposed implant surface (**Figure 2**). Whenever there is a persistent supra-crestal bone defect (Class II bone defect, classified by Schwarz [71]), implantoplasty appears to be the most effective treatment. Among the benefits of implantoplasty there is a very low bacteria adhesion and recolonization rate.

Due to the implant surface roughness, it could not be possible to remove bacteria and their waste products completely. Therefore, it is recommended to be combined with antiseptics and antibiotics. Various chemical agents such as chlorhexidine gluconate (CHX), hydrogen peroxide (H_2O_2), citric acid, and phosphoric acid have been proposed as means to decontaminate titanium implant surfaces in both non-surgical and surgical therapies.

The CHX is a commonly used antiseptic agent that is considered a 'gold standard' in various treatment procedures. It is a time-dependent chemical agent which exhibits both bactericidal and bacteriostatic effects. With increasing CHX concertation, in both pure titanium discs and titanium-zirconium alloy discs there was a decrease in the mean number of colony-forming units indicating antibacterial dose–response and biofilm control [72]. Even so, the clinical and microbiological outcomes in one of RCTs had not shown statistical differences when two CHX concentrations (2% vs. 0.12% CHX + 0.5% CPC) were used for the decontamination of commercially available implant surfaces during peri-implantitis resective surgery [73]. These results were consistent with our prior published study in which implant surface decontamination was performed by applying 1% gel of CHX followed by saline solution irrigation during regenerative surgery. Our study concluded that this chemical procedure had insufficient effectiveness in clinical and microbiological results [57]. Under *in vitro* conditions, CHX can remain on implant surfaces gradually releasing and acting within 24 hours against bacteria without harming the surface. Nevertheless, a special caution needs to be taken during implant surface decontamination due to CHX cytotoxic effects on osteoblastic, endothelium, and fibroblastic cells [74]. Irrigation by saline solution for

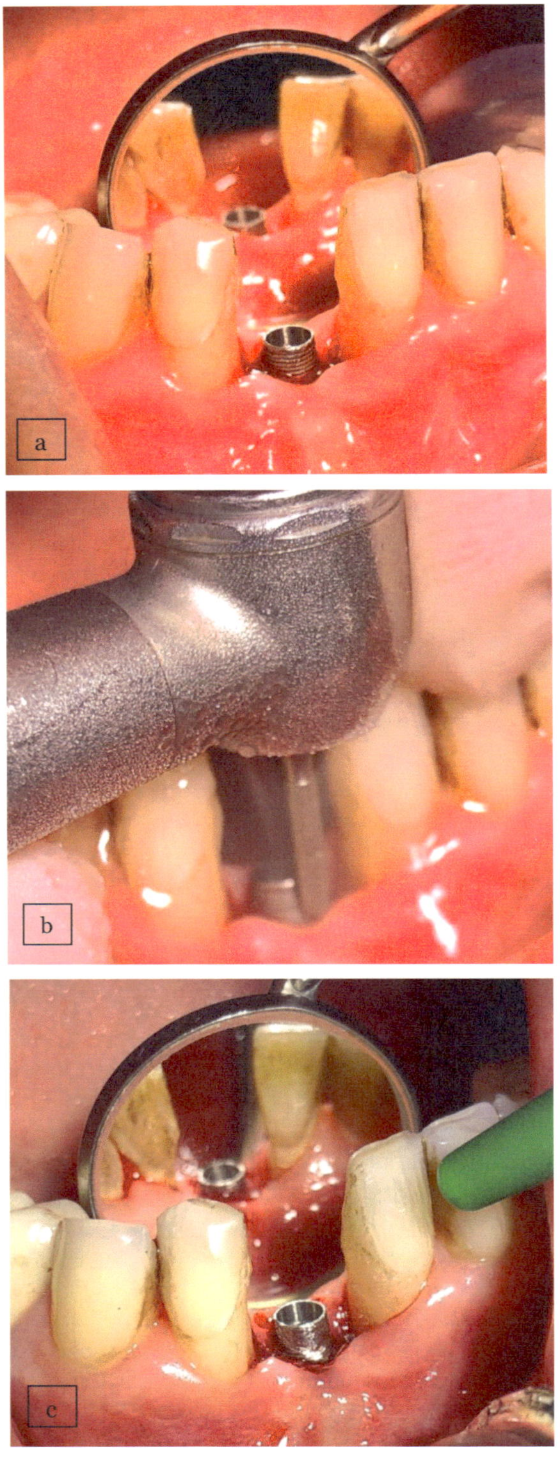

Figure 2.
Implantoplasty as a mechanical method for implant surface decontamination: Exposed implant surface (a), implantoplasty procedure (b), smooth implant surface (c).

approximately a minute could alleviate the negative effect of CHX; however, it should be noted that this irrigation might reduce CHX-substantivity. Furthermore, because of CHX's low cleaning capacity, gauze soaked in saline solution should be taken after CHX application to mechanically remove debris and death cells that might act as a substrate for recolonization, and consequently, disease reappearance.

The use of adjuvant systemic or local antibiotic therapy could also be affected by implant surface topography in peri-implantitis therapy. A successful treatment outcome was documented in only 45% of treated implants by Carcuac et al. In this study, 79% of implants with non-modified surface features and 34% of implants with modified surfaces had successful treatment after peri-implant surgery [75]. In the Heitz-Mayfield et al. study, a significant improvement of clinical parameters was achieved within 12 months after an open-flap surgical procedure of moderate and advance peri-implantitis followed by adjuvant systemic antibiotics administration (amoxicillin and metronidazole) and antiseptic solution (0.12% CHX). Approximately 47% of implants with various surface topographies completely resolved inflammation post-operatively. However, within 12 months of implant surgery, bone continues to lose on implants with porous anodized, titanium plasma-sprayed, and machine surfaces [54]. Systemic antibiotics had limited penetration into the biofilm attached to the titanium implant surface. These findings would support the recommendation that implant surface should be carefully evaluated prior to adjuvant systemic antibiotics administration. Apart from this, broad-spectrum antibiotics' excessive use, their side effects, and allergic reactions have led to bacterial-resistance development, thus additional care should be taken in their administration.

In order to overcome these drawbacks of chemical and mechanical methods, novel methods such as laser or photodynamic therapy were introduced to improve implant surface decontamination.

2.2 Application of laser and photodynamic therapy in peri-implantitis treatment

2.2.1 Laser use in peri-implantitis therapy

In the late 1980's, a laser system was introduced in dentistry [76] increasing laser popularity in dental implantology considerably. Due to the laser's capacity to achieve satisfactory cutting, induce good coagulation, and antibacterial effect, the laser is widely used in dental implantology for the safe second stage surgery of submerging implants, peri-implant soft tissue plastic surgery, and implant surface decontamination. Lasers have been described to possess ability to facilitate implant site preparation enhancing bone healing and osseointegration [56, 77, 78].

The lasers' use in non-surgical and surgical peri-implantitis therapy was widely examined, especially its effects on implant surface decontamination and re-osseointegration. Titanium implant surfaces have greater absorption characteristics resulting in the surface overheating and alteration, so special consideration should be given when they are exposed to the laser. A literature review has recommended a few types of lasers for decontaminating implant surfaces [56].

Er: YAG laser is suggested for successful implant surface decontamination with a tendency to achieve re-osseointegration (**Figure 3**). Safe irradiation settings for this laser should be above 300 mJ/10 Hz for 10s achieving efficiently a bactericide effect, and not increasing implant temperature or altering the surface of polished or SLA implants [79]. Favorable long-term outcomes following treatment of peri-implantitis with Er: YAG lasers were observed in a few clinical studies [80, 81]. A case report

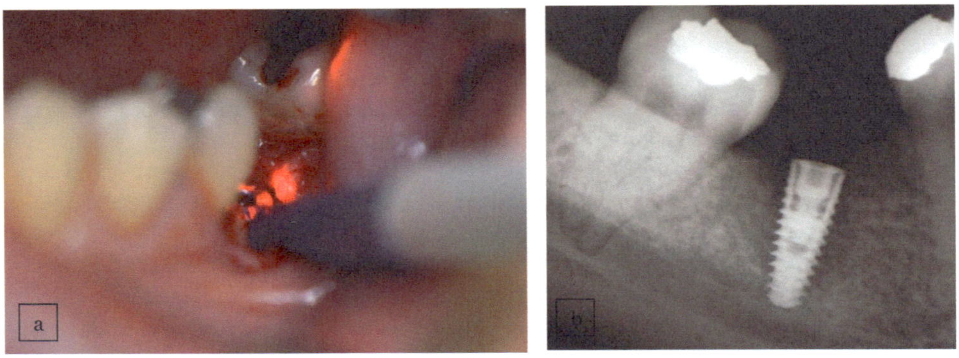

Figure 3.
Implant surface decontamination by performing laser therapy in the treatment of early peri-implantitis stage (LightWalker, Fotona, Slovenia) (a) implant radiography before laser therapy (b).

study on zirconium implants found that Er: YAG led to improvements in clinical parameters (PPD and BOP) six months after peri-implantitis surgery [82].

CO2 (carbon dioxide laser) and gallium-aluminum-arsenide lasers (one of the diode lasers) are introduced as safe methods for implant decontamination with antibacterial effects. Depending on implant surface topography, special attention should be taken considering the time of laser exposure, power, and irradiation mode (continues, CW, or pulse, PW, mode). *In vitro* study had shown that CO2 and diode laser with lower settings and at 810 nm wavelength could effectively destroy *P. gingivalis* on zirconium and titanium surfaces, whereas a higher setting of diode laser is required in order to eliminate *S. sanguis* and *P. gingivalis* adhered to zirconium surface [83]. Furthermore, diode laser of 810 nm and 4 W power showed a slight alteration on moderate roughness sandblasting implant surface compared to 3 W power laser settings [68]. On the polished and SLA implant surfaces, CO2 laser set in CW mode, up to 4 W, and diode laser set at 810 nm, CW mode, and 1 W–3 W showed no alteration [79], and thereby could be recommended as safe implant surface decontamination method in peri-implantitis treatment. To determine the influence of these recommended parameters on implant surface decontamination methods for different peri-implantitis stages and implant topographies, further experiments and clinical studies are required.

On the other hand, Nd: YAG lasers could induce surface alteration by causing surface melt and increasing its roughness. This type of laser is contraindicated for any dental implant surgical interventions. Application of diode lasers with other wavelengths or fiber systems should be used with special care as the laser light directly contacting the bone may cause thermal damage.

2.2.2 Photodynamic therapy assessment in peri-implantitis therapy

A novel antimicrobial treatment modality, photodynamic therapy (PDT) was introduced for the various oral infection treatments. The PDT mechanism is based on a suitable wavelength low-energy single-frequency diode laser activating a photoactive material (photosensitiser) that binds a target cell. In this mechanism, the photochemical oxygen-dependent reaction is induced producing very reactive superoxide radicals, such as single oxygen that causes photogenic species death.

Studies demonstrated the PDT efficiency in treating peri-implantitis with a particular emphasis on implant surfaces decontamination using the procedure (**Figure 4**).

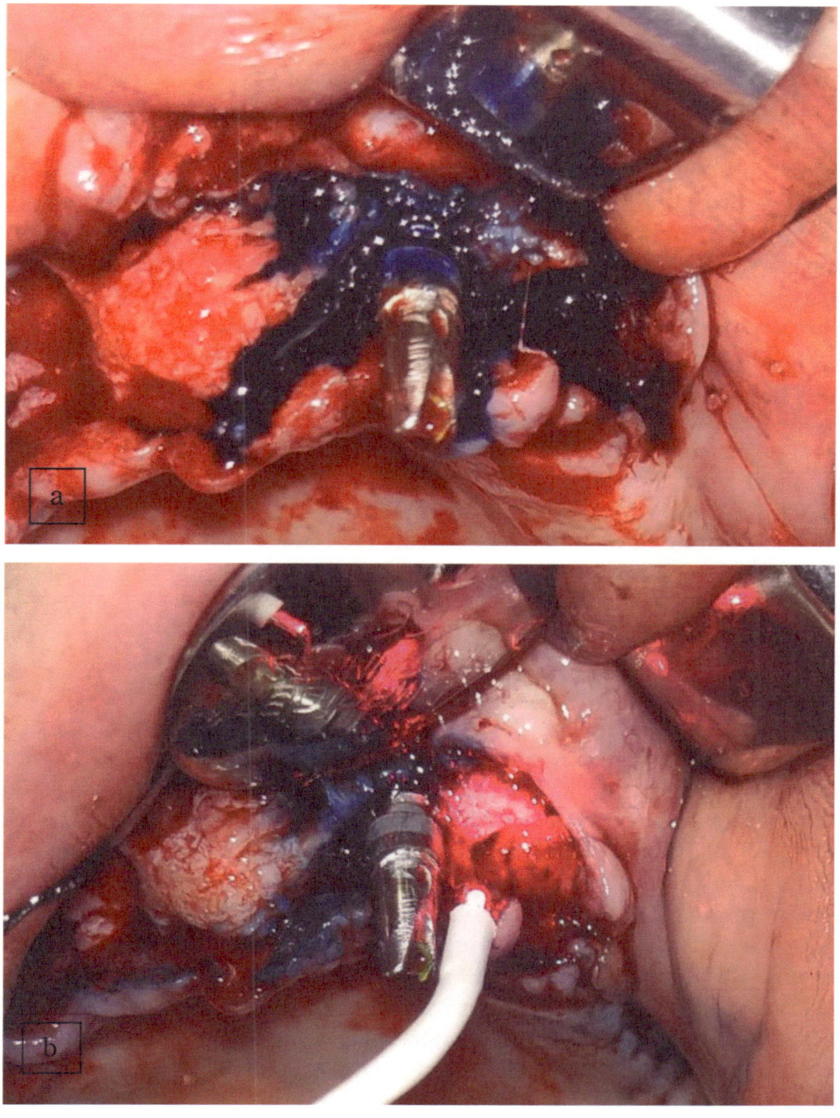

Figure 4.
Photodynamic therapy (HELBO, photodynamic systems GmbH, Bredent medical GmbH & Co KG) performed for implant surface decontamination during peri-implantitis surgery: Photosensitizer- phenothiazine chloride application (HELBO® blue photosensitizer) on implant surface and surrounding tissue (a) followed by diode laser irradiation with 2D fiber optic probe (b).

A few *in vitro* studies have demonstrated a reduction and elimination of bacteria from implant surfaces performing PDT [58, 60, 84, 85]. Haas et al. achieved a significant reduction in number of periodontopathogen bacteria (*P. gingivalis, P. intermedia* and *A. actinomycetemcomitans*) from machined, plasma-flame-sprayed, etched, and hydroxy-apatite-coated implant surfaces [85]. Other *in vitro* studies also showed a significant reduction in the total number of bacteria on titanium implants (Bredent, Sedan, Germany) [58], zirconium implants [84], and anodized rough implant surface (TiUnite, Nobel) without any implant surface changes. Considering implant topography on zirconium surfaces, PDT has revealed greater efficiency in eliminating a total number of bacteria compared to titanium surfaces [86].

In our previous clinical study, the positive effects of PDT on microbiological reduction and clinical outcomes improvement after peri-implantitis surgery were assessed three months postoperatively [57]. PDT proved to be a very effective decontamination method for various titanium implant surfaces according to the research. Additionally, the further follow-up observation aimed to show the maintenance results achieved by performing PDT, six and 12 months postoperatively. Patients' inclusion criteria, follow-up parameters and surgical treatment procedures have previously been reported in detail [57]. In brief, the surgical regenerative treatment procedure was performed on each patient with early or moderate peri-implantitis. During the surgery, after careful mucoperiosteal flap elevation, granulation tissue removal, patients were randomly divided into two groups. In one group (21 systemically healthy patients), PDT (HELBO, Photodynamic Systems GmbH, Wels, Austria) was performed for implant surface decontamination, while in another group (19 systemically healthy patients), CHX was used as a chemical decontamination method. Clinical and microbiological outcomes were used to assess treatment success. Microbiological samples were taken both from the pockets around the implant prior to any procedure and during follow-ups, and during surgical procedures before and immediately after surface decontamination. Samples were cultured and biochemically analyzed using standard procedures for anaerobic bacteria diagnosis. Detailed microbiological sample collecting and analyses were explained in the previous study [57]. The results were examined using SPSS 20.0.

Different pathogenic bacteria (**Table 1**) were isolated either from various examined implant surfaces (**Table 2**) during the surgical therapy or from the peri-implant pockets prior to any treatment. The presence of *S. aureus* on implant surfaces confirmed the earlier statements of bacteria affinity to colonize the titanium implant surface [41, 42]. This could emphasize the possible influence of *S. aureus* on the onset and progression of peri-implantitis. Furthermore, *C. albicans* was isolated from peri-implant pockets indicating a possible role of *Candida species* in peri-implantitis onset. This observation reported that mechanical implant surface decontamination followed by PDT along with regenerative surgical therapy successfully reduced pathogenic bacteria (**Table 1**) and improved clinical parameters in terms of PPD and BOP reduction three, six and 12 months postoperatively (**Table 3**). Similar clinical parameters' improvements and pathogen reduction in peri-implantitis treatment were recorded in other clinical and experimental studies [87–89]. Performing either PDT or titanium brushes combined with PDT for implant surface decontamination in *in vitro* study, *S. aureus* was successfully reduced from polished, SLA, and SLAactive implant surfaces [41].

One of the goals in peri-implantitis therapy is the total elimination of pathogens allowing the tissue to regenerate. As a final result, re-osseointegration is considered to be an essential outcome of peri-implantitis treatment that may be affected by different implant surface decontamination protocols. Experimental outcomes demonstrated partial peri-implant defect reconstruction and re-osseointegration after performing PDT for SLA implant surface decontamination combined with or without guide bone regeneration (GBR) and collagen membrane [90]. One of the earliest experimental studies evaluated the ability of PDT to re-osseointegrate peri-implantitis defects around a variety of implant surfaces utilizing GBR and polytetrafluoroethylene membrane [91]. Study results indicated that the TPS surface showed a greater re-osseointegration rate than HA

	T_0	S_1	S_2	T_1	T_2	T_3
P.g.	4 (14)	8 (29)	0 (0)[¥]	0 (0)[¥]	0 (0)	0 (0)
P.i.	5 (17.9)	6 (21.4)	0 (0)[¥]	0 (0)[¥]	0 (0)	0 (0)
P.s.	5 (17.9)	3 (10.7)	0 (0)[¥]	0 (0)[¥]	0 (0)[¥]	2 (7.1)
F.n.	1 (3.6)	4 (14.3)	0 (0)[¥]	0 (0)	0 (0)	0 (0)
A.n.	2 (7.1)	8 (29)	0 (0)[¥]	3 (10.7)	2 (10.7)	3 (10.7)
V.	9 (32.1)	9 (32.1)	2 (7.1)[¥]	2 (7.1) [¥]	5 (17.9)	7 (28)
S.a.	0 (0)	3 (10.7)	0 (0)	0 (0)	0 (0)	0 (0)
A.o.	1 (3.6)	0 (0)	0 (0)	3 (10.7)	3 (10.7)	2 (7.1)

[¥]Statistically significant change from baseline, three, six and 12 months after therapy, and also before and after implant surface decontamination during surgical procedure by Cochran Test, $p < 0.05$;
T_0 – isolated bacteria form peri-implant pocket before any treatment; T_1, T2, T3- isolated bacteria form peri-implant pocket three, six and 12 months postoperatively; S_1 and S_2– isolated bacteria from implant surface decontamination before and immediately after decontamination followed by PDT during surgical therapy;
P.g. - Porphyromonas gingivalis; P.i.- Prevotella intermedia; P.s. - Peptostreptococcus spp.; F.n.- Fusobacterium nucleatum; A.n.- A. naeslundii; V.- Veillonella spp.; S.a.- Staphylococcus aureus; A.o.- A. odontolyticus.

Table 1.
Number (n) of culture-positive implants at baseline and culture-negative after selected bacteria decontamination with photodynamic therapy.

Implant surface	Number (N)
Acid washed surface, MTX	10%
Titanium-oxide layer, TiUnit	47%
Osseospeed surface	16%
Machined polished surface	27%

Table 2.
Percentage of various implant topographies decontaminated by photodynamic therapy.

Parameter	Baseline	3 months	6 months	12 months	p-value
PPD (mm)	5.74 ± 1.55	3.26 ± 0.79	2.52 ± 0.92	2.52 ± 0.54	<0.001*
BOP	86 ± 19.5	0.67 ± 3.3	0.3 ± 1.1	0.67 ± 3.1	<0.001*

**Significant statistical difference measured before and after surgical therapy by T test;*

Table 3.
Mean pocket probing depth (PPD) ± SD, and mean bleeding on probing (BOP) for each implant at baseline and three, six and 12 months later.

implant surface. Based on these findings, PDT may have potential effects in peri-implantitis treatment with a potential to lead to re-osseointegration. Different bone grafts application in filling peri-implant defects might contribute to clinical outcomes improvement that may be an explanation for earlier interpreted clinical results.

Nevertheless, decontamination of implant surfaces aims to recreate the conditions that existed before infection or after the implant was placed and integrated. Hence, in order to achieve re-integration, and considering implant topography as well, both micro- and macro-design need to be almost identical to what existed before the implant was placed enhancing osteoblast stimulation and creating re-novel BIC. Accordingly, peri-implantitis requires special consideration in determining the appropriate decontamination methods since there are no standard treatment protocols. Consequently, more clinical trials are required to determine the efficacy of proposed decontamination methods for implant surfaces, with or without regenerative and resective methods.

3. Conclusion

Implant micro- and macro-design could be possible risk factors in peri-implantits onset or progression. Various implant surfaces may lead to peri-implantitis. In addition, choosing the right decontamination method could be influenced by the very implant surface. Mechanical methods coupled with PDT or a chemical method such as CHX and H_2O_2 may be effective in peri-implantitis treatment. Antibiotics administration in peri-implant treatment, on the other hand, must be taken with caution. Laser decontamination of implant surfaces is indicated provided that all parameters necessary for successful treatment are respected.

Conflict of interest

The authors declare no conflict of interest.

Author details

Dragana Rakašević[1]* and Dragana Gabrić[2,3]

1 Department of Periodontology and Oral Medicine, Faculty of Dental Medicine, University of Belgrade, Belgrade, Serbia

2 Department of Oral Surgery, School of Dental Medicine, University of Zagreb, Croatia

3 Clinical Hospital Center Zagreb, University Dental Clinic, Zagreb, Croatia

*Address all correspondence to: dr.rakasevic@gmail.com

References

[1] Albrektsson, T., et al., *Osseointegrated titanium implants. Requirements for ensuring a long-lasting, direct bone-to-implant anchorage in man.* Acta Orthop Scand, 1981. **52**(2): p. 155-70.

[2] Ryu, H.S., et al., *The influence of thread geometry on implant osseointegration under immediate loading: a literature review.* J Adv Prosthodont, 2014. **6**(6): p. 547-54.

[3] Albrektsson, T. and A. Wennerberg, *Oral implant surfaces: Part 1--review focusing on topographic and chemical properties of different surfaces and in vivo responses to them.* Int J Prosthodont, 2004. **17**(5): p. 536-43.

[4] Javed, F., et al., *Role of primary stability for successful osseointegration of dental implants: Factors of influence and evaluation.* Interv Med Appl Sci, 2013. **5**(4): p. 162-7.

[5] Wennerberg, A. and T. Albrektsson, *Effects of titanium surface topography on bone integration: a systematic review.* Clin Oral Implants Res, 2009. **20 Suppl 4**: p. 172-84.

[6] Novaes, A.B., Jr., et al., *Influence of implant surfaces on osseointegration.* Braz Dent J, 2010. **21**(6): p. 471-81.

[7] Schwarz, F., G. Iglhaut, and J. Becker, *Quality assessment of reporting of animal studies on pathogenesis and treatment of peri-implant mucositis and peri-implantitis. A systematic review using the ARRIVE guidelines.* J Clin Periodontol, 2012. **39 Suppl 12**: p. 63-72.

[8] Schwarz, F., et al., *Peri-implantitis.* J Periodontol, 2018. **89 Suppl 1**: p. S267-s290.

[9] Misch, C.E., M.W. Bidez, and M. Sharawy, *A bioengineered implant for a predetermined bone cellular response to loading forces. A literature review and case report.* J Periodontol, 2001. **72**(9): p. 1276-86.

[10] Berglundh, T., et al., *Peri-implant diseases and conditions: Consensus report of workgroup 4 of the 2017 World Workshop on the Classification of Periodontal and Peri-Implant Diseases and Conditions.* J Clin Periodontol, 2018. **45 Suppl 20**: p. S286-s291.

[11] Lang, N.P., T.G. Wilson, and E.F. Corbet, *Biological complications with dental implants: their prevention, diagnosis and treatment.* Clin Oral Implants Res, 2000. **11 Suppl 1**: p. 146-55.

[12] Mombelli, A., *Microbiology and antimicrobial therapy of peri-implantitis.* Periodontol 2000, 2002. **28**: p. 177-89.

[13] Heitz-Mayfield, L.J. and N.P. Lang, *Comparative biology of chronic and aggressive periodontitis vs. peri-implantitis.* Periodontol 2000, 2010. **53**: p. 167-81.

[14] Dalago, H.R., et al., *Risk indicators for Peri-implantitis. A cross-sectional study with 916 implants.* Clin Oral Implants Res, 2017. **28**(2): p. 144-150.

[15] Heitz-Mayfield, L.J., et al., *Group 4 ITI Consensus Report: Risks and biologic complications associated with implant dentistry.* Clin Oral Implants Res, 2018. **29 Suppl 16**: p. 351-358.

[16] Heitz-Mayfield, L.J.A., F. Heitz, and N.P. Lang, *Implant Disease Risk Assessment IDRA-a tool for preventing peri-implant disease.* Clin Oral Implants Res, 2020. **31**(4): p. 397-403.

[17] Mombelli, A., N. Muller, and N. Cionca, *The epidemiology of peri-implantitis.* Clin Oral Implants Res, 2012. **23 Suppl 6**: p. 67-76.

[18] Zandim-Barcelos, D.L., et al., *Implant-based factor as possible risk for peri-implantitis.* Braz Oral Res, 2019. **33**(suppl 1): p. e067.

[19] Abuhussein, H., et al., *The effect of thread pattern upon implant osseointegration.* Clin Oral Implants Res, 2010. **21**(2): p. 129-36.

[20] Misch and S. C.E., T. & Bidez, M.W., *Scientifific rationale for dental implant design*, in *Contemporary Implant Dentistry*, Misch and C.E., Editors. 2008: St Louis: Mosby. p. 200-229.

[21] Hansson, S. and M. Werke, *The implant thread as a retention element in cortical bone: the effect of thread size and thread profile: a finite element study.* J Biomech, 2003. **36**(9): p. 1247-58.

[22] Albrektsson, T., et al., *Statements from the Estepona consensus meeting on peri-implantitis, February 2-4, 2012.* Clin Implant Dent Relat Res, 2012. **14**(6): p. 781-2.

[23] Aguirre-Zorzano, L.A., et al., *Prevalence of peri-implant inflammatory disease in patients with a history of periodontal disease who receive supportive periodontal therapy.* Clin Oral Implants Res, 2014.

[24] Serino, G. and A. Turri, *Extent and location of bone loss at dental implants in patients with peri-implantitis.* J Biomech, 2011. **44**(2): p. 267-71.

[25] Dvorak, G., et al., *Peri-implantitis and late implant failures in postmenopausal women: a cross-sectional study.* J Clin Periodontol, 2011. **38**(10): p. 950-5.

[26] Korsch, M., U. Obst, and W. Walther, *Cement-associated peri-implantitis: a retrospective clinical observational study of fixed implant-supported restorations using a methacrylate cement.* Clin Oral Implants Res, 2014. **25**(7): p. 797-802.

[27] Linkevicius, T., et al., *Does residual cement around implant-supported restorations cause peri-implant disease? A retrospective case analysis.* Clin Oral Implants Res, 2013. **24**(11): p. 1179-84.

[28] Quesada-García, M.P., et al., *Dental Implant Stability Is Influenced by Implant Diameter and Localization and by the Use of Plasma Rich in Growth Factors.* Journal of Oral and Maxillofacial Surgery, 2012. **70**(12): p. 2761-2767.

[29] De Bruyn, H., et al., *Implant surface roughness and patient factors on long-term peri-implant bone loss.* Periodontology 2000, 2017. **73**(1): p. 218-227.

[30] Li, D., et al., *Biomechanical comparison of the sandblasted and acid-etched and the machined and acid-etched titanium surface for dental implants.* J Biomed Mater Res, 2002. **60**(2): p. 325-32.

[31] Zitzmann, N.U. and T. Berglundh, *Definition and prevalence of peri-implant diseases.* J Clin Periodontol, 2008. **35** (8 Suppl): p. 286-91.

[32] Polizzi, G., F. Gualini, and B. Friberg, *A two-center retrospective analysis of long-term clinical and radiologic data of TiUnite and turned implants placed in the same mouth.* Int J Prosthodont, 2013. **26**(4): p. 350-8.

[33] Albouy, J.P., et al., *Spontaneous progression of peri-implantitis at different types of implants. An experimental study in dogs. I: clinical and radiographic observations.* Clin Oral Implants Res, 2008. **19**(10): p. 997-1002.

[34] Albouy, J.P., et al., *Implant surface characteristics influence the outcome of treatment of peri-implantitis: an experimental study in dogs.* J Clin Periodontol, 2011. **38**(1): p. 58-64.

[35] Fickl, S., et al., *Experimental Peri-Implantitis around Different Types of Implants - A Clinical and Radiographic Study in Dogs.* Clin Implant Dent Relat Res, 2015. **17 Suppl 2**: p. e661-9.

[36] Susin, C., et al., *Safety and efficacy of a novel, gradually anodized dental implant surface: A study in Yucatan mini pigs.* Clinical Implant Dentistry and Related Research, 2019. **21**(S1): p. 44-54.

[37] Teughels, W., et al., *Effect of material characteristics and/or surface topography on biofilm development.* Clin Oral Implants Res, 2006. **17 Suppl 2**: p. 68-81.

[38] Weerkamp, A.H., et al., *The Role of Surface Free Energy in the Early In vivo Formation of Dental Plaque on Human Enamel and Polymeric Substrata.* Microbial Ecology in Health and Disease, 1989. **2**(1): p. 11-18.

[39] Conserva, E., et al., *Plaque accumulation on titanium disks with different surface treatments: an in vivo investigation.* Odontology, 2018. **106**(2): p. 145-153.

[40] Meza-Siccha, A.S., et al., *In Vitro Evaluation of Bacterial Adhesion and Bacterial Viability of Streptococcus mutans, Streptococcus sanguinis, and Porphyromonas gingivalis on the Abutment Surface of Titanium and Zirconium Dental Implants.* Int J Dent, 2019. **2019**: p. 4292976.

[41] Widodo, A., et al., *An in vitro study on disinfection of titanium surfaces.* Clinical Oral Implants Research, 2016. **27**(10): p. 1227-1232.

[42] Salvi, G.E., et al., *One-year bacterial colonization patterns of Staphylococcus aureus and other bacteria at implants and adjacent teeth.* Clin Oral Implants Res, 2008. **19**(3): p. 242-8.

[43] Leonhardt, A., S. Renvert, and G. Dahlen, *Microbial findings at failing implants.* Clin Oral Implants Res, 1999. **10**(5): p. 339-45.

[44] Souza, J.G.S., et al., *Biofilm Interactions of Candida albicans and Mitis Group Streptococci in a Titanium-Mucosal Interface Model.* Appl Environ Microbiol, 2020. **86**(9).

[45] Souza, J.G.S., et al., *Targeting implant-associated infections: titanium surface loaded with antimicrobial.* iScience, 2021. **24**(1): p. 102008.

[46] Ferraris, S. and S. Spriano, *Antibacterial titanium surfaces for medical implants.* Mater Sci Eng C Mater Biol Appl, 2016. **61**: p. 965-78.

[47] Koo, H., et al., *Targeting microbial biofilms: current and prospective therapeutic strategies.* Nat Rev Microbiol, 2017. **15**(12): p. 740-755.

[48] *Academy Report: Peri-Implant Mucositis and Peri-Implantitis: A Current Understanding of Their Diagnoses and Clinical Implications.* Journal of Periodontology, 2013. **84**(4): p. 436-443.

[49] Schwarz, F., et al., *Influence of different treatment approaches on non-submerged and submerged healing of ligature induced peri-implantitis lesions: an experimental study in dogs.* J Clin Periodontol, 2006. **33**(8): p. 584-95.

[50] Louropoulou, A., D.E. Slot, and F.A. Van der Weijden, *Titanium surface alterations following the use of different mechanical instruments: a systematic review.*

[51] Levin, L., et al., *Water jet with adjunct chlorhexidine gel for nonsurgical treatment of peri-implantitis.* Quintessence Int, 2014.

[52] Schwarz, F., et al., *Impact of the method of surface debridement and decontamination on the clinical outcome following combined surgical therapy of peri-implantitis: a randomized controlled clinical study.* J Clin Periodontol, 2011. **38**(3): p. 276-84.

[53] Carcuac, O., et al., *The effect of the local use of chlorhexidine in surgical treatment of experimental peri-implantitis in dogs.* J Clin Periodontol, 2014.

[54] Heitz-Mayfield, L.J., et al., *Anti-infective surgical therapy of peri-implantitis. A 12-month prospective clinical study.* Clin Oral Implants Res, 2012. **23**(2): p. 205-10.

[55] Valderrama, P. and T.G. Wilson, Jr., *Detoxification of implant surfaces affected by peri-implant disease: an overview of surgical methods.* Int J Dent, 2013. **2013**: p. 740680.

[56] Romanos, G.E., et al., *Lasers use in dental implantology.* Implant Dent, 2013. **22**(3): p. 282-8.

[57] Rakašević, D., et al., *Efficiency of photodynamic therapy in the treatment of peri-implantitis – A three-month randomized controlled clinical trial.* Srp Arh Celok Lek, 2016. **144**(9-10): p. 478-84.

[58] Azizi, B., et al., *Antimicrobial Efficacy of Photodynamic Therapy and Light-Activated Disinfection Against Bacterial Species on Titanium Dental Implants.* Int J Oral Maxillofac Implants, 2018. **33**(4): p. 831-837.

[59] de Waal, Y.C., et al., *Implant decontamination during surgical peri-implantitis treatment: a randomized, double-blind, placebo-controlled trial.* J Clin Periodontol, 2013. **40**(2): p. 186-95.

[60] Marotti, J., et al., *Decontamination of dental implant surfaces by means of photodynamic therapy.* Lasers Med Sci, 2013. **28**(1): p. 303-9.

[61] Louropoulou, A., D.E. Slot, and F. Van der Weijden, *The effects of mechanical instruments on contaminated titanium dental implant surfaces: a systematic review.* Clin Oral Implants Res, 2014. **25**(10): p. 1149-60.

[62] Mengel, R., et al., *An in vitro study of the treatment of implant surfaces with different instruments.* Int J Oral Maxillofac Implants, 1998. **13**(1): p. 91-6.

[63] Louropoulou, A., D.E. Slot, and F.A. Van der Weijden, *Titanium surface alterations following the use of different mechanical instruments: a systematic review.* Clin Oral Implants Res, 2012. **23**(6): p. 643-658.

[64] Schwarz, F., et al., *Influence of plaque biofilm removal on reestablishment of the biocompatibility of contaminated titanium surfaces.* J Biomed Mater Res A, 2006. **77**(3): p. 437-44.

[65] Fox, S.C., J.D. Moriarty, and R.P. Kusy, *The effects of scaling a titanium implant surface with metal and plastic instruments: an in vitro study.* J Periodontol, 1990. **61**(8): p. 485-90.

[66] Karring, E.S., et al., *Treatment of peri-implantitis by the Vector system.* Clin Oral Implants Res, 2005. **16**(3): p. 288-93.

[67] Louropoulou, A., D.E. Slot, and F. Van der Weijden, *Influence of mechanical instruments on the biocompatibility of titanium dental implants surfaces: a systematic review.* Clin Oral Implants Res, 2015. **26**(7): p. 841-50.

[68] Lollobrigida, M., et al., *The Prevention of Implant Surface Alterations in the Treatment of Peri-Implantitis: Comparison of Three Different Mechanical and Physical Treatments.* Int J Environ Res Public Health, 2020. **17**(8).

[69] de Tapia, B., et al., *The adjunctive effect of a titanium brush in implant surface decontamination at peri-implantitis surgical regenerative interventions: A randomized controlled clinical trial.* J Clin Periodontol, 2019. **46**(5): p. 586-596.

[70] Ratka, C., et al., *The Effect of In Vitro Electrolytic Cleaning on Biofilm-Contaminated Implant Surfaces.* J Clin Med, 2019. **8**(9).

[71] Schwarz, F., et al., *Surgical therapy of advanced ligature-induced peri-implantitis defects: cone-beam computed tomographic and histological analysis.* J Clin Periodontol, 2011. **38**(10): p. 939-49.

[72] Souza, J.G.S., et al., *Dose-response effect of chlorhexidine on a multispecies oral biofilm formed on pure titanium and on a titanium-zirconium alloy.* Biofouling, 2018. **34**(10): p. 1175-1184.

[73] de Waal, Y.C., et al., *Implant decontamination with 2% chlorhexidine during surgical peri-implantitis treatment: a randomized, double-blind, controlled trial.* Clin Oral Implants Res, 2014.

[74] Giannelli, M., et al., *Effect of chlorhexidine digluconate on different cell types: a molecular and ultrastructural investigation.* Toxicol In Vitro, 2008. **22**(2): p. 308-17.

[75] Carcuac, O., et al., *Adjunctive Systemic and Local Antimicrobial Therapy in the Surgical Treatment of Peri-implantitis: A Randomized Controlled Clinical Trial.* J Dent Res, 2016. **95**(1): p. 50-7.

[76] Myers, T.D., W.D. Myers, and R.M. Stone, *First soft tissue study utilizing a pulsed Nd:YAG dental laser.* Northwest Dent, 1989. **68**(2): p. 14-7.

[77] Schwarz, F., et al., *Influence of different treatment approaches on the removal of early plaque biofilms and the viability of SAOS2 osteoblasts grown on titanium implants.* Clin Oral Investig, 2005. **9**(2): p. 111-7.

[78] Schwarz, F., et al., *Influence of implant bed preparation using an Er:YAG laser on the osseointegration of titanium implants: a histomorphometrical study in dogs.* J Oral Rehabil, 2007. **34**(4): p. 273-81.

[79] Stubinger, S., et al., *Surface alterations of polished and sandblasted and acid-etched titanium implants after Er:YAG, carbon dioxide, and diode laser irradiation.* Int J Oral Maxillofac Implants, 2010. **25**(1): p. 104-11.

[80] Schwarz, F., et al., *Four-year follow-up of combined surgical therapy of advanced peri-implantitis evaluating two methods of surface decontamination.* J Clin Periodontol, 2013. **40**(10): p. 962-7.

[81] Schwarz, F., et al., *Combined surgical therapy of advanced peri-implantitis evaluating two methods of surface decontamination: a 7-year follow-up observation.* J Clin Periodontol, 2017. **44**(3): p. 337-342.

[82] Schwarz, F., et al., *Non-surgical treatment of peri-implant mucositis and peri-implantitis at zirconia implants: a prospective case series.* J Clin Periodontol, 2015. **42**(8): p. 783-788.

[83] Hauser-Gerspach, I., S. Stübinger, and J. Meyer, *Bactericidal effects of different laser systems on bacteria adhered to dental implant surfaces: an in vitro study comparing zirconia with titanium.* Clinical

Oral Implants Research, 2010. **21**(3): p. 277-283.

[84] Azizi, B., et al., *Antimicrobial efficacy of photodynamic therapy and light-activated disinfection on contaminated zirconia implants: An in vitro study.* Photodiagnosis Photodyn Ther, 2018. **21**: p. 328-333.

[85] Haas, R., et al., *Elimination of bacteria on different implant surfaces through photosensitization and soft laser. An in vitro study.* Clin Oral Implants Res, 1997. **8**(4): p. 249-54.

[86] Gabrić, D., et al., *Evaluation of the Antimicrobial Efficacy of Different Types of Photodynamic Therapy on the Main Pathogenic Bacteria of Peri-Implantitis*. 2020.

[87] Dortbudak, O., et al., *Lethal photosensitization for decontamination of implant surfaces in the treatment of peri-implantitis.* Clin Oral Implants Res, 2001. **12**(2): p. 104-8.

[88] Wang, H., et al., *Adjunctive photodynamic therapy improves the outcomes of peri-implantitis: a randomized controlled trial.* Aust Dent J, 2019. **64**(3): p. 256-262.

[89] Hayek, R.R., et al., *Comparative study between the effects of photodynamic therapy and conventional therapy on microbial reduction in ligature-induced peri-implantitis in dogs.* J Periodontol, 2005. **76**(8): p. 1275-81.

[90] Ramos, U.D., et al., *Comparison between two antimicrobial protocols with or without guided bone regeneration in the treatment of peri-implantitis. A histomorphometric study in dogs.* Clin Oral Implants Res, 2017. **28**(11): p. 1388-1395.

[91] Shibli, J.A., et al., *Treatment of ligature-induced peri-implantitis by lethal photosensitization and guided bone regeneration: a preliminary histologic study in dogs.* J Periodontol, 2003. **74**(3): p. 338-45.

Chapter 13

Peri-Implantitis Revisited

Amer Shatta and Sukumaran Anil

Abstract

Dental implants have become a well-accepted treatment option for patients with partial or complete edentulism. The long-term success of the endosseous dental implant depends not only on osseointegration, but on the healthy soft tissue interface that surrounds the implant. Peri-implantitis is defined as an inflammatory process affecting the supporting hard and soft tissue around an implant in function, leading to loss of supporting bone. Peri-implant mucositis has been defined as a reversible inflammatory reaction in the peri-implant mucosa surrounding an osseointegrated dental implant. Peri-implant mucositis is assumed to precede peri-implantitis. Data indicate that patients diagnosed with peri-implant mucositis may develop peri-implantitis, especially in the absence of regular maintenance care. However, the features or conditions characterizing the progression from peri-implant mucositis to peri-implantitis in susceptible patients have not been identified. The most common etiological factors associated with the development of peri-implantitis are the presence of bacterial plaque and host response. The risk factors associated with peri-implant bone loss include smoking combined with IL-1 genotype polymorphism, a history of periodontitis, poor compliance with treatment and oral hygiene practices, the presence of systemic diseases affecting healing, cement left behind following cementation of the crowns, lack of keratinized gingiva, and previous history of implant failure There is strong evidence that there is an increased risk of developing peri-implantitis in patients who have a history of severe periodontitis, poor plaque control, and no regular maintenance care after implant therapy. Management of peri-implantitis generally works on the assumption that there is a primary microbial etiology. Furthermore, it is assumed that micro-organisms and/or their by-products lead to infection of the surrounding tissues and subsequent destruction of the alveolar bone surrounding an implant. A combination of surgical, open debridement, and antimicrobial treatment has been advocated for the treatment of peri-implantitis. Surgical intervention is required once a patient has bleeding on probing, greater than 5 mm of probing depth, and severe bone loss beyond that expected with remodeling. Access flaps require full-thickness elevation of the mucoperiosteum, facilitating debridement and decontamination of the implant surface *via* hand instruments, ultrasonic tips, or lasers. When necessary, surgical procedures may be used in conjunction with detoxification of the implant surface by mechanical devices, such as high-pressure air powder abrasion or laser.

Keywords: dental implant, peri-implant disease, peri-implant mucositis, peri-implantitis, periodontitis, risk factors

1. Introduction

Dental implants have become a well-accepted treatment option for patients with partial or complete edentulism. The long-term success of the endosseous dental implant depends not only on osseointegration, but on the healthy soft tissue interface that surrounds the implant [1]. Dental implants are susceptible to disease, and they might develop inflammatory reactions, which might lead to peri-implant mucositis and/or peri-implantitis.

Peri-implant disease progresses quietly without pain and often starts with marginal bone loss. The factors responsible can be broadly classified as biological factors and biomechanical factors. The biological factors include progressive bone loss, bacterial infections, and microbial plaque [2]. Biological complications are grouped as early biological failures and late implant failures. The early failures are applied to inappropriate aseptic measures of the surgical implant [3], and late complications are typically infections caused by peri-implantitis and bacterial plaque. Peri-implantitis due to biomechanical factors are either prosthesis-related factors such as occlusal overload, residual cement, inadequate prosthetic placement, or inappropriate abutment angle and bruxism [4].

2. Definitions

2.1 Peri-implant mucositis

Peri-implant mucositis is defined as inflammation of the peri-implant mucosa around an osseointegrated implant without loss of the supporting bone. Clinical signs of peri-implant inflammation are bleeding and/or suppuration on probing, with or without increased probing depths [5, 6].

2.2 Peri-implantitis

Peri-implantitis is defined as a pathological condition characterized by inflammation in the peri-implant mucosa/connective tissue and progressive loss of the supporting bone around a dental implant. Clinical signs of peri-implantitis are bleeding and/or suppuration on probing, increasing probing depths, and/or recession of the mucosal margin, in addition to radiographic bone loss compared to previous examinations. When a previous radiograph is not available, the following is indicative for the diagnosis of peri-implantitis: bone loss >3 mm in combination with bleeding on probing and pocket depth > 6 mm [5].

3. Diagnosis of peri-implantitis

The advanced case of peri-implantitis can be identifiable with the evidence of radiographic bone loss, mobility, and clinical signs of infection. The challenge is to diagnose the early stage of peri-implantitis that will aid in the prevention of further bone resorption and subsequent loss of the implant. Diagnosing peri-implant diseases using periodontal probing and radiographs may be inaccurate and only provides a historical record of past disease rather than current disease activity (**Figure 1**).

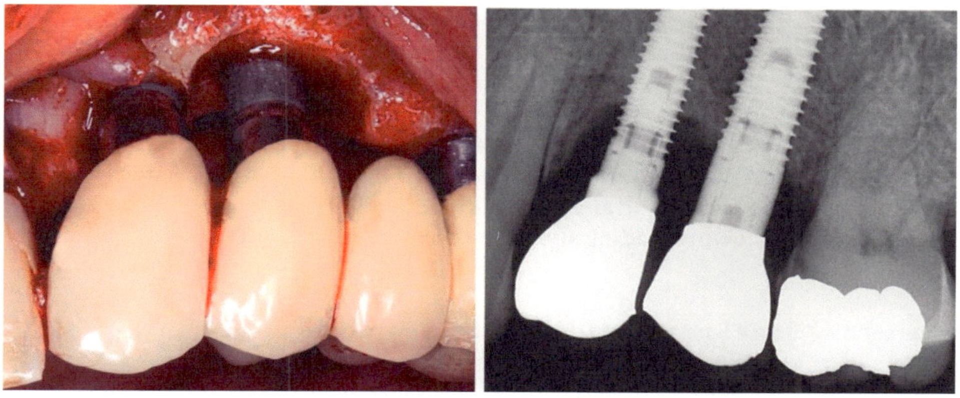

Figure 1.
The clinical and radiographic appearance of peri-implantitis.

Some of the clinical parameters used for the diagnosis are as follows [7]:

- Vertical destruction of the crestal bone,
- Formation of a peri-implant pocket >4 mm,
- Bleeding or suppuration after gently probing,
- Tissue redness and swelling,
- Mobility.

Developing biomarker technologies may offer possibilities in the diagnostic application. Although more research is needed, the assessment of proinflammatory cytokines (IL-1β, TNFα, MMP-8) in the peri-implant crevicular fluid may be of value to diagnose peri-implantitis and peri-implant mucositis but are, at this time, inappropriate to predict peri-implantitis because of the limited evidence of controlled longitudinal clinical trials. MMP-8 is a promising biomarker as an early signal of peri-implant inflammation [8]. Commercially available chair-side diagnostic tests for MMP-8 to detect peri-implant diseases are promising. Elevated levels of MMP-8 in peri-implant crevicular fluid (PICF) are associated with peri-implant inflammation, while low MMP-8 levels (<20 ng/mL) indicate healthy peri-implant tissues. Pathologically elevated levels of MMP-8 (>20 ng/mL) can be detected by a quantitative MMP-8 chair-side device, ImplantSafe® [9].

4. Classification peri-implantitis

Currently, there is no standard classification system to classify the parameters and the severity of the peri-implant disease. Froum and Rosen [10] proposed a classification for peri-implant disease based on the disease severity. This classification includes three clinical stages:

Early: Pocket depth (PD) $\geq$ 4 mm (bleeding and/or suppuration on probing) Bone loss <25% of the implant length.

Moderate: PD ≥ 6 mm (bleeding and/or suppuration on probing) bone loss 25–50% of the implant length.

Advanced: PD ≥ 8 mm (bleeding and/or suppuration on probing) bone loss >50% of the implant length.

Bleeding on probing should be noted on two or more aspects of the implant, and bone loss is measured on the radiographs from the time of prosthetic loading to the current time. If the radiograph at prosthetic loading is not available, the earliest available radiograph following loading should be used [11].

5. Pattern of bone loss in peri-implantitis

The pattern of bone loss in peri-implantitis is classified into vertical, horizontal, and combined bone loss. The most common pattern of bone loss is vertical (65%) and then horizontal (22%), and the least common pattern is combined (13%) [11].

6. Prevalence of peri-implantitis

The prevalence of peri-implant mucositis and peri-implantitis has ranged from 19 to 65% and 1 to 47%, respectively [12, 13]. A systematic review revealed that the frequency of peri-implant mucositis was 63.4% on the patient level and 30.7% on the implant level. The peri-implantitis prevalence was 18.8 and 9.6%. In smokers, the frequency of peri-implantitis increased to 36.3% [11]. The prevalence of peri-implant mucositis at the patient level varied between 1.1 and 80% [14–19]. The prevalence of peri-implantitis at the patient level ranged from 1.4 to 53.3% [14, 15, 17–26].

7. Etiology of peri-implantitis

Peri-implantitis is a result of biofilm-induced inflammation in the soft tissue that subsequently triggers a host response, with possible tissue degradation [27]. Peri-implantits inflammation is initiated by the accumulated bacterial biofilm. The development of disease was initially studied in an experimental gingivitis model in animals (dogs) and humans, and a cause-effect relationship between *de novo* plaque formation and peri-implant mucositis was observed [28, 29].

Histopathological, the early biofilm-induced inflammatory host response in mucositis is comparable to that in gingivitis, but the lesion of the inflammatory connective tissue (ICT) is larger and extends apically to the junctional epithelium. The established biofilm results in a more pronounced host response, and the extension of the ICT lesion is even larger in size than that in gingivitis, with the increased amounts of inflammatory cells in peri-implant mucositis [30]. The inflammation is reversible after biofilm removal, and no difference between implant systems has been observed [29, 31, 32]. Peri-implantitis lesions investigated in experimental ligature-induced peri-implantitis in a dog model presented more aggressive tissue degradation at the implant site than teeth with periodontitis. A larger inflammatory infiltrate extending close to the crestal bone and more bone-resorbing osteoclasts were observed at the implant site. Spontaneous progression after ligature removal varied with different implant surfaces [33, 34]. Peri-implant inflammation develops when microbes activate the host's innate and adaptive immune responses. Several cell types, such as epithelial cells, fibroblasts, stromal cells, endothelial cells, and osteoblasts, release pro-inflammatory mediators, such as cytokines and chemokines, to recruit leukocytes. Leukocytes are recruited from blood vessels and tissues. Human biopsies revealed that the proportion of vascular structures was smaller within the peri-implant ICT lesion and greater lateral to the peri-implant ICT than reported for periodontitis lesions. Neutrophil granulocytes (polymorphonuclear neutrophils [PMNs]) and monocytes/macrophages are prevalent close to the sulcus epithelium in the peri-vascular area and the center of the ICT. Although the ICT lesion is dominated by T and B lymphocytes and plasma cells, the inflammatory lesion has a more acute character in peri-implantitis than in chronic periodontitis, with a larger proportion of PMNs and macrophages [35–37].

8. Risk factors associated with peri-implantitis

8.1 Poor plaque control and lack of regular supportive therapy

Poor plaque control and a lack of regular supportive therapy constitute the risk factors for developing peri-implantitis. A 5-year follow-up revealed a lower incidence of peri-implantitis with regular supportive care [20]. A 10-year follow-up study also revealed that patients on a regular maintenance program had less chances of developing peri-implantitis [38].

8.2 History of periodontitis

Patients who have lost teeth from periodontitis are treated with implants, and these patients may be more at risk of peri-implantitis disease. There is strong evidence from longitudinal and cross-sectional studies that a history of periodontitis constitutes a risk factor for peri-implantitis. Systematic reviews have indicated that subjects with a history of periodontitis are at greater risk of peri-implant disease. Long-term follow-up studies also revealed a correlation between peri-implantitis development with periodontitis [38–40].

8.3 Genetic traits

Genetic trait studies are scarce, and the overall evidence is limited and inconclusive. The most thoroughly investigated genetic factor is interleukin (IL)-1 composite gene polymorphism [41]. The genetic traits can influence susceptibility to peri-implantitis development in periodontitis patients, even if the inflammatory condition is under control at the time of implant placement. IL-1RN gene polymorphism was proposed as a risk factor for peri-implantitis [42]. The IL-1 genotype in combination with smoking was observed to affect implant failure [43]. The vascular endothelial growth factor (VEGF) may play a protective role in marginal bone loss, that is, peri-implantitis [36].

8.4 Diabetes mellitus

Based on the available data, no association was found between diabetes and peri-implantitis. Although the role of distinct physiological mediators in pathogenesis is not fully understood, evidence suggests that pro-inflammatory gene expression in peri-implantitis regions is affected by glycemic control [44]. Patients with diabetes mellitus are more prone to peri-implantitis than non-diabetic subjects, and the poor metabolic control has been shown to provide a more favorable environment for infection and loss of implants [45]. Controlling the blood sugar level is critical in increasing the implant success rate in diabetic patients [46].

8.5 Smoking

Smoking has a detrimental effect on tissue healing. Nicotine can reduce the nutrition to the tissues as a result of its vasoconstrictive effect on the blood vessels during the early osseointegration phase. Based on the available studies, smoking can be considered as a greatest identifiable risk factor for peri-implantitis. The extent of osseointegration as well as the plaque accumulation around dental implants was compromised among csmokers. A 10-year cohort study reported that peri-implantitis developed for 28% of all implants in smokers, while the corresponding incidence was 6% of all implants in non-smokers [39]. Several cross-sectional studies also showed a higher prevalence of peri-implantitis among smokers [15, 47, 48]. A systematic review of prospective and retrospective studies indicated an enhanced risk of biological complications among smokers; similarly, a meta-analysis indicated an enhanced risk of implant failure among smokers [49]. Studies indicate smoking as the greatest identifiable and most often cited risk.

8.6 Keratinized mucosa

Compared to sites with a keratinized mucosa of greater than 2 mm, sites with a keratinized mucosa of less than 2 mm are associated with plaque accumulation followed by peri-implant inflammation in the soft tissue and radiographic bone loss [50]. The evidence is limited and controversial that the absence of a keratinized mucosa is a risk factor for peri-implantitis, but this factor may negatively affect self-performed oral hygiene (**Figure 2**) [50].

8.7 Excess cement and over-contoured supra-structures

Potential risk indicators that are indirectly related to plaque accumulation have been proposed; for example, constructions with excess cement may result in a higher prevalence of peri-implantitis than screw-retained constructions [51]; similar results were

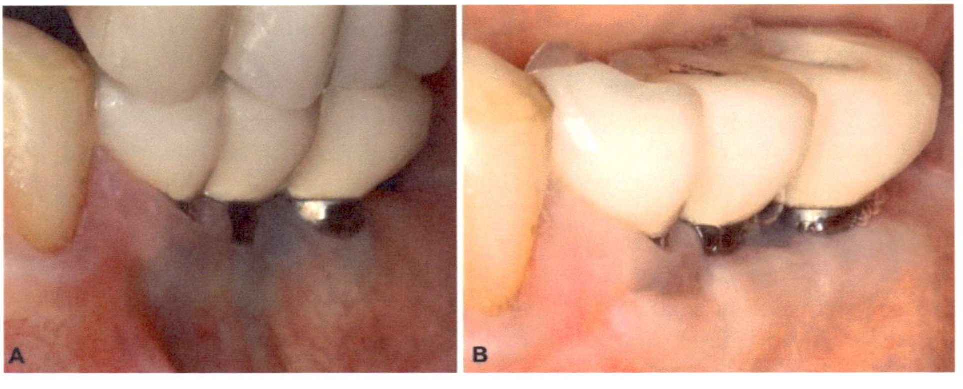

Figure 2.
A. Case showing lack of keratinized gingiva in the implant site. B. After gingival augmentation.

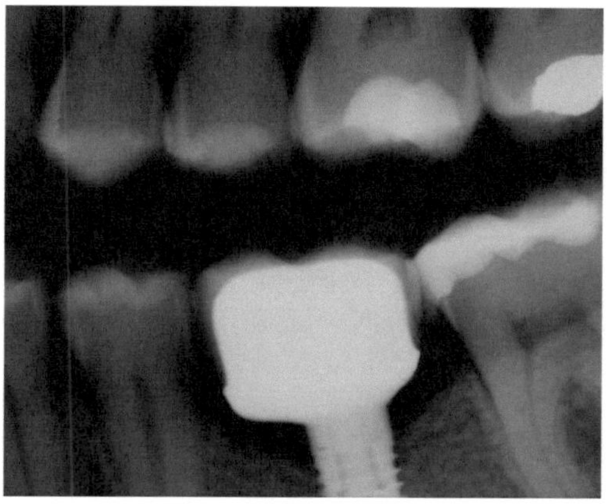

Figure 3.
A case of peri-implantitis consequent to over-contoured restoration.

reported for over contoured crowns and supra-structures [52]. A wide emergence profile in the restoration contour was reported to cause an unhealthy state (**Figure 3**) [53].

8.8 Implant-related factors

The titanium particles from the implant surface may be present in the tissues after implant placement and may enhance infection-induced inflammation and activate macrophages [54]. Implant surface characteristics vary in terms of topography, surface roughness, and chemical composition. Currently, most implants have a moderately rough surface with improved bone responses during initial healing after implant placement [55]. Marginal bone loss was found to be greater when implants with rough surfaces were used, and turned surfaces generally demonstrated the smallest marginal bone loss [56, 57].

8.8.1 Implant platform switching

The platform switch concept might influence the marginal bone loss. The theory is that the micro-gap is displaced medially causing less bone loss (**Figure 4**) [58–60].

8.8.2 Implant installation

It is advisable to have a minimum thickness of 2-mm bone in the anterior region and at least 1 mm in the posterior region to reduce soft and hard tissue loss. The quality of bone in the region of implant placement is an important factor for the success [61].

8.9 Overload

Clinical signs of occlusal overloads, such as abutment fracture, loss of retention and/or signs of abrasive forces on supra-structures, seem to be an indirect but potential risk. The factors related to occlusal overload are probably related to the location of the implant, the deviation of the axis of the implant, and the incompatibility of the implant dimensions and the prosthesis. Occlusal overload can lead to bone loss around the osseo-integrated implants [4]. However, the evidence is limited concerning overload and its influence on the onset or progression of peri-implantitis [41, 62]. In a dog model, occlusal overload did not induce marginal bone loss in implants with a healthy mucosa [63].

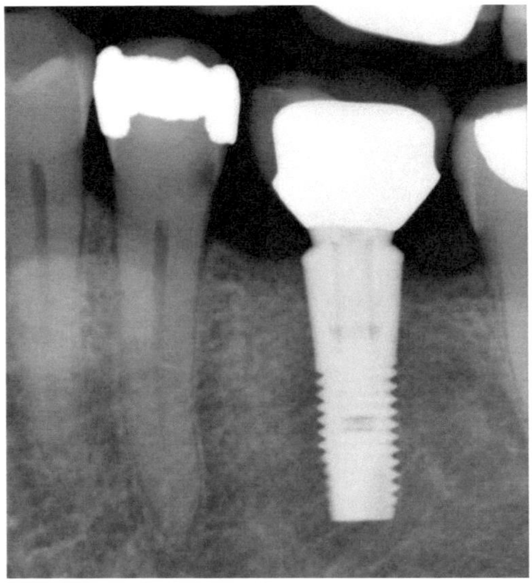

Figure 4.
Platform switching to prevent marginal bone loss and peri-implantitis.

8.10 Parafunctional habits-bruxism

Bruxism is a movement disorder of the masticatory system that is characterized among others by teeth grinding and clenching during sleep as well as during wakefulness. Since there is no periodontal ligament between the implant and surrounding bone, the occlusal load is directly transmitted [64]. Even though bruxism is likely to be a risk factor for mechanical complications in the implant periphery, it is unlikely to be a potential risk factor for biological complications [65].

8.11 Alcohol consumption

Alcohol consumption was investigated in one prospective study, which showed that an intake of more than 10 g of alcohol per day was related to peri-implantitis bone loss, as well as tobacco use, plaque, and inflammation [66].

8.12 Iatrogenic factors

The proposed potential risk of iatrogenic factors for the initiation and progression of peri-implantitis caused by implant mal-positioning, surgical trauma, and inadequate restoration abutment seating has not yet been clearly investigated [67].

9. Treatment

9.1 Treatment of peri-implant mucositis

The main goal is to detoxify the contaminated implant surface. Peri-implant mucositis can be managed by non-surgical methods. Methods such as mechanical implant cleaning with titanium or plastic curettes, ultrasonics, or air polishing can be used. Photodynamic therapy as well as local antiseptic medication such as chlorhexidine gluconate, hydrogen peroxide, sodium percarbonate, and povidone-iodine can be used [68–70].

9.2 Treatment of peri-implantitis

The management of peri-implantitis relies on strategies of disinfection such as debridement with curettes and use of local/systemic broad-spectrum antibiotics associated or not with anti-infective solutions, such as used for chemical plaque control. The strategy is to disinfect and to reduce the inflammation as well as restoration of the peri-implant tissue lost due to the disease progression, usually with regenerative approaches using biologics and/or growth factors. The treatment of peri-implant infections comprises conservative and surgical approaches. Depending on the severity of the peri-implant disease, either a nonsurgical therapy alone or a combined with the surgical method can be used to resolve the situation.

9.3 Non-surgical therapy

Manual treatment approaches using curettes, ultrasonic and air polishing systems, laser-supported, and photodynamic therapy are used along with medications.

9.4 Mechanical therapy

The bleeding from the site can be controlled either with piezoelectric scalers as well as with hand instruments [71]. The manual curetting of the area can be done using special curettes made of Teflon, carbon, plastic, and titanium curettes than the conventional curettes to protect the implant surfaces [72, 73]. The efficiency of the ultrasonic curettage can be supplemented with the air polishing systems [74–77]. Though the abrasive air polishing medium can modify the surface of implants, the cell response and healing were compromised probably due to the contamination of the implant surface [74, 76]. The extent of re-osseointegration of titanium implants after air polishing therapy has been reported between 39 and 46% with increased clinical implant attachment and pocket depth reduction [75]. The air polishing systems such as hydroxylapatite/tricalcium phosphate, hydroxylapatite, glycine, titanium dioxide, water and air, phosphoric acid can be used depending on the surface topography of implants [74, 77].

9.5 Decontamination of the surface of the implant

Decontamination of the root surface is done by various methods such as air powder flow, saline wash, citric acid, laser, and hydrogen peroxide [78]. The electrochemical decontamination of the surface of the implant is an innovative technique that is being tested in preclinical studies [79]. Rubber cups have been shown to smoothen the titanium surface and significantly decrease roughness by removing surface debris. Polishing the implant surfaces with pumice and a rubber cup combined with irrigation with chlorhexidine and systemic antibiotics results in the reduction of anaerobic bacteria and bleeding scores in patients with peri-implantitis [80].

9.6 Laser therapy

Laser treatment using CO_2, diode-, Er:YAG- (erbium-doped: yttrium-aluminum-garnet), and Er, Cr: YSGG- (erbium, chromium-doped:

yttrium-scandium-gallium-garnet) lasers are used in the treatment of peri-implant diseases [81, 82]. The use of Er:YAG lasers showed significantly better results than mechanical methods in terms of bleeding at peri-implantitis [83]. Er:YAG and Er, Cr: YAG with a wavelength of 3 microns can reduce biofilms up to 90%, but in contrast to most mechanical therapies, any biological compatibilities and cell stimulatory properties cannot be re-induced [84]. The CO_2 excimer laser was effective in reducing the anaerobic bacteria [85].

9.7 Photodynamic therapy

Photodynamic therapy has to be considered as an additional treatment option in peri-implantitis. Photodynamic therapy generates reactive oxygen species by multiplicity with help of a high-energy single-frequency light in combination with photosensitizers. In a wavelength range of 580–1400 nm and toluidine blue-concentrations between 10 and 50 μg/mL, photodynamic therapy generates bactericide effects against aerobic and anaerobic bacteria such as *Aggregatibacter actinomycetemcomitans*, *Porphyromonas gingivalis*, *Prevotella intermedia*, *Streptococcus mutans*, *Enterococcus faecalis* [86, 87]. An improvement in both clinical attachment and the bleeding index was observed on a moderate and severe peri-implantitis with phototherapy [88]. Photodynamic therapy has been tried as an adjunctive to manual debridement and local chemotherapeutic agents [89].

9.8 Surgical therapy

Surgical techniques may include open flap debridement with removal of the inflammatory tissue as well as mechanical and chemical decontamination of the exposed implant surface. Recontouring of the bony architecture and smoothing of the implant surface may improve infection control [90]. The surgical flap helps in comprehensive debridement and decontamination of the affected implant. The surgical resection is generally confined to implants placed in non-esthetic sites [91].

9.9 Regenerative approaches

Regenerative procedures using a membrane and bone graft substitutes attempting to partially fill the bony defects caused by peri-implantitis can be successful [92].

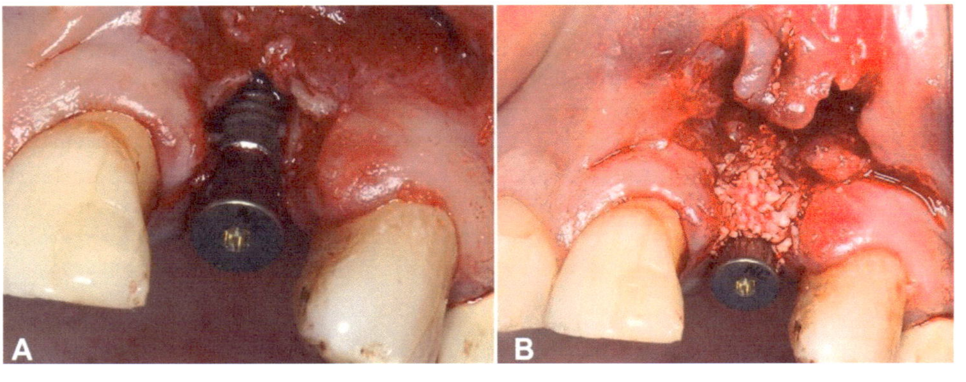

Figure 5.
A case of peri-implantitis treated with bone augmentation.

Therapy of peri-implantitis followed by regular supportive care resulted in favorable clinical improvements and stable peri-implant bone levels in the majority of patients according to a systematic review (**Figure 5**) [93].

9.10 Resective therapy

Resective surgery has been shown to be effective in the reduction of BOP, probing depths and clinical signs of inflammation. The basic principles include the elimination of the peri-implant osseous defect using ostectomy and osteoplasty as well as bacterial decontamination. Additionally, smoothening and polishing of the supracrestal implant surface may be done. Surgical pocket elimination and bone recontouring in combination with plaque control before and after surgery showed effective in treating peri-implantitis [94].

10. Prevention and maintenance

Besides, a maintenance program with regular evaluation of the peri-implant probing depths, supportive professional implant cleaning, and oral hygiene training should be an integral part of every post-operative care after implant insertion [95]. The establishment of an adequate oral hygiene should, therefore, be considered as the key issue of the prevention of peri-implantitis infections.

11. Conclusion

Peri-implantitis is an inflammatory disease of microbial origin causing bone loss around the implant, which could lead to the loss of the implant. The etiology of peri-implantitis is associated with a complex microbial biofilm and risk factors such as smoking and diabetes. Occlusal overloading, osteoporosis, and other factors compromising the surgical site might adversely affect the severity of the destruction of the peri-implant tissue. Several surgical and non-surgical therapeutic approaches have been proposed to manage this complex-multifactorial condition. Anti-infective and regenerative therapeutic strategies were used to restore the peri-implant health as well as to achieve new bone-to-implant contact.

Conflict of interest

The authors declare no conflict of interest.

Author details

Amer Shatta[1*] and Sukumaran Anil[1,2]

1 Department of Dentistry, Oral Health Institute, Hamad Medical Corporation, Doha, Qatar

2 College of Dental Medicine, Qatar University, Doha, Qatar

*Address all correspondence to: ashatta@hamad.qa

References

[1] Bouri A Jr, Bissada N, Al-Zahrani MS, Faddoul F, Nouneh I. Width of keratinized gingiva and the health status of the supporting tissues around dental implants. The International Journal of Oral & Maxillofacial Implants. 2008;**23**(2):323-326

[2] Shatta A, Bissada NF, Ricchetti P, Paes A, Demko C. Impact of implant and site characteristics on the pattern of bone loss in peri-implantitis. The International Journal of Oral & Maxillofacial Implants. 2019;**34**(6):1475-1481

[3] Esposito M, Hirsch JM, Lekholm U, Thomsen P. Biological factors contributing to failures of osseointegrated oral implants. (II). Etiopathogenesis. European Journal of Oral Sciences. 1998;**106**(3):721-764

[4] Quirynen M, De Soete M, van Steenberghe D. Infectious risks for oral implants: A review of the literature. Clinical Oral Implants Research. 2002;**13**(1):1-19

[5] Lindhe J, Meyle J. Group DoEWoP: Peri-implant diseases: Consensus Report of the Sixth European Workshop on Periodontology. Journal of Clinical Periodontology. 2008;**35**(8 Suppl):282-285

[6] Berglundh T, Armitage G, Araujo MG, Avila-Ortiz G, Blanco J, Camargo PM, et al. Peri-implant diseases and conditions: Consensus report of workgroup 4 of the 2017 World Workshop on the Classification of Periodontal and Peri-Implant Diseases and Conditions. Journal of Clinical Periodontology. 2018;**45**(S20):S286-S291

[7] Mombelli A, Lang NP. The diagnosis and treatment of peri-implantitis. Periodontology 2000. 1998;**17**:63-76

[8] Sorsa T, Tervahartiala T, Leppilahti J, Hernandez M, Gamonal J, Tuomainen AM, et al. Collagenase-2 (MMP-8) as a point-of-care biomarker in periodontitis and cardiovascular diseases. Therapeutic response to non-antimicrobial properties of tetracyclines. Pharmacological Research. 2011;**63**(2):108-113

[9] Alassiri S, Parnanen P, Rathnayake N, Johannsen G, Heikkinen AM, Lazzara R, et al. The ability of quantitative, specific, and sensitive point-of-care/chair-side oral fluid immunotests for aMMP-8 to detect periodontal and peri-implant diseases. Disease Markers. 2018;**2018**:1306396

[10] Froum SJ, Rosen PS. A proposed classification for peri-implantitis. The International Journal of Periodontics & Restorative Dentistry. 2012;**32**(5):533-540

[11] Atieh MA, Alsabeeha NH, Faggion CM Jr, Duncan WJ. The frequency of peri-implant diseases: A systematic review and meta-analysis. Journal of Periodontology. 2013;**84**(11):1586-1598

[12] Derks J, Tomasi C. Peri-implant health and disease. A systematic review of current epidemiology. Journal of Clinical Periodontology. 2015;**42**(Suppl 16):S158-S171

[13] Rakic M, Galindo-Moreno P, Monje A, Radovanovic S, Wang HL, Cochran D, et al. How frequent does peri-implantitis occur? A systematic review and meta-analysis. Clinical Oral Investigations. 2018;**22**(4):1805-1816

[14] Casado PL, Villas-Boas R, de Mello W, Duarte ME, Granjeiro JM. Peri-implant disease and chronic periodontitis: is interleukin-6 gene promoter polymorphism the common

risk factor in a Brazilian population? The International Journal of Oral & Maxillofacial Implants. 2013;**28**(1):35-43

[15] Rinke S, Ohl S, Ziebolz D, Lange K, Eickholz P. Prevalence of periimplant disease in partially edentulous patients: a practice-based cross-sectional study. Clinical Oral Implants Research. 2011;**22**(8):826-833

[16] Charalampakis G, Leonhardt A, Rabe P, Dahlen G. Clinical and microbiological characteristics of peri-implantitis cases: a retrospective multicentre study. Clinical Oral Implants Research. 2012;**23**(9):1045-1054

[17] Mir-Mari J, Mir-Orfila P, Figueiredo R, Valmaseda-Castellon E, Gay-Escoda C. Prevalence of peri-implant diseases. A cross-sectional study based on a private practice environment. Journal of Clinical Periodontology. 2012;**39**(5):490-494

[18] Marrone A, Lasserre J, Bercy P, Brecx MC. Prevalence and risk factors for peri-implant disease in Belgian adults. Clinical Oral Implants Research. 2013;**24**(8):934-940

[19] Corbella S, Del Fabbro M, Taschieri S, De Siena F, Francetti L. Clinical evaluation of an implant maintenance protocol for the prevention of peri-implant diseases in patients treated with immediately loaded full-arch rehabilitations. International Journal of Dental Hygiene. 2011;**9**(3):216-222

[20] Costa FO, Takenaka-Martinez S, Cota LO, Ferreira SD, Silva GL, Costa JE. Peri-implant disease in subjects with and without preventive maintenance: A 5-year follow-up. Journal of Clinical Periodontology. 2012;**39**(2):173-181

[21] Cecchinato D, Parpaiola A, Lindhe J. A cross-sectional study on the prevalence of marginal bone loss among implant patients. Clinical Oral Implants Research. 2013;**24**(1):87-90

[22] Cecchinato D, Parpaiola A, Lindhe J. Mucosal inflammation and incidence of crestal bone loss among implant patients: A 10-year study. Clinical Oral Implants Research. 2014;**25**(7):791-796

[23] Dvorak G, Arnhart C, Heuberer S, Huber CD, Watzek G, Gruber R. Peri-implantitis and late implant failures in postmenopausal women: A cross-sectional study. Journal of Clinical Periodontology. 2011;**38**(10):950-955

[24] Gotfredsen K. A 10-year prospective study of single tooth implants placed in the anterior maxilla. Clinical Implant Dentistry and Related Research. 2012;**14**(1):80-87

[25] Casado PL, Pereira MC, Duarte ME, Granjeiro JM. History of chronic periodontitis is a high risk indicator for peri-implant disease. Brazilian Dental Journal. 2013;**24**(2):136-141

[26] Meyle J, Gersok G, Boedeker RH, Gonzales JR. Long-term analysis of osseointegrated implants in non-smoker patients with a previous history of periodontitis. Journal of Clinical Periodontology. 2014;**41**(5):504-512

[27] Heitz-Mayfield LJ, Lang NP. Comparative biology of chronic and aggressive periodontitis vs. peri-implantitis. Periodontology 2000. 2010;**53**:167-181

[28] Berglundh T, Lindhe J, Ericsson I, Liljenberg B. Enhanced gingivitis in the deciduous and permanent dentition. An experimental study in the dog. Journal of Clinical Periodontology. 1992;**19**(2):135-142

[29] Pontoriero R, Tonelli MP, Carnevale G, Mombelli A, Nyman SR,

Lang NP. Experimentally induced peri-implant mucositis. A clinical study in humans. Clinical Oral Implants Research. 1994;**5**(4):254-259

[30] Ericsson I, Berglundh T, Marinello C, Liljenberg B, Lindhe J. Long-standing plaque and gingivitis at implants and teeth in the dog. Clinical Oral Implants Research. 1992;**3**(3):99-103

[31] Salvi GE, Aglietta M, Eick S, Sculean A, Lang NP, Ramseier CA. Reversibility of experimental peri-implant mucositis compared with experimental gingivitis in humans. Clinical Oral Implants Research. 2012;**23**(2):182-190

[32] Abrahamsson I, Berglundh T, Glantz PO, Lindhe J. The mucosal attachment at different abutments. An experimental study in dogs. Journal of Clinical Periodontology. 1998;**25**(9):721-727

[33] Carcuac O, Abrahamsson I, Albouy JP, Linder E, Larsson L, Berglundh T. Experimental periodontitis and peri-implantitis in dogs. Clinical Oral Implants Research. 2013;**24**(4):363-371

[34] Lindhe J, Berglundh T, Ericsson I, Liljenberg B, Marinello C. Experimental breakdown of peri-implant and periodontal tissues. A study in the beagle dog. Clinical Oral Implants Research. 1992;**3**(1):9-16

[35] Berglundh T, Zitzmann NU, Donati M. Are peri-implantitis lesions different from periodontitis lesions? Journal of Clinical Periodontology. 2011;**38**(s11):188-202

[36] Carcuac O, Berglundh T. Composition of human peri-implantitis and periodontitis lesions. Journal of Dental Research. 2014;**93**(11):1083-1088

[37] Gualini F, Berglundh T. Immunohistochemical characteristics of inflammatory lesions at implants. Journal of Clinical Periodontology. 2003;**30**(1):14-18

[38] Roccuzzo M, Bonino F, Aglietta M, Dalmasso P. Ten-year results of a three arms prospective cohort study on implants in periodontally compromised patients. Part 2: Clinical results. Clinical Oral Implants Research. 2012;**23**(4):389-395

[39] Karoussis IK, Salvi GE, Heitz-Mayfield LJ, Bragger U, Hammerle CH, Lang NP. Long-term implant prognosis in patients with and without a history of chronic periodontitis: A 10-year prospective cohort study of the ITI Dental Implant System. Clinical Oral Implants Research. 2003;**14**(3):329-339

[40] Derks J, Schaller D, Hakansson J, Wennstrom JL, Tomasi C, Berglundh T. Peri-implantitis—Onset and pattern of progression. Journal of Clinical Periodontology. 2016;**43**(4):383-388

[41] Schwarz F, Derks J, Monje A, Wang HL. Peri-implantitis, 45. Journal of Clinical Periodontology, Suppl. 2018;**20**(S20):S246-S266

[42] Laine ML, Leonhardt A, Roos-Jansaker AM, Pena AS, van Winkelhoff AJ, Winkel EG, et al. IL-1RN gene polymorphism is associated with peri-implantitis. Clinical Oral Implants Research. 2006;**17**(4):380-385

[43] Feloutzis A, Lang NP, Tonetti MS, Burgin W, Bragger U, Buser D, et al. IL-1 gene polymorphism and smoking as risk factors for peri-implant bone loss in a well-maintained population. Clinical Oral Implants Research. 2003;**14**(1):10-17

[44] Venza I, Visalli M, Cucinotta M, De Grazia G, Teti D, Venza M.

Proinflammatory gene expression at chronic periodontitis and peri-implantitis sites in patients with or without type 2 diabetes. Journal of Periodontology. 2010;**81**(1):99-108

[45] Ferreira SD, Silva GL, Cortelli JR, Costa JE, Costa FO. Prevalence and risk variables for peri-implant disease in Brazilian subjects. Journal of Clinical Periodontology. 2006;**33**(12):929-935

[46] Naujokat H, Kunzendorf B, Wiltfang J. Dental implants and diabetes mellitus—A systematic review. International Journal of Implant Dentistry. 2016;**2**(1):5

[47] Schwarz F, Becker K, Sahm N, Horstkemper T, Rousi K, Becker J. The prevalence of peri-implant diseases for two-piece implants with an internal tube-in-tube connection: A cross-sectional analysis of 512 implants. Clinical Oral Implants Research. 2017;**28**(1):24-28

[48] Roos-Jansaker AM, Lindahl C, Renvert H, Renvert S. Nine- to fourteen-year follow-up of implant treatment. Part I: Implant loss and associations to various factors. Journal of Clinical Periodontology. 2006;**33**(4):283-289

[49] Strietzel FP, Reichart PA, Kale A, Kulkarni M, Wegner B, Kuchler I. Smoking interferes with the prognosis of dental implant treatment: A systematic review and meta-analysis. Journal of Clinical Periodontology. 2007;**34**(6):523-544

[50] Roccuzzo M, Grasso G, Dalmasso P. Keratinized mucosa around implants in partially edentulous posterior mandible: 10-year results of a prospective comparative study. Clinical Oral Implants Research. 2016;**27**(4):491-496

[51] Staubli N, Walter C, Schmidt JC, Weiger R, Zitzmann NU. Excess cement and the risk of peri-implant disease—A systematic review. Clinical Oral Implants Research. 2017;**28**(10):1278-1290

[52] Becker CM, Kaldahl WB. Current theories of crown contour, margin placement, and pontic design. The Journal of Prosthetic Dentistry. 1981;**45**(3):268-277

[53] Katafuchi M, Weinstein BF, Leroux BG, Chen YW, Daubert DM. Restoration contour is a risk indicator for peri-implantitis: A cross-sectional radiographic analysis. Journal of Clinical Periodontology. 2018;**45**(2):225-232

[54] Pettersson M, Pettersson J, Johansson A, Molin Thoren M. Titanium release in peri-implantitis. Journal of Oral Rehabilitation. 2019;**46**(2):179-188

[55] Albrektsson T, Wennerberg A. Oral implant surfaces: Part 1—Review focusing on topographic and chemical properties of different surfaces and in vivo responses to them. The International Journal of Prosthodontics. 2004;**17**(5):536-543

[56] Baelum V, Ellegaard B. Implant survival in periodontally compromised patients. Journal of Periodontology. 2004;**75**(10):1404-1412

[57] Wennerberg A, Albrektsson T, Chrcanovic B. Long-term clinical outcome of implants with different surface modifications. European Journal of Oral Implantology. 2018;**11**(Suppl 1):S123-S136

[58] Nguyen-Hieu T, Borghetti A, Aboudharam G. Peri-implantitis: From diagnosis to therapeutics. Journal of Investigative and Clinical Dentistry. 2012;**3**(2):79-94

[59] Cappiello M, Luongo R, Di Iorio D, Bugea C, Cocchetto R, Celletti R.

Evaluation of peri-implant bone loss around platform-switched implants. The International Journal of Periodontics & Restorative Dentistry. 2008;**28**(4):347-355

[60] Lazzara RJ, Porter SS. Platform switching: A new concept in implant dentistry for controlling postrestorative crestal bone levels. The International Journal of Periodontics & Restorative Dentistry. 2006;**26**(1):9-17

[61] Quoc JB, Vang A, Evrard L. Peri-implant bone loss at implants placed in preserved alveolar bone versus implants placed in native bone: A retrospective radiographic study. The Open Dentistry Journal. 2018;**12**:529-545

[62] Klinge B, Meyle J, Working G. Peri-implant tissue destruction. The Third EAO Consensus Conference 2012. Clinical Oral Implants Research. 2012;**23**(Suppl 6):108-110

[63] Heitz-Mayfield LJ, Schmid B, Weigel C, Gerber S, Bosshardt DD, Jonsson J, et al. Does excessive occlusal load affect osseointegration? An experimental study in the dog. Clinical Oral Implants Research. 2004;**15**(3):259-268

[64] Kahramanoglu E, Kulak-Ozkan Y. Marginal and internal adaptation of different superstructure and abutment materials using two different implant systems for five-unit implant-supported fixed partial dentures: An in vitro study. The International Journal of Oral & Maxillofacial Implants. 2013;**28**(5):1207-1216

[65] Zupnik J, Kim SW, Ravens D, Karimbux N, Guze K. Factors associated with dental implant survival: A 4-year retrospective analysis. Journal of Periodontology. 2011;**82**(10):1390-1395

[66] Galindo-Moreno P, Fauri M, Avila-Ortiz G, Fernandez-Barbero JE, Cabrera-Leon A, Sanchez-Fernandez E. Influence of alcohol and tobacco habits on peri-implant marginal bone loss: A prospective study. Clinical Oral Implants Research. 2005;**16**(5):579-586

[67] Lang NP, Berglundh T. Working Group 4 of Seventh European Workshop on P: Periimplant diseases: Where are we now?—Consensus of the Seventh European Workshop on Periodontology. Journal of Clinical Periodontology. 2011;**38**(Suppl 11):178-181

[68] Heitz-Mayfield LJ, Salvi GE, Botticelli D, Mombelli A, Faddy M, Lang NP, et al. Anti-infective treatment of peri-implant mucositis: A randomised controlled clinical trial. Clinical Oral Implants Research. 2011;**22**(3):237-241

[69] Hallstrom H, Persson GR, Lindgren S, Olofsson M, Renvert S. Systemic antibiotics and debridement of peri-implant mucositis. A randomized clinical trial. Journal of Clinical Periodontology. 2012;**39**(6):574-581

[70] Zeza B, Pilloni A. Peri-implant mucositis treatments in humans: A systematic review. Annali di Stomatologia (Roma). 2012;**3**(3-4):83-89

[71] Renvert S, Samuelsson E, Lindahl C, Persson GR. Mechanical non-surgical treatment of peri-implantitis: A double-blind randomized longitudinal clinical study. I: Clinical results. Journal of Clinical Periodontology. 2009;**36**(7):604-609

[72] Augthun M, Tinschert J, Huber A. In vitro studies on the effect of cleaning methods on different implant surfaces. Journal of Periodontology. 1998;**69**(8):857-864

[73] Unursaikhan O, Lee JS, Cha JK, Park JC, Jung UW, Kim CS, et al. Comparative evaluation of roughness of

titanium surfaces treated by different hygiene instruments. Journal of Periodontal and Implant Science. 2012;**42**(3):88-94

[74] Tastepe CS, Liu Y, Visscher CM, Wismeijer D. Cleaning and modification of intraorally contaminated titanium discs with calcium phosphate powder abrasive treatment. Clinical Oral Implants Research. 2013;**24**(11):1238-1246

[75] Tastepe CS, van Waas R, Liu Y, Wismeijer D. Air powder abrasive treatment as an implant surface cleaning method: A literature review. The International Journal of Oral & Maxillofacial Implants. 2012;**27**(6):1461-1473

[76] Sahm N, Becker J, Santel T, Schwarz F. Non-surgical treatment of peri-implantitis using an air-abrasive device or mechanical debridement and local application of chlorhexidine: A prospective, randomized, controlled clinical study. Journal of Clinical Periodontology. 2011;**38**(9):872-878

[77] Louropoulou A, Slot DE, Van der Weijden F. The effects of mechanical instruments on contaminated titanium dental implant surfaces: A systematic review. Clinical Oral Implants Research. 2014;**25**(10):1149-1160

[78] Ntrouka V, Hoogenkamp M, Zaura E, van der Weijden F. The effect of chemotherapeutic agents on titanium-adherent biofilms. Clinical Oral Implants Research. 2011;**22**(11):1227-1234

[79] Mohn D, Zehnder M, Stark WJ, Imfeld T. Electrochemical disinfection of dental implants—A proof of concept. PLoS One. 2011;**6**(1):e16157

[80] Schwarz F, Schmucker A, Becker J. Efficacy of alternative or adjunctive measures to conventional treatment of peri-implant mucositis and peri-implantitis: A systematic review and meta-analysis. International Journal of Implant Dentistry. 2015;**1**(1):22

[81] Schwarz F, Sculean A, Rothamel D, Schwenzer K, Georg T, Becker J. Clinical evaluation of an Er:YAG laser for nonsurgical treatment of peri-implantitis: A pilot study. Clinical Oral Implants Research. 2005;**16**(1):44-52

[82] Mailoa J, Lin GH, Chan HL, MacEachern M, Wang HL. Clinical outcomes of using lasers for peri-implantitis surface detoxification: A systematic review and meta-analysis. Journal of Periodontology. 2014;**85**(9):1194-1202

[83] Persson GR, Roos-Jansaker AM, Lindahl C, Renvert S. Microbiologic results after non-surgical erbium-doped:yttrium, aluminum, and garnet laser or air-abrasive treatment of peri-implantitis: A randomized clinical trial. Journal of Periodontology. 2011;**82**(9):1267-1278

[84] Yamamoto A, Tanabe T. Treatment of peri-implantitis around TiUnite-surface implants using Er:YAG laser microexplosions. The International Journal of Periodontics & Restorative Dentistry. 2013;**33**(1):21-30

[85] Deppe H, Horch HH, Schrodl V, Haczek C, Miethke T. Effect of 308-nm excimer laser light on peri-implantitis-associated bacteria: An in vitro investigation. Lasers in Medical Science. 2007;**22**(4):223-227

[86] Al-Ahmad A, Tennert C, Karygianni L, Wrbas KT, Hellwig E, Altenburger MJ. Antimicrobial photodynamic therapy using visible light plus water-filtered infrared-A (wIRA).

Journal of Medical Microbiology. 2013;**62**(Pt 3):467-473

[87] Meisel P, Kocher T. Photodynamic therapy for periodontal diseases: State of the art. Journal of Photochemistry and Photobiology. B. 2005;**79**(2):159-170

[88] Deppe H, Mucke T, Wagenpfeil S, Kesting M, Sculean A. Nonsurgical antimicrobial photodynamic therapy in moderate vs severe peri-implant defects: A clinical pilot study. Quintessence International. 2013;**44**(8):609-618

[89] Bassetti M, Schar D, Wicki B, Eick S, Ramseier CA, Arweiler NB, et al. Anti-infective therapy of peri-implantitis with adjunctive local drug delivery or photodynamic therapy: 12-month outcomes of a randomized controlled clinical trial. Clinical Oral Implants Research. 2014;**25**(3):279-287

[90] Schou S, Berglundh T, Lang NP. Surgical treatment of peri-implantitis. The International Journal of Oral & Maxillofacial Implants. 2004;**19**(Suppl):140-149

[91] Prathapachandran J, Suresh N. Management of peri-implantitis. Dental Research Journal. 2012;**9**(5):516-521

[92] Roccuzzo M, Layton DM, Roccuzzo A, Heitz-Mayfield LJ. Clinical outcomes of peri-implantitis treatment and supportive care: A systematic review. Clinical Oral Implants Research. 2018;**29**(Suppl 16):331-350

[93] Sahrmann P, Attin T, Schmidlin PR. Regenerative treatment of peri-implantitis using bone substitutes and membrane: A systematic review. Clinical Implant Dentistry and Related Research. 2011;**13**(1):46-57

[94] Serino G, Strom C. Peri-implantitis in partially edentulous patients: association with inadequate plaque control. Clinical Oral Implants Research. 2009;**20**(2):169-174

[95] Khammissa RA, Feller L, Meyerov R, Lemmer J. Peri-implant mucositis and peri-implantitis: Clinical and histopathological characteristics and treatment. SADJ. 2012;**67**(3):122, 124-126

Section 4

Prosthodontic Trends in Dental Implantology

Chapter 14

Prosthetic Concepts in Dental Implantology

Ivica Pelivan

Abstract

This chapter will address evidence-based prosthetic concepts in dental implantology as well as clinical evidence with focus on appropriate logic and technical skills. Those prosthetic factors are as just important as surgical factors, and long-term success can only be achieved if both of those factors are considered, respected, and strictly followed from planning to prosthetic phase of treatment. This chapter will deal with materials selection for prosthetic part, shape, size, and design of supra-crestal parts of abutments and their influence on soft tissue and bone stability around dental implants. Furthermore, one of most important decisions is about choosing the proper way of retention: screw- vs. cement-retained restorations, and it will be discussed in detail. Additionally, emergence profile and its function in soft tissues adaptation and adhesion to different prosthetic materials also have important role in long-term success of dental implant restorations.

Keywords: materials selection, dental implant abutment, screw-retained restoration, cement-retained restoration, emergence profile

1. Introduction

In contemporary implant prosthodontics, proper treatment planning prior to dental implant placement is equally important as the prosthetic factors. The good work of oral surgeon could be easily ruined by poor prosthodontic execution, thus changing the dental implant therapy success into therapy failure.

For decades, the scientific literature identified the following criteria for the survival and success of dental implant-based prosthetic rehabilitation:

1. Implant survival: At the time of measurement, the implant is in situ and loaded.

2. Implant success is determined using the Albrektsson criteria [1] with the following modifications: Adell [2], Buser et al. [3], Mombelli and Lang [4], and Misch et al. [5].

    - Implant placed in situ and loaded; no chronic discomfort; no nerve lesion; no peri-implant infection with suppuration; no mobility; no continuous peri-implant radiolucency [1, 3].

- No probing depth greater than 5 mm in the presence of a bleeding index of 3 [4].

Absence of radiographic peri-implant bone resorption greater than 1.5 mm in the first year of function [2] and greater than 0.2 mm in subsequent years (i.e. 1.7 mm after 2 years); alternative cut-off values for radiographic bone resorption after 2 years of 2 mm (I. Success) and 4 mm (II. Satisfactory Survival) were also evaluated [5].

Currently, implant success is defined by these three criteria [6]:

1. Annual bone lose not more than 0.2 mm,

2. Periodontal probing depth (PPD) no greater than 5–7 mm,

3. No bleeding on probing.

These criteria are based on older studies, previous dental implant designs and restorations that are not biocompatible, and they might need to be re-evaluated. Porcelain fused to metal (PFM) restorations lack the biocompatibility of zirconia, which is widely used today, and current concepts allow bone stability or even growth over time. Therefore, the expected 1.5 mm loss after 1 year and subsequent gradual resorption can be considered relicts of the past [6].

2. Cemented vs. screw-retained restorations

The debate between cemented and screw-retained dental implant restorations is old as the implant prosthodontics itself. There are also different opinions in the scientific literature. Studies have shown that there are no significant differences in survival between the two methods, but screw connection has shown a total of fewer technical and biological complications [7]. But, from the clinical perspective, all cemented dental implant restorations should be checked very meticulously for any cement remnants. Even after many years of function, cement remnants can cause peri-implant mucositis which if undetected and untreated can lead to peri-implantitis with severe crestal bone loss around dental implants (**Figure 1**). This bone loss is the

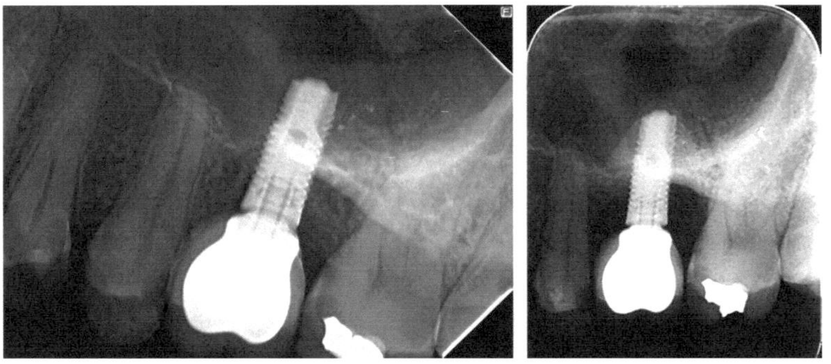

Figure 1.
Dental implant with cement-retained PFM crown; left image—immediately after delivery with no cement remnants visible on the radiograph; right image—patient did not come for regular follow-ups until he noticed bleeding while using dental floss, 9 years later. Unfortunately, dental implant needed to be removed due to severe bone loss.

clinical issue which we are trying to avoid by careful treatment planning and precise execution of clinical and laboratory procedures.

Even when using screw-retained restoration, we can witness crestal bone loss around dental implants. This can be caused by the inappropriate size and/or shape of titanium base. Too short or too wide titanium base profile for screw-retained crown can compromise transitional zone of connective tissue and junctional epithelium around dental implant restoration leading to crestal bone loss (**Figure 2**).

The difference in two titanium base height and screw-retained crowns is clearly visible in **Figure 3**. The impact of different titanium base as well the slight changes in emergence profile shape on the crestal bone level and density in a period of 3 months is shown in **Figure 4**.

Nevertheless, the clinical success of dental reconstructions is determined not only by survival rates, but also by the number of technical or biological complications that develop during clinical function. The optimum materials and techniques for

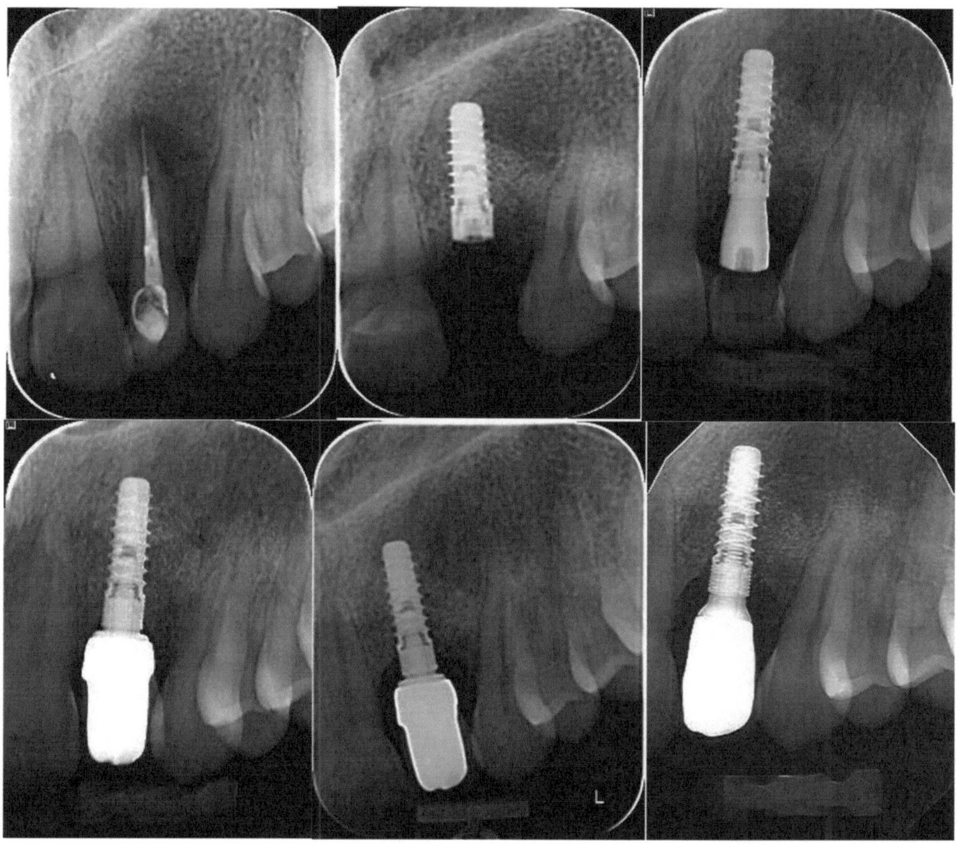

Figure 2.
The story of dental implant system, which was newly introduced to the market, with only one available titanium base height at that time (0.5 mm). Subsequent radiographs from top left to bottom right: initial situation; immediately after dental implant placement in augmented socket (two-stage surgery); second stage surgery and healing abutment; at the time of crown delivery (highly polished CAD/CAM zirconia abutment with laboratory cemented screw-retained lithium disilicate crown); 2 years follow-up with crestal bone loss; final radiograph at the time of new crown delivery (1.5 mm high titanium base was available on the market and micro-layered screw-retained zirconia crown with polished subgingival part was made in hope to prevent further crestal bone loss).

Figure 3.
Left: screw-retained crown with 0.5 mm high titanium base; right: screw-retained crown with 1.5 mm high titanium base for the patient in ***Figure 2****.*

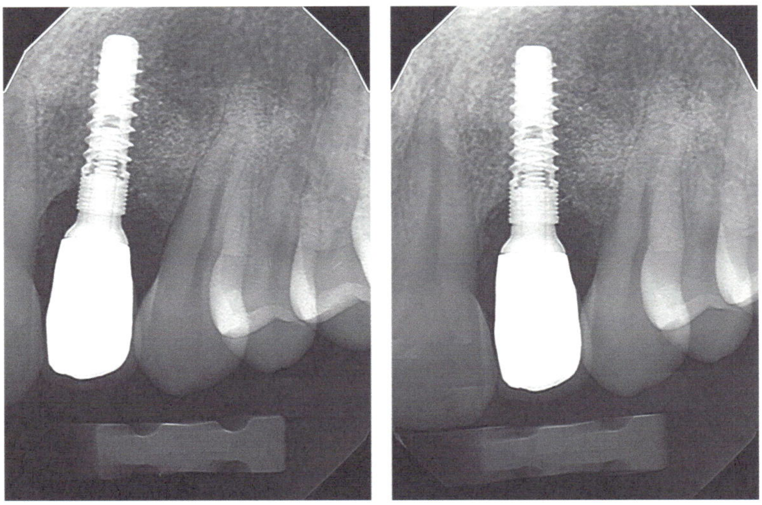

Figure 4.
Left: final radiograph at the time of new crown delivery; right: 3 months' follow-up radiograph with clearly visible bone remineralization and bone density increase around dental implant neck.

implant-borne reconstructions are frequently debated to increase clinical outcomes. One of the current discussions is about the best fixation method between the implant and the reconstruction. For a patient-centred clinical approach, it is currently uncertain whether cementation or screw retention is the superior option for restoring dental implants. In clinical practice, both cementation and screw retention appear to have advantages and disadvantages. Clinically and technically, cemented implant reconstructions are quite similar to tooth-borne reconstructions. As a result, they may be easier to make and handle in the mouths of patients. However, prefabricated cement-onto or even custom abutments are required. Recently, CAD/CAM (computer-aided design/computer-aided manufacture) technologies enable a wide range of customized abutments to be used, and cemented reconstructions have become the preferred choice in many clinical settings. The difficulty in removing extra cement from cemented crowns and FDPs is one of their drawbacks. More worrying, excess cement has been demonstrated to cause peri-implantitis in the clinical setting [8]. Another notable disadvantage of cemented reconstructions is that, in the event of a problem, they are difficult or impossible to remove without causing damage, such as in the case of technical complications.

The retrievability of screw-retained reconstructions, on the other hand, is a big advantage. Furthermore, biological issues are extremely unlikely to arise if the reconstruction is well-fitting. Because the position of the screw access hole and the surrounding material parameters of the suprastructure must be considered, the horizontal and angular positioning of the implant is more delicate and has less tolerance than when employing screw-retained reconstructions. The fixation screw opening should ideally be located in a non-visible palatal or oral location, which is only possible if a suitable implant site and angulation are available. Furthermore, screw-retained reconstructions require more technical production because the reconstruction core must constantly be customized. Technical issues such as retaining screw loosening or veneering ceramic fracture have been clinically observed.

It is indeed difficult to choose between the two types of reconstructions, and it quite often comes down to personal preference rather than scientific data.

In a systematic review published by Sailer et al. [9], it was discovered that cemented restorations cause much higher bone loss than screw-retained restorations. From a total of 4511 titles, 59 clinical studies were chosen for this review, and the data were retrieved and analysed. For cemented single crowns, the estimated 5-year reconstruction survival was 96.5%, for screw-retained single crowns it was 89.3% ($P = 0.091$ for difference). The 5-year survival for cemented partial fixed dental prostheses was 96.9%, similar to the one for screw-retained partial fixed dental prostheses with 98% ($P = 0.47$). For cemented full-arch partial fixed dental prostheses, the 5-year survival was 100%, which was somewhat higher than that for screw-retained FDPs with 95.8% ($P = 0.54$). The projected cumulative incidence of technical problems over a 5-year period was 11.9% for cemented single crowns and 24.4% for screw-retained crowns. In comparison to the cemented partial fixed dental prostheses, a tendency towards decreased complication was observed with the screw-retained partial fixed dental prostheses (partial fixed dental prostheses cemented 24.5%, screw-retained 22.1%; full-arch partial fixed dental prostheses cemented 62.9%, screw-retained 54.1%). Biological problems such as marginal bone loss greater than 2 mm occurred more frequently with cemented crowns (incidence: 2.8%) than with screw-retained crowns (5-year incidence: 2.8%) (5-year incidence: 0%).

This study found that both types of reconstructions had varied effects on clinical outcomes and that neither fixation approach was clearly superior to the other. Screw-retained reconstructions had more technical issues, while cemented reconstructions had more substantial biological consequences (implant loss, bone loss >2 mm). Screw-retained reconstructions are more easily retrievable than cemented reconstructions, allowing for easier treatment of technical and biological difficulties. These reconstructions appear to be preferred for this reason, as well as their apparent higher biological compatibility.

In contrary, Nissan et al. published a study that compared the long-term outcomes of cement versus screw-retained implant supported partial dentures in a randomized controlled trial and found that cement-retained FPDs had a better outcome [10]. The study group consisted of consecutive patients with bilateral partial posterior edentulism. In a split-mouth design, implants were placed and cemented or screw-retained restorations were randomly assigned to the patients. Examinations for follow-up (up to 15 years) were done every 6 months in the first year and every 12 months in the following years. Ceramic fracture, abutment screw loosening, metal frame fracture, Gingival Index and marginal bone loss were all assessed and reported at each recall appointment. Total of 221 implants were used to support partial prosthesis in 38 individuals. No implants were lost throughout the follow-up period (mean follow-up, 66 47 months [range, 18–180 months] for screw-retained restorations and 61 ± 40 months [range, 18–159 months] for cemented restorations). Ceramic fracture occurred substantially more frequently (P.001) in screw-retained restorations (38% ± 0.3%) than in cemented restorations (4% ± 0.1%). Abutment screw loosening occurred statistically substantially more frequently (P = .001) in screw-retained restorations (32% ± 0.3%) than in cement-retained restorations (92% ± 0.2%). Neither technique of restoration resulted in metal framework fractures. The mean Gingival Index scores for screw-retained (0.48 ± 0.5) restorations were statistically substantially higher (P.001) than for cemented (0.09 ± 0.3) restorations. The mean marginal bone loss was statistically considerably greater (P.001) for screw-retained restorations (1.4 ± 0.6 mm) than for cemented restorations (0.69 ± 0.5 mm).

The long-term clinical and biological outcomes of cemented implant-supported restorations were found to be better to screw-retained restorations in this study. With such contradictory facts, it is difficult to determine which technique is superior. The choice between cement-retained and screw-retained restorations might be philosophical. By opting for cemented restorations, the clinician accepts responsibility for removing all cement residues. Peri-implantitis caused by cement remnants is entirely an iatrogenic condition with no delegation of responsibility to the patient's oral hygiene habits.

Whether we use standard abutments or custom CAD/CAM abutments, the cementation margin is critical. One of the most common causes of cement residues in soft tissues around dental implant restorations is the widespread clinical practice of setting the implant restoration margin too deep subgingival for aesthetic reasons.

This is typically done to conceal the abutment-crown interface and to allow for eventual peri-implant soft tissue recession. When the margin is deeper than 1.5 mm below the soft tissue level, according to one of the Academy of Osseointegration's consensus statements, the risk of cement residues is significant [11]. Furthermore, the American Academy of Periodontology recently included residual cement to the list of risk factors for peri-implant mucositis and peri-implantitis [12]. The key challenge is where to put the cementation margin and how deep it should be?

According to the literature, the margin depth should be deep enough to conceal the margin yet shallow enough to allow residual cement to be removed. Because it is difficult to identify the exact ideal cementation margin depth, this statement does not provide sufficient information for safe and successful everyday clinical practice. To identify a safe margin for cementation, several laboratory and clinical trials were conducted.

The study conducted by Linkevicius et al. sought to determine the amount of cement that remained undiscovered following cementation and cleaning of implant-supported restorations [13]. Fifty-three single implant-supported metal-ceramic restorations were used to treat 53 patients. A periodontal probe was used to assess the subgingival location of each implant's margin mesially, distally, buccaly and lingually, giving 212 measurements. The data were separated into four groups: tissue level (14 samples), 1 mm subgingivally (56 samples), 2 mm (74 samples) and 3 mm (68 samples) below the tissues contour. Metal-ceramic restorations with occlusal holes were made and resin-reinforced glass-ionomer was used to bond them to conventional abutments. After cleaning, a radiograph was taken to determine if all of the cement had been removed. After that, the abutment and crown complex were unscrewed for testing. Adobe Photoshop was used to analyse the photographs of all quadrants of the specimens and peri-implant tissues. Two proportions were determined: (1) the area of cement remnants relative to the overall area of the abutment/restoration; and (2) the area of cement remnants relative to the total area of the implant soft tissue contour.

Excess on the crown groups were group-1 (0.002 ± 0.001); group-2 (0.024 ± 0.005); group-3 (0.036 ± 0.004) and group-4 (0.055 ± 0.007). The amount of undetected excess grew as the margin became deeper subgingivally (P = 0.000), and there was a significant difference between all groups (P 0.05). The soft tissue groups had the following remnants: group-1 (0.014 0.006), group-2 (0.052 0.011), group-3 (0.057 0.009) and group-4 (0.071 0.012). The increase in cement remnants was statistically significant as well as the difference between groups 1 and 2. Radiographic examination revealed cement residues mesially in four cases of 53, or 7.5 %, and distally in six cases of 53, or 11.3 %.

According to the findings of this investigation, the deeper the position of the margin, the more undetected cement was revealed. Dental radiographs should not be considered as a reliable method for cement excess evaluation.

Another study done by Linkevicius et al had the purpose to determine the relationship between patients with a history of periodontitis and development of cement-related peri-implant disease [14]. Between 2006 and 2011, in private practice, 77 patients with 129 implants were selected for this retrospective study from completed implant cases that were scheduled for routine maintenance or had mechanical or biological issues. Researchers analysed implants with extracoronal cement residues and implants without cement residues. The selected cases were then separated into two groups: implants in patients with a history of periodontitis (1) and implants in persons without a history of periodontitis (2). These groups were chosen based on the patient's treatment history and orthopantomogram. As a control group, a set of 238 screw-retained implant restorations was investigated that were delivered to 66 patients throughout the same period. The incidence of peri-implant disease was assessed in all implant groups.

In 62 of 73 implants with cement residues, peri-implant disease was seen (85%). All implants in group 1 developed peri-implantitis—four cases of early disease and 35 cases of delayed disease. Twenty-one of 30 implants in the periodontally healthy group were diagnosed with peri-implant mucositis, 3 implants developed early peri-implantitis and 11 implants with cement remnants did not develop biological problems. Peri-implant illness was identified in 17 of 56 cases of implants without cement remains (30%). In comparison, just two occurrences of peri-implant disease were discovered in the control group of screw-retained restorations (1.08%).

This study concluded that implants with cement remnants may be more likely to develop peri-implantitis in individuals with a history of periodontitis than in patients without a history of periodontitis.

The literature established that each retention method has a number of advantages and disadvantages. However, there are some clinical situations in which one method of retention is preferable to the other. Shadid and Sadaqa's review of the literature on screw-retained versus cement-retained fixed implant supported reconstruction identifies several clinical situations in which one method of retention is preferable to the other [15].

Clinical situations that prefer screw-retained restoration:

- Screw-retained large-arch implant reconstructions are preferred, as complications with these long-span prostheses are more common than with short-span prostheses.

- Screw-retained cantilevered prostheses are preferred, as some maintenance of restorative structures or implants is likely to be required during the life of such prostheses.

- Screw-retained restorations are preferred in patients who are at a high risk of developing gingival recession. This enables their uncomplicated removal and subsequent modification of the restorations to reflect the changed circumstances.

- Screw-retained restorations are preferred in patients who are expected to lose additional teeth in the future. This is to facilitate the removal of the restorations and subsequent modification of the restorations.

- In situations where there is little interocclusal space, adequate retention for cement-retained restorations may be impossible, as these restorations require a vertical component of at least 5mm to provide retention and resistance form. However, screw-retained restorations can be used with as little as 4 mm of interocclusal space. Additionally, screw-retained restorations can be directly attached to implants without the use of an intermediate abutment, reducing the amount of interocclusal space required for these restorations.

- In situations where it is difficult or impossible to remove excess cement (e.g. if the final restorative margin will be greater than 3 mm subgingivally, the use of screw-retained restoration is indicated). In this situation, an alternative to screw-retained restoration is to fabricate a custom abutment for cement retention with a restorative margin that follows the gingival contours.

- Screw-retained restorations are preferred in cases where technical or biologic complications are anticipated, as they allow for easy removal of the restorations, thereby resolving the issues.

Clinical situations that prefer cemented restoration:

- Cement-retained restorations are preferred for single-unit and short-span implant restorations, assuming that implant table size, implant number and abutment screw torque can be optimized. In such cases, screw retention would be used only if the implant's long axis was excessively palatal in the anterior region.

- Cement-retained crowns are preferred in cases involving small diameter crowns where screw access may jeopardize the crown's integrity.

- Cement-retained restorations are preferred in situations where the occlusal surface will be compromised in terms of aesthetics or occlusal stability as a result of the presence of a restorative material sealing the screw access.

- If the divergence between the implant axis and the retaining screw of the angled abutment receiving the restoration is less than 17 degrees, conventional screw retention of the restoration using premachined abutments is not possible.

Very valuable information for clinicians was identified in a more recent review by Hamed et al, which comprised 12 clinical research (randomized controlled trials, clinical trials, prospective studies and retrospective cohort studies) with at least 2 years' follow-up time and published between 2010 and 2020 [16]. One of the most important advantages of cement-retained restorations is it's the passivity and simplicity in manufacturing process in comparison with screw-retained restorations. This feature comes to light especially when zirconia is used as material for framework. The review indicates that the cement-retained implant approach is appropriate when enhanced predictability, a patient's desire for superior aesthetic outcomes and a cost-effective method are present. Due to the significant complications associated with screw-retained restorations in terms of technical and prosthetic outcomes, cement-retained implant restoration results in more successful outcomes. Whereas a biological complication associated with the cemented implant promotes the use of screw-based implant reconstruction. Additionally, the screw-retained repair is more suitable for multiple unit implantation for patients with restricted inter-arch space. For instance, screw retention reconstruction is advised when inter-arch space is restricted (less than 4 mm) and retrievability is necessary. Similarly, cement retention can be used to compensate for inappropriately angled implants and when occlusion is easier to control without the hole.

It must be emphasized that prosthodontics plays a crucial role in maintaining mucosal homeostasis. Plaque accumulation and the soft tissue reaction are directly related to design, structural connections (screw-retained or cement-retained) and characteristics of materials. Proper prosthetic design with an appropriate emergence profile that promotes excellent oral hygiene and prevents plaque accumulation is unquestionably critical in preventing peri-implant mucositis [17]. According to de Tapia et al, when peri-implant tissue inflammation arises, the prosthetic design should be evaluated and, if necessary, adjusted to correct design issues that may obstruct good hygiene and to reduce biomechanical stress factors that may be involved [18].

3. Emergence profile

The ninth edition of the Glossary of Prosthodontic Terms (GPT9) defines 'emergence profile' and 'emergence angle' identically for natural teeth and implant prosthesis [19]. Emergence profile is defined as the contour of a tooth or restoration, such as the crown on a natural tooth, dental implant or dental implant abutment, as it relates to the emergence from circumscribed soft tissues. Emergence angle is the angle between the average tangent of the transitional contour relative to the long axis of a tooth, dental implant or dental implant abutment.

However, extrapolating these words to implant prostheses remains ambiguous at the moment, as there are no established outcome metrics or protocols to support quantitative measurements. Emergence profile and emergence angle are currently defined in terms of 'circumscribed soft tissues'. While these can be clearly characterized and quantified in the relatively narrow periodontal sulcus, they present considerable complications when it comes to implant measurements [20].

The term 'implant supracrestal complex' has been recently proposed in order to describe the anatomic complex of human tissue, mechanical components and bacteria extending through the transmucosal part of an implant prosthesis. The paradigm of the 'implant supracrestal complex' aims to describe the human tissue in parallel with the design features of the implant-abutment-prosthesis complex and assists in identifying the role of design elements in health and disease of the peri-implant tissue [21]. The review article by Mattheos et al. investigated seven focus questions regarding emergence profile, emergence angle and/or 'implant supracrestal complex' [21]:

1. Is any particular design of the implant supracrestal complex's emergence profile or emergence angle associated with an increased risk of peri-implant mucositis or peri-implantitis?

2. Is there evidence that peri-implant mucositis and peri-implantitis are more prevalent in bone-level implants than in tissue-level implants?

3. Is there evidence that certain components of the implant supracrestal complex increase the incidence of peri-implant mucositis or peri-implantitis by obstructing oral hygiene access?

4. Is there evidence that an increased risk of peri-implant mucositis or peri-implantitis is associated with the 'implant supracrestal complex' tissue height (total vertical tissue height and/or peri-implant sulcus depth)?

5. Is there evidence linking the material used in the abutment and/or prosthesis to an increased risk of peri-implant mucositis or peri-implantitis?

6. Is there evidence that the design and placement of implant-abutment-prosthesis junctions are associated with an increased incidence of peri-implant mucositis or peri-implantitis?

7. Is there evidence that the kind of prosthesis retention (cement or screw) increases the incidence of peri-implant mucositis or peri-implantitis?

The conclusions from this review article can be summarized as follows:

1. The highest rate of peri-implantitis (37.8%) occurred when a convex profile was combined with a restoration emergence angle of >30 degrees for the bone-level implants, but the same was not confirmed for tissue-level implants. The highest prevalence of peri-implantitis occurred in the combination of bone-level implants, emergence angle ≥30, convex profile and splinted-middle implant prosthesis.

2. Most of analysed studies did not find any significant difference in the prevalence of peri-implant mucositis/peri-implantitis or the respective clinical outcomes measures between tissue-and bone-level implants. Few of the analysed studies reported different prevalence of peri-implantitis between bone-level and tissue-level implants, yet no statistical comparison was attempted or if then being statistically insignificant.

3. The complete resolution of inflammation in cases affected by peri-implant mucositis was achieved in 66.6% of the patients who were treated with additional prosthesis contour modification versus only in 9.6% of the patients who received standard peri-implant mucositis treatment. Modifying the contour of the prostheses to improve access for oral hygiene significantly improved the clinical outcomes after standard mechanical treatment of peri-implant mucositis.

4. Sites with a shallow mucosal tunnel showed greater and faster resolution of inflammation after treatment compared with the deep ones.

5. Analysis of abutment material (titanium, zirconia or gold) and peri-implant tissue health outcomes measures reported no, or insignificant, differences.

6. Results from different studies concluded that the use or not of intermediary abutments on an external connection implant was not found to have any influence on the prevalence of peri-implantitis after 5 years. Marginal bone loss was significantly lower at superstructures connected to abutments compared with those at implant level. No significant difference was found between abutments with different surface topography.

7. Of the five analysed papers which suggested a difference, two papers found cement-retained restorations to be related to higher risk of peri-implantitis, while two found cement-retained restorations to be related to higher risk of peri-implant mucositis and one found screw-retained restorations to be related to higher risk of peri-implant mucositis.

Additionally, the authors state that there are insufficient data with bone-level implants to conclude that a large emergence angle in combination with a convex abutment or prosthesis may result in peri-implantitis. Additional study is necessary to characterize the emerging profile in respect to the real degree of peri-implant soft tissue and to interpret these results more accurately. A single randomized clinical study found no difference in the risk of peri-implant mucositis between tissue- and bone-level implants. Prosthesis modification may be an effective and necessary adjunct to anti-infective therapy for peri-implant mucositis in implant-supported prostheses with limited access to oral hygiene. At the moment, there are no data to suggest that increasing the vertical height of the peri-implant soft tissues alone increases the risk of peri-implantitis. However, it has been shown that treating established peri-implant mucositis is more difficult in the presence of a deep peri-implant sulcus. It has not been shown that the presence or absence of a prosthetic abutment, or the material of the abutment (Titanium or Zirconia), alters the risk of peri-implantitis. The evidence relating the kind of prosthesis retained and the risk of developing peri-implantitis is equivocal.

From a clinical standpoint, properly shaped dental implant restorations are critical for the treatment's aesthetics and biological success. The primary challenge is the shift from a round dental implant to the cervical shape of the missing tooth. This transition is accomplished through the use of implant abutments. Su et al. [22] characterized this contour as having two adjacent but distinct zones within the dental implant abutment and crown, an apically located subcritical contour zone and a coronally located critical zone. The critical zone refers to the portion of the dental implant abutment and crown that lies between the free gingival margin and the deeper subcritical zone. This zone is circumferential in form, approximately 1 mm wide in the apicocoronally direction and is often convex or flat in shape. The critical zone may or may not contain a variety of restorative materials, depending on the kind of restoration (cemented or screw-retained). The subcritical zone is positioned apically to the critical zone and may be concave, convex or flat in shape. Changes in the shape of the critical and subcritical contour zones should be planned carefully in accordance with the dental implant site, soft tissue thickness and materials used. If the crown form cannot be adjusted, reshaping the subcritical zone can improve both the aesthetic and biological success of the treatment.

There are numerous strategies for peri-implant soft tissue conditioning, including immediate temporary restorations, custom-made healing abutments and gradual remodelling of soft tissues through modification of critical and subcritical zones of the temporary implant crown. **Figure 5** shows the emergence profile shaping with custom-made temporary PMMA crown on PEEK abutment after the implant was integrated.

In clinical cases like the one shown in **Figure 5**, additional challenge may emerge during copying and transferring emergence profile shape to either digital or conventional stone cast model. In both ways, the clinician needs to act fast due to fast tissue begin to collapse immediately after removing temporary crown (or custom-made healing abutment). In conventional prosthodontics impression, fast and predictable

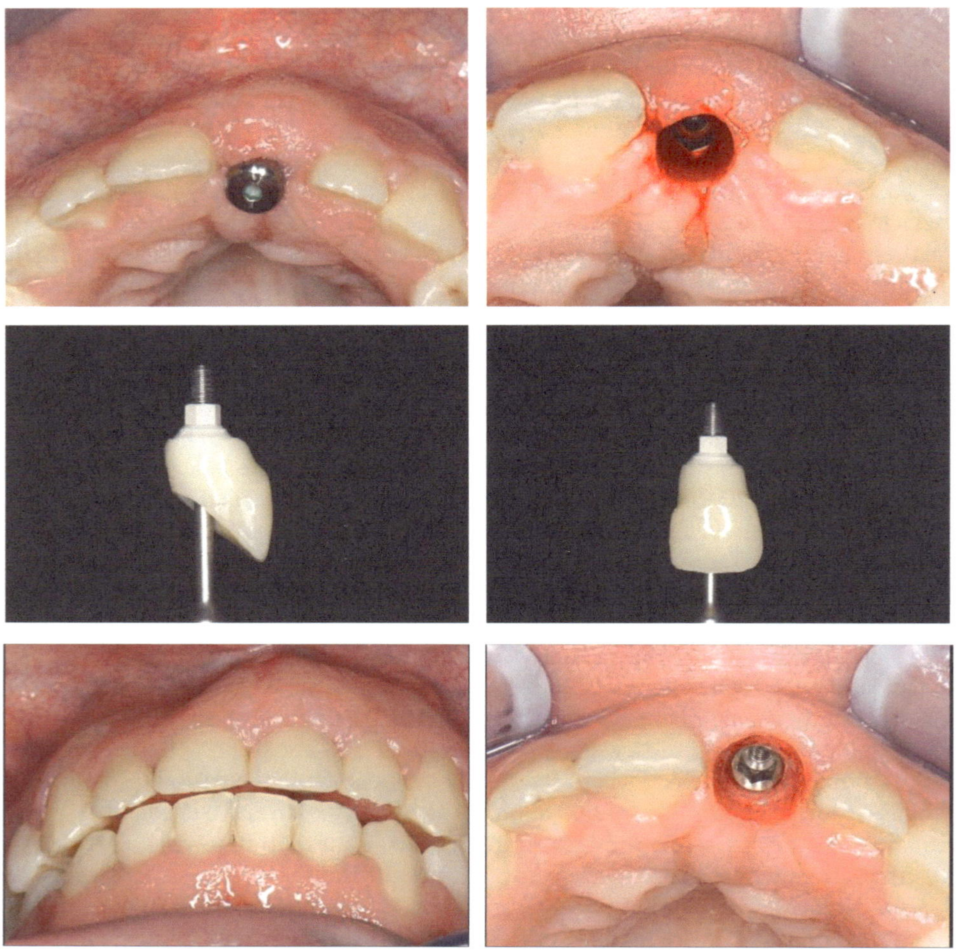

Figure 5.
Emergence profile shaping with temporary PMMA crown on PEEK abutment. Upper-left: initial clinical appearance with stock healing abutment; upper-right: size and shape of soft tissue emergence profile after removal of stock healing abutment; middle-left: lateral view of temporary PMMA crown on PEEK abutment; middle-right: frontal view of temporary PMMA crown on PEEK abutment; lower-left: clinical appearance 2 months after temporary crown delivery; lower-right: newly formed and shaped emergence profile with soft tissue maturation.

way is open tray pick-up transfer customization intraorally or extra orally with flowable composite resin material. This technique with intra oral customization with flowable composite resin material is shown in **Figure 6**.

Additionally, the significance of the emergence profile and the interest of clinicians and researchers have increased significantly in recent years. Gomez-Meda et al. [23] defined a more detailed classification of emergence profile surfaces and areas. This article discusses the esthetic biological contour concept (EBC), which consists of distinguishing important zones of emergence profiles and recommending detailed design principles for those zones. The clinical significance of EBC is that it promotes aesthetic outcomes and a favourable biological response to implant-supported restorations when designed properly. The EBC concept denotes three zones that correspond to the subgingival contour of an implant restoration's emergence profile (**Figure 7**). Each of these zones will come into contact with a distinct type of tissue and therefore must be designed differently.

The EBC concept is divided into three zones:

- E Zone (esthetic zone) is a subgingival area that is 1 mm wide and located apical to the free gingival margin. It should be shaped similarly to the crown of the extracted or contralateral tooth to resemble a natural crown. Its contour should be convex and support the free gingival margin in the proper

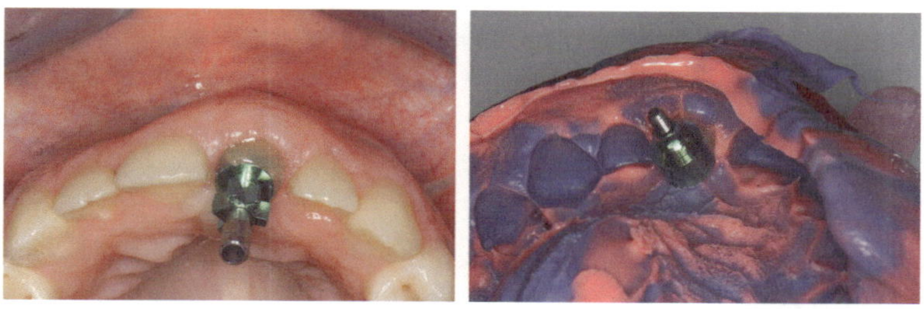

Figure 6.
Left: intraoral customization of open tray pick-up transfer and final impression with preserved emergence profile size and shape for final crown fabrication.

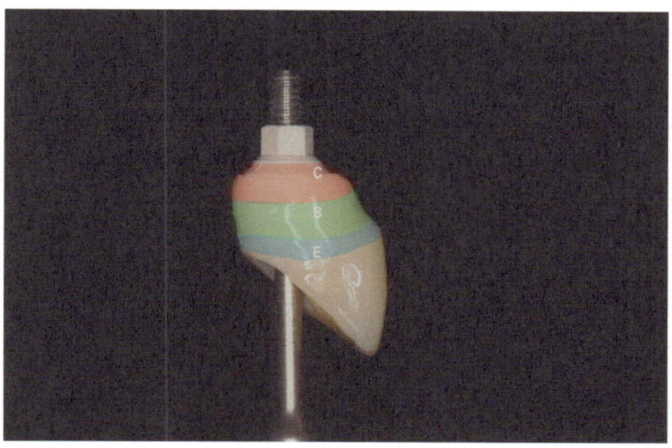

Figure 7.
Schematic presentation of three zones of EBC concept: E—esthetic zone (blue), B—bounded zone (green) and C—crestal zone (red).

position, establishing the implant crown's cervical morphology. This zone is adjacent to sulcular epithelium, a type of stratified squamous epithelium.

- B Zone (bounded zone) is the emergence profile area apical to the E zone that is approximately 1–2 mm wide in cases where the dental implant is ideally placed 3–4 mm apical from the free gingival margin zenith point. Although the B zone is normally concave, in patients with deficient soft tissues, connective tissue graft may be required to improve gingival phenotype, crestal stability and aesthetics. This biologic boundary zone is in contact with junctional epithelium, which is a non-keratinized epithelium.

- C Zone (crestal zone) is a 1–1.5 mm wide area immediately coronal to the implant neck. However, its dimensions vary depending on the depth of the integrated dental implant. In this area, the abutment contour should be flat or slightly concave to avoid putting pressure on the bone tissue surrounding the restoration. **Figure 2** illustrates the detrimental effect of this pressure on crestal bone stability. Additionally, certain dental implant designs (i.e. tissue level implants) incorporate this zone into the implant body. This zone is critical for the stability of the crestal bone because it is in contact with connective tissue.

Each of the zones described in the EBC concept serves a distinct purpose in the emergence profile's design. Understanding the significance and unique design features of the EBC zones enables the provision of aesthetic and biologically sound interim and definitive implant restorations.

4. Materials selection

Several new dental materials have entered the market over the last decade. They offer an aesthetic, functional and economical alternative to metal-ceramics, the most frequently used material for prosthodontic restorations. This is especially true for zirconium oxide and lithium disilicate ceramics. The incorporation of CAD/CAM manufacturing technology into daily work has resulted in a significant reduction in dental technicians' labour costs. Furthermore, these increased aesthetic standards have resulted in an increase in the use of metal-free restorations at the expense of metal-ceramic restorations. These events also influenced the materials used and the manufacturing process for custom-made dental implant abutments, effectively eradicating stock dental implant abutments. Additionally, the titanium bases for implant abutments have been redesigned to incorporate anti-rotation properties and a cylindrical shape, allowing for more efficient extraoral cementation of prosthodontic restorations. Such prosthodontic restorations, particularly following the introduction of angulated screw access to the abutment screw, resulted in an increase in the proportion of screw-retained restorations versus cemented restorations. All these advancements are now being used more frequently in clinical practice, but they have also prompted scientists to explore new materials and techniques. Given the time, material, human and technical resources required to conduct a high-quality long-term prospective or retrospective study, there is still insufficient solid evidence of these new materials and technologies' clinical benefits and effectiveness. However, prior research and the subjective clinical experience of numerous clinicians indicate that the new materials will eventually justify their partially uncritical use in clinical practice.

From the clinician's perspective, 5- or 10-year success or survival rates are not the only criterion to consider when planning and implementing implant-prosthodontic treatment. Additionally, the clinician should consider the frequency with which technical and biological issues may emerge when specific materials are used.

With so much conflicting information and data, clinicians may depend on review articles that structurally describe and analyse more scientific studies on a given subject. Pjetursson et al. recently published a statement paper about material selection for implant-supported restorations [24].

4.1 Metal-ceramic implant-supported restorations

For a long period of time, metal frameworks veneered with feldspathic ceramic have been used in dentistry. They are well-researched and documented restorations that can be used for single crowns and fixed partial dentures. The metal framework provides a high-strength core, protecting the whole restoration against tensile and flexural stress during chewing function. Besides the conventional casting technique, metal framework nowadays can be produced by milling or an additive laser printing process. There are two important published meta-review papers that examine the clinical outcomes, success and survival rates of metal-ceramic implant-supported restorations, as well as the complications rates.

The meta-review analysing metal-ceramic single crowns [25] included 30 studies with a total of 4542 crowns, with 83% of cement-retained crowns and 17% of screw-retained crowns, respectively. The meta-analysis estimated an annual failure rate of 0.35% (95% CI: 0.19%–0.66%), which corresponds to a 5-year survival rate of 98.3%. The respective complication rates were 13.3%, which means that one out of eight metal-ceramic single crowns showed some technical, biologic or aesthetic complication or failure. Only 86.7% of the metal-ceramic implant-supported single crowns showed no complications over the 5-year follow-up period. The 5-year incidence rate of peri-implantitis and soft-tissue complications was 5.1%, and significant bone loss of more than 2 mm at marginal bone level was 3.3%. Technical complications, including fracture of abutments or abutment screws, were rare complications, with an incidence rate of 0.2%. Abutment screws loosening was more frequent, with a 5-year complication rate of 3.6%. The incidence of ceramic fractures and chipping was 2.9%, and framework fractures were only reported to be 0.2%.

Another meta-review by Sailer et al was analysing multiple-unit metal-ceramic fixed partial dentures [26] and included 16 studies with a total of 993 fixed partial dentures supported by 2289 dental implant abutments, with 73% of cement-retained fixed partial dentures and 27% of screw-retained fixed partial dentures, respectively. The annual failure rate for metal-ceramic fixed partial dentures was 0.26% (95% CI: 0.10%–0.64%), corresponding to a 5-year survival rate of 98.7%. The respective complication rates were 15.1%, meaning that one out of six fixed partial dentures had some kind of complication. Hence, 84.9% of fixed partial dentures were free of any complications over the 5-year follow-up observation period. The 5-year rate of peri-implantitis and soft tissue complications was estimated to be 8.5%. The significant bone loss incidence rate was reported to be 2.6%. Among technical complications, the incidence rate was reported as follows: abutment screws loosening was 5.3%, ceramic fractures or chipping was 11.6% and framework fractures were 0.5%.

Both metal-ceramic single crowns and multiple-unit fixed partial dentures are well researched with very good long-term success rates. They can be used as a treatment option in a wide spectrum of clinical indications, especially in clinical cases with high clinical implant crowns, cantilever types of implant restorations and implant-supported fixed partial dentures with distal units extending more than 8 mm, fixed partial dentures with more than two pontics and in cases with small connector height due to limited interocclusal space.

4.2 Zirconia-ceramic implant-supported restorations

Increasing aesthetic demands have led to the development of different subtypes of zirconia ceramics. With their appearance, they adequately imitate not only the appearance but also the structure of hard dental tissues. In addition, new generations of zirconia ceramics have excellent biocompatibility and improved mechanical properties. Previous generations of zirconia ceramics had an opaque whitish appearance and had to be veneered to make the restoration look aesthetically pleasing. Newer generations of zirconia ceramics come in multilayer blanks or blocks with different levels of translucency and can be used as monolithic restorations.

The previously mentioned meta-reviews also analysed zirconia-ceramic implant-supported single crowns and fixed partial dentures.

The review by Pjetursson et al [25] analysed eight studies with a total of 912 zirconia-ceramic implant supported single crowns for an average 5-year follow-up period. Of all the included single crowns, 51% were cement retained and 49% were screw retained. The annual failure rate for implant-supported zirconia-ceramic single crowns was 0.49% (95% CI: 0.21%–1.18%), which corresponds to a respective 5-year survival rate of 97.6%. The estimated 5-year complication rate was 16.2%, meaning that only 83.8% of implant-supported zirconia-ceramic single crowns were free of any complications over the complete 5-year observation period. The most frequent complication rates were: 5.3% for peri-implantitis and soft tissue complications, 4.4% for marginal bone loss of more than 2 mm, 2.8% for ceramic fractures or chipping and 2.1% for framework fracture.

Another meta-review by Sailer et al [26] included three studies with a total of 175 zirconia-ceramic fixed partial dentures and an average follow-up period of 5.1 years. Only 15% of all restorations were cement-retained and 75% were screw-retained. The annual failure rate for implant-supported fixed partial dentures was 1.455 (95% CI: 1.06%–1.98%), which corresponds to a respective 5-year survival rate of 93.0%. The most frequent complications were soft tissue complications with a 10.1% incidence rate and framework fracture with a 4.7% rate.

According to the previously mentioned research and numerous other published articles, today we cannot consider veneered zirconia-ceramic as the material of choice for implant-supported fixed partial dentures. They show a high degree of risk of chipping or catastrophic fracture of the restoration framework. The study by Larsson et al. [27] states that the frequency of chipping and framework fractures of fixed partial dentures is up to 50%, which is a clinically unacceptable value. These problems are largely eliminated by the use of monolithic zirconia-ceramic, which with its aesthetic properties satisfies everyday clinical applications. In addition to the lack of chipping, implant-supported restorations of monolithic zirconia-ceramic show greater fracture resistance because the framework of such structures has larger dimensions compared with the framework of coated veneered zirconia-ceramic restorations. Evidence of this is a recent systematic review paper by Pjetursonn et al. [28] that analysed the 3-year survival and failure rates of veneered and monolithic zirconia-ceramic implant-supported restorations. The estimated 3-year survival rates were 96.3% (95% CI: 93.9%–97.7%) for veneered zirconia-ceramic single crowns and 96.1% (95% CI:

93.4%–97.8%) for monolithic zirconia single crowns. Veneered single crowns showed significantly ($p = 0.017$) higher annual ceramic chipping rates (1.65%) compared with monolithic single crowns (0.39%). Interestingly, the location of the single crowns, anterior vs. posterior, did not influence survival and chipping rates.

When a clinician needs to choose between veneered or monolithic zirconia-ceramic implant-supported restorations, the following factors must be considered: aesthetic demands, location in the dental arch, physical properties of the material, possibility for surface modification and abrasion (wear) properties of the material [24].

4.3 Lithium-disilicate reinforced glass-ceramic implant-supported restorations

To improve the physical properties of glass-ceramic and make it more suitable for prosthetic restorations, lithium disilicate or, in rare cases, leucite fillers were added. Nowadays, there are several techniques for the production of lithium-disilicate reinforced glass-ceramic, such as heat pressing and CAD/CAM milling from prefabricated blanks. Due to its mechanical properties, lithium-disilicate reinforced glass-ceramic can be used for both implant-supported single crowns and short-span fixed partial dentures in the anterior region of the dental arch. A systematic review article by Pjetursson et al. [28] evaluated five studies reporting on veneered leucite or lithium-disilicate reinforced glass-ceramic implant-supported single crowns (a total of 110 crowns) and 14 studies on monolithic leucite or lithium-disilicate reinforced glass-ceramic implant-supported single crowns (a total of 484 crowns). The mean follow-up period for veneered single crowns was 8.1 years and 2.6 years for monolithic single crowns, respectively. Results show a low annual failure rate of 0.80% (95% CI: 0.14%–4.64%) for veneered crowns and 1.02% (95% CI: 0.51%–2.05%) for monolithic reinforced glass-ceramic single crowns. This means that 3-year survival rates were 97.6% for veneered single crowns and 97.0% for monolithic single crowns. The study also reported that monolithic reinforced glass-ceramic crowns had the lowest annual complication rate of 1.7%, and veneered reinforced glass-ceramic crowns had an annual complication rate of 2.6%. In comparison, annual complication rates for monolithic zirconia-ceramic single crowns were 3.6% and for veneered zirconia-ceramic single crowns were 4.5%.

Considering these meta-review results, it is reasonable to conclude that lithium-disilicate reinforced glass-ceramic implant-supported crowns are the treatment of choice for high aesthetic-demanding clinical cases in the maxillary anterior region **Figure 8** shows such a clinical case with tooth #21 replaced by a dental implant where the implant-supported crown was made on a titanium base abutment customized

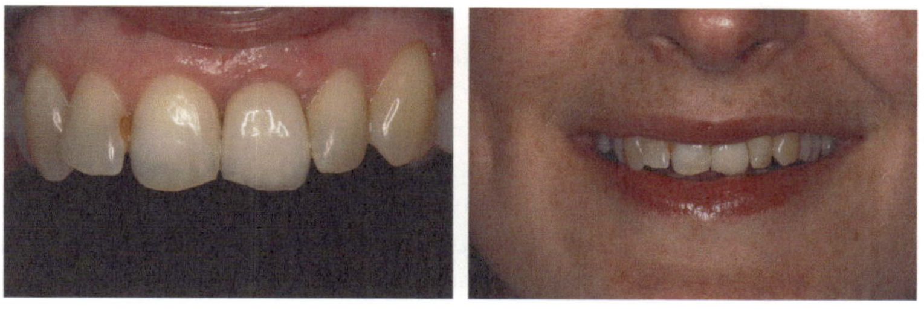

Figure 8.
Clinical case with tooth #21 replaced by a dental implant where the implant-supported crown was made on a titanium base abutment customized with a zirconia CAD/CAM abutment and a lithium-disilicate reinforced glass-ceramic crown.

with a zirconia CAD/CAM abutment and a lithium-disilicate reinforced glass-ceramic crown.

5. Conclusions

Proper treatment planning prior to dental implant implantation is just as critical in current implant prosthodontics as the prosthetic components. The wonderful work of the oral surgeon may quickly be destroyed by inadequate prosthodontic execution, resulting in the failure of dental implant treatment.

The controversy between cemented and screw-retained dental implant restorations is as ancient as implant prosthodontics itself. Additionally, there are divergent views in the scientific literature. Although no substantial difference in survival has been shown between the two procedures, screw connection has demonstrated a total of less technical and biological problems. It is presently unknown whether cementation or screw retention is the preferable choice for restoring dental implants from a patient-centred clinical perspective. Both cementation and screw retention seem to have benefits and downsides in practical practice. Choosing between cement-retained and screw-retained restorations may be a matter of philosophy. By choosing cemented restorations, the physician is responsible for completely eliminating all cement residue. Peri-implantitis induced by cement remains is a completely iatrogenic disease with no blame assigned to the patient's oral hygiene practices.

The emergence profile of a tooth or restoration, such as a crown on a natural tooth, a dental implant or a dental implant abutment, is described as the shape of the tooth or restoration in relation to its emergence from restricted soft tissues. Clinically, appropriately designed dental implant restorations are crucial for both the aesthetics and biological effectiveness of the procedure. The biggest difficulty is adapting the circular dental implant to the cervical form of the lost tooth. This shift is made possible by implant abutments. Changes in the critical and subcritical contour zones should be carefully considered in relation to the dental implant location, soft tissue thickness and materials employed. If the crown shape cannot be altered, altering the subcritical zone may significantly enhance the treatment's cosmetic and biological success.

Over the recent decade, many innovative dental materials have reached the market. They provide an attractive, practical and cost-effective alternative to metal-ceramic restorations, the most often used material in prosthodontics. This is particularly true for ceramics made of zirconium oxide and lithium disilicate. Both metal-ceramic single crowns and multi-unit fixed partial dentures have a lengthy track record of success. They can be used to treat a wide variety of clinical indications but are particularly useful in cases requiring high clinical implant crowns, cantilever-type implant restorations, implant-supported fixed partial dentures with distal units extending beyond 8 mm, fixed partial dentures with more than two pontics and cases requiring a small connector height due to limited interocclusal space. When a clinician must choose between veneered and monolithic zirconia-ceramic implant-supported restorations, the following factors must be considered: aesthetic requirements, location in the dental arch, material physical properties, surface modification capability and material abrasion (wear) properties. Considering the findings of this meta-analysis, it is acceptable to infer that lithium-disilicate reinforced glass-ceramic implant-supported crowns are the treatment of choice for clinical situations requiring a high level of aesthetics in the maxillary anterior area.

Conflict of interest

The author declares no conflict of interest.

Author details

Ivica Pelivan
School of Dental Medicine, University of Zagreb, Zagreb, Croatia

*Address all correspondence to: pelivan@sfzg.hr

References

[1] Albrektsson T, Zarb G, Worthington P, Eriksson AR. The long-term efficacy of currently used dental implants: A review and proposed criteria of success. The International Journal of Oral & Maxillofacial Implants. 1986;**1**:11-25

[2] Adell R, Lekholm U, Rockler B, Branemark PI. A 15-yearstudy of osseointegrated implants in the treatment of the edentulous jaw. International Journal of Oral Surgery. 1981;**10**:387-416

[3] Buser D, Weber HP, Lang NP. Tissue integration of non-submerged implants. 1-year results of a prospective study with100 ITI hollow-cylinder and hollow-screw implants. Clinical Oral Implants Research. 1990;**1**:33-40

[4] Mombelli A, Lang NP. Clinical parameters for the evaluation of dental implants. Periodontology. 2000;**4**:81-86

[5] Misch CE, Perel ML, Wang HL, Sammartino G, Galindo-Moreno P, Trisi P, et al. Implant success, survival, and failure: The International Congress of Oral Implantologists (ICOI) Pisa Consensus Conference. Implant Dentistry. 2008;**17**:5-15. DOI: 10.1097/ID.0b013e31816760599

[6] Linkevicius T. Zero Bone Loss Concepts. 1st ed. Batavia: Quintessence Publishing USA; 2019. p. 114

[7] Wittneben JG, Millen C, Brägger U. Clinical performance of screw - versus cement-retained fixed implant-supported reconstructions: A systematic review. The International Journal of Oral & Maxillofacial Implants. 2014;**29**(Suppl):84-98. DOI: 10.11607/jomi.2014suppl.g2.1

[8] Wilson TG Jr. The positive relationship between excess cement and peri-implant disease: A prospective clinical endoscopic study. Journal of Periodontology. 2009;**80**(9):1388-1392. DOI: 10.1902/jop.2009.090115

[9] Sailer I, Mühlemann S, Zwahlen M, Hämmerle CHF, Schneider D. Cemented and screw-retained implant reconstructions: A systematic review of the survival and complication rates. Clinical Oral Implants Research. 2012;**23**(Suppl. 6):163-201. DOI: 10.1111/j.1600-0501.2012.02538.x

[10] Nissan J, Narobai D, Gross O, Ghelfan O, Chaushu G. Long-term outcome of cemented versus screw-retained implant-supported partial restorations. The International Journal of Oral & Maxillofacial Implants. 2011;**26**(5):1102-1107

[11] Belser U, Buser D, Higginbottom F. Consensus statements and recommended clinical procedures regarding esthetics in implant dentistry. The International Journal of Oral & Maxillofacial Implants. 2004;**19**(Suppl): 73-74

[12] Peri-implant mucositis and peri-implantitis: A current understanding of their diagnoses and clinical implications. Journal of Periodontology. 2013;**84**(4):436-443. DOI: 10.1902/jop.2013.134001

[13] Linkevicius T, Vindasiute E, Puisys A, Linkeviciene L, Maslova N, Puriene A. The influence of the cementation margin position on the amount of undetected cement. A prospective clinical study. Clinical Oral Implants Research. 2013;**24**(1):71-76. DOI: 10.1111/j.1600-0501.2012.02453.x

[14] Linkevicius T, Puisys A, Vindasiute E, Linkeviciene L, Apse P.

Does residual cement around implant-supported restorations cause peri-implant disease? A retrospective case analysis. Clinical Oral Implants Research. 2013;**24**(11):1179-1184. DOI: 10.1111/j.1600-0501.2012.02570.x

[15] Shadid R, Sadaqa N. A comparison between screw- and cement-retained implant prostheses: A literature review. Journal of Oral Implantology. 2012;**38**(3):298-307. DOI: 10.1563/AAID-JOI-D-10-00146

[16] Hamed MT, Abdullah Mously H, Khalid Alamoudi S, Hossam Hashem AB, Hussein NG. A systematic review of screw versus cement-retained fixed implant supported reconstructions. Clinical, Cosmetic and Investigational Dentistry. 2020;**12**:9-16. DOI: 10.2147/CCIDE.S231070

[17] Lo Bianco L, Montevecchi M, Ostanello M, Checchi V. Recognition and treatment of peri-implant mucositis: Do we have the right perception? A structured review. Dental Medical Problem. 2021;**58**(4):545-554. DOI: 10.17219/dmp/136359

[18] de Tapia B, Mozas C, Valles C, Nart J, Sanz M, Herrera D. Adjunctive effect of modifying the implant-supported prosthesis in the treatment of peri-implant mucositis. Journal of Clinical Periodontology. 2019;**46**(10):1050-1060. DOI: 10.1111/jcpe.13169

[19] Ferro KJ, Morgano SM, Driscoll CF, Freilich MA, Guckes AD, Knoernschild KL, et al. The glossary of prosthodontic terms: Ninth Edition. The Journal of Prosthetic Dentistry. 2017;**117**:e1-e105. DOI: 10.1016/j.prosdent.2016.12.001

[20] Mattheos N, Janda M, Acharya A, Pekarski S, Larsson C. Impact of design elements of the implant supracrestal complex (ISC) on the risk of peri-implant mucositis and peri-implantitis: A critical review. Clinical Oral Implants Research. 2021;**32**(Suppl. 21):181-202. DOI: 10.1111/clr.13823

[21] Mattheos N, Vergoullis I, Janda M, Miseli A. The implant supracrestal complex and its significance for long-term successful clinical outcomes. The International Journal of Prosthodontics. 2021;**34**(1):88-100

[22] Su H, Gonzalez-Martin O, Weisgold A, Lee E. Considerations of implant abutment and crown contour: Critical contour and subcritical contour. The International Journal of Periodontics & Restorative Dentistry. 2010;**30**:335-343

[23] Gomez-Meda R, Esquivel J, Blatz MB. The esthetic biological contour concept for implant restoration emergence profile design. Journal of Esthetic and Restorative Dentistry. 2021;**33**(1):173-184. DOI: 10.1111/jerd.12714

[24] Pjetursson BE, Fehmer V, Sailer I. EAO Position Paper: Material selection for implant-supported restorations. The International Journal of Prosthodontics. 2022;**35**(1):7-16

[25] Pjetursson BE, Valente NA, Strasding M, Zwahlen M, Liu S, Sailer I. A systematic review of the survival and complication rates of zirconia-ceramic and metal-ceramic single crowns. Clinical Oral Implants Research. 2018;**29**(Suppl. 16):199-214. DOI: 10.1111/clr.13306

[26] Sailer I, Strasding M, Valente NA, Zwahlen M, Liu S, Pjetursson BE. A systematic review of the survival and complication rates of zirconia-ceramic and metal-ceramic multiple-unit fixed dental prostheses. Clinical Oral Implants Research. 2018;**29**(Suppl. 16):184-198. DOI: 10.1111/clr.13277

[27] Larsson C, Vult von Steyern P. Ten-year follow-up of implant-supported all-ceramic fixed dental prostheses: A Randomized, Prospective Clinical Trial. The International Journal of Prosthodontics. 2016;**29**(1):31-34

[28] Pjetursson BE, Sailer I, Latyshev A, Rabel K, Kohal RJ, Karasan D. A systematic review and meta-analysis evaluating the survival, the failure, and the complication rates of veneered and monolithic all-ceramic implant-supported single crowns. Clinical Oral Implants Research. 2021;**32**(Suppl. 21): 254-288. DOI: 10.1111/clr.13863

Chapter 15

A Review of Current Concepts in Full Arch Rehabilitation with Dental Implants

Leandro Díez-Suárez

Abstract

Various causes can be responsible for tooth loss. In general, caries, periodontal disease, facial trauma, pathology of the jaws, among other causes, could lead to the loss of a tooth or a group of teeth. As a consequence, the stimuli that participate in bone maintenance are compromised and bone reduction occurs gradually, making it difficult to use conventional prostheses. Fortunately, technological advances applied to dental implantology have allowed us to perform full-arch prosthetic treatments, managing to rehabilitate the form, function, esthetics and lost self-esteem in patients with severe atrophy of the jaws. The objective of this chapter is to describe the key and current aspects in full-arch rehabilitation with dental implants.

Keywords: dental implants, buttress implant, hybrid prosthesis, full arch, all on X, zygomatic implants

1. Introduction

Edentulism is a state of oral health that consists of the loss of teeth. Although the causes of tooth loss are diverse, dental cavity and periodontal disease are the main causes. Despite the decrease in edentulism in developed countries, edentulism continues to have a high prevalence affecting multiple functions such as chewing, nutrition, speech, self-esteem and quality of life [1].

After tooth loss, the physiological stimuli that give mechanical and cellular maintenance to the alveolar bone disappear. As a consequence, there is a reduction in the quantity and quality of bone, which we define as bone atrophy. The International Journal of Oral & Maxillofacial Implants defines alveolar atrophy as "decrease in the volume of the alveolar process occurring after tooth loss, drecased fuction and/or localized overloading from an improperly fitting removable partial or complete denture" [2].

Conventional full arch rehabilitation treatments achieved stability, support and retention at the expense of remaining teeth or residual bone anatomy. However, when a patient has edentulism and bone atrophy, conventional rehabilitative treatment does not meet the treatment goals, expectations, and comfort for the patient.

Dental implants are biocompatible alloplastic devices that are inserted into a residual bone ridge. The use of osseointegrated endosteal implants was introduced in

North America in 1982 thanks to the research of Dr. Branemar. His results established the guidelines for contemporary implantology [3].

To replace missing teeth there are different prosthodontic options. Which include implant-supported crowns (ISCs), implant-supported fixed dental prostheses (IFDPs), implant-supported removable dental prostheses (IRDPs), tooth-supported fixed dental prostheses (TFDPs), and removable partial dentures (RPDs). In patients with several missing teeth, implant-supported fixed dental prostheses (IFDPs) have shown excellent results in the short and medium term, positively impacting quality of life [4].

The objective of this chapter was to describe the key and current aspects in full-arch rehabilitation with dental implants. The purpose is to guide professionals in the diagnosis and rehabilitation treatment of the full arch with dental implants in the patient with edentulism.

2. Diagnosis of the patient with bone atrophy, selection of the patient

As mentioned, dental extraction induces a series of physiological changes in the hard and soft tissue of the dental socket. These local alterations arise as a natural healing process that aims to achieve a secondary closure of the wound and the dental socket. The healing phases of an alveolus include an inflammatory phase, a proliferation phase, and a remodeling phase. After multiple tooth extractions with or without the use of dentures, people may suffer from extensive vertical and horizontal reduction in their alveolar bone process. A reduction of up to 50% of the original bone table can be expected, being greater in the buccal aspect than in its lingual/palatal counterpart [5]. This process of bone resorption continues and determines the morphological configuration of the alveolar process and the severity of the bone atrophy of the jaws. Occasionally, bone resorption is so severe that the alveolar process may be non-existent, compromising important anatomical structures such as the maxillary sinus, the piriformis notch, the nasopalatine nerve, the inferior alveolar nerve, among others (**Figure 1**).

Currently there are multiple classifications that describe alveolar bone atrophy. The two most used are the Seibert classification and the Cawood and howell classification. The Seibert's nomenclature divides alveolar bone loss into three types: Class 1: Loss of vestibule/lingual tissue with normal bone crest height, Class 2: Loss of apical/coronal tissue with normal vestibule/lingual dimension, Class 3: Loss combined horizontal and vertical bone [6].

The Cawood and Howell classification evaluates the post-extraction socket and the edentulous crest for a subsequent restoration treatment, it is divided as follows: Class I: toothed, Class II: post-extraction, Class III: convex shaped process, with width and height adequate, Class IV: sharp edge with adequate height, insufficient width of alveolar process, Class V: flat shape with loss of alveolar process, Class VI: loss of basal bone [7].

Regardless of the degree and severity of bone atrophy, the patient's selection for full arch rehabilitation treatment with dental implants depends on his or her expectations. During the consultation, it is essential to carry out an adequate questioning and understand the reason for our patient's consultation. Esthetic, functional and personal needs. In general, when a patient requires a complete rehabilitative treatment, he has undergone multiple treatments throughout his life, his mentality towards treatment, although in most cases it is "philosophical", sometimes we could have demanding patients with "hysterical" mentality.

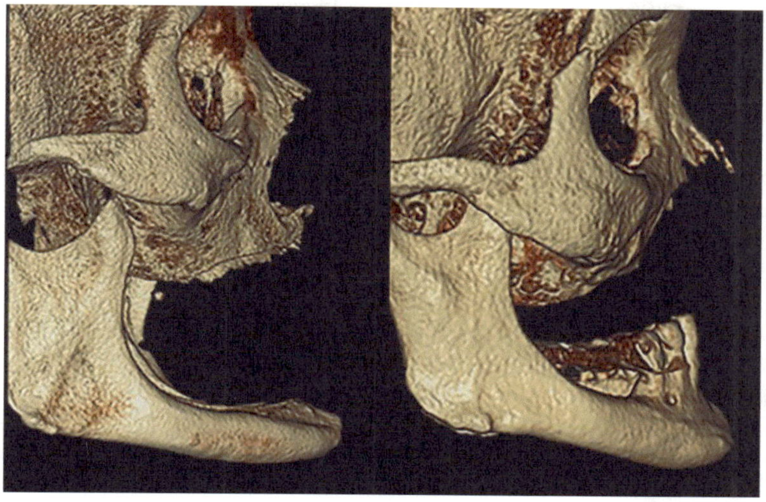

Figure 1.
Different degrees of bone atrophy. The first patient presents a mild/moderate maxillary atrophy, however, he presents a severe mandibular atrophy at the level of the inferior alveolar nerve. The second patient presented severe maxillary atrophy with loss of the premaxilla. The atrophy extends posteriorly to the floor of the maxillary sinus, making it impossible to place conventional implants. In the mandible it presents a mild/moderate atrophy in the posterior sector.

Understanding the attitude of patients and their expectations is important for the success of full arch rehabilitation and to offer the best rehabilitative treatment [8].

In general, indications for a full arch rehabilitative treatment with dental implants include:

- Complete edentulism of one or both jaws.
- Partial edentulism with poor periodontal and prosthetic prognosis for existing teeth.
- Failure or denial of fixed prosthetic treatment or conventional prosthodontics.
- Moderate and severe atrophy that does not achieve retention with the use of conventional prostheses [9].
- Xerostomy or hypersensitivity of the mucosa that prevents the use of conventional prostheses [10, 11].

There are few contraindications to dental implant treatment, most are relative and not absolute.

- Uncontrolled systemic disease: Systemic compromises such as cancer, radiotherapy, chemotherapy, autoimmune diseases, HIV, bisphosphonates and bone diseases could contraindicate treatment if the patient does not have a pharmacological control with adequate response to treatment. However, when these conditions are medically controlled and performed with established protocols, they can have a high success rate and are not an absolute contraindication to dental implant treatment [12–14].

- Alcoholics, drug addicts or patients with psychosis: these are patients who have no commitment and good control of treatment. This could lead to complications and a low success rate. Smoking patients may have a higher failure rate for dental implant treatment. However, it is not an absolute contraindication to treatment [15].

- Allergy to titanium: Although allergy to titanium is extremely low (0.6%), this can explain a failure of implants or previous treatments in an inexplicable way. Currently, zirconia implants have been manufactured that can satisfactorily solve this situation [16, 17].

- Pregnancy: Rehabilitation treatments with dental implants should be postponed during the gestation period. During treatment, advanced imaging studies are needed in addition to the pharmacological implications during and after surgery.

3. Therapeutic options: bone grafting versus buttress implant concept

There are different surgical techniques used in the rehabilitation of atrophic jaws that are divided into two large groups: Non-grafted versus Grafted treatments. Graft procedures include: bone regeneration with bone substitutes with or without the use of membranes, maxillary sinus lift and platelet-rich plasma [18, 19].

Procedures that do not use grafts, use skeletal anchors with long and conventional implants in the different anatomical points of the facial bones.

For both techniques there is a high success rate of 90–95% at 5 years with no statistically significant difference in implant survival [20].

Currently there are multiple classifications with diagnostic and therapeutic criteria in rehabilitation with dental implants. However, there is no classification that unites all implant alternatives with diagnostic, surgical and implant criteria.

The buttress implant concept is a classification that I have designed and is based on the bony buttresses of the face. These areas offer adequate quality and quantity of bone where the placement and functional load of osseointegrated implants is feasible.

The classification for the patient with jaws atrophy is divided into 6 zones: Zone I/maxillary alveolar buttress, Zone II/nasomaxillary buttress, Zone III/zygomatico-maxillary buttress, Zone IV/pterygomaxillary buttress, Zone V/mandibular alveolar buttress and Zone VI mandibular/basal buttress (**Figure 2**).

- Zone I/alveolar buttress: In the alveolar buttress of the maxilla we can anchor osseointegrated implants in the bone process. In this area we can place implants axially or tilted. Tilted implants with an angle between 17° and 45° perform as well as axial implants. Among our options, in this buttress we find conventional and short implants ≤8 mm, nasopalatine duct implant, tilted implants such as those described in the All on 4 techniques, and tuberosity implants [21].

- Zone II/nasomaxillary buttress: Although the term "Nasomaxillary implant" has not been defined in the Glossary of Oral and Maxillofacial Implants (GOMI) [22]. I define it as "Implant placement through the alveolar process and into the nasomaxillary buttress". Nasomaxillary implants can be used as an anchorage point in a location anterior to the prosthetic arch. With this, we achieve anterior stability and the reduction of work forces in posterior implants.

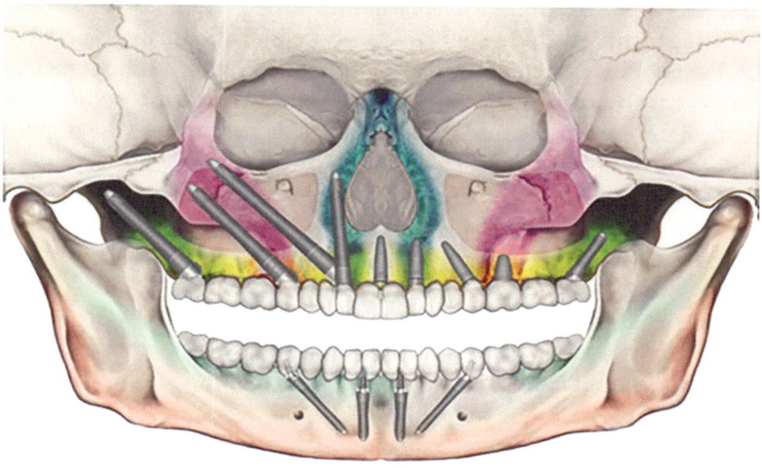

Figure 2.
Buttress implant concept and classification for the patient with jaws atrophy: Zone I/maxillary alveolar buttress, zone II/nasomaxillary buttress, zone III/zygomaticomaxillary buttress, zone IV/pterygomaxillary buttress, zone V/ mandibular alveolar buttress and zone VI mandibular/basal buttress.

- Zone III/zygomaticomaxillary buttress: In 1998 Dr. P. I Branemark described zygomatic implants as a bone anchorage alternative with a design between 30 and 52.5 mm long that are inserted into the body of the malar bone [23]. Zygomatic implants offer adequate insertion torque. Immediate loading is usually more feasible compared to conventional implants. Up to 3 zygomatic implants can be placed on each side offering a full arch rehabilitation with an adequate polygonal distribution within the prosthetic arch.

- Zone IV/pterygomaxillary buttress: Tulasne and Tessier in 1989 were the first to describe the technique for the placement of pterygoid implants [24]. Pterygoid implants are implants between 15 and 20 mm long that allow a bone anchorage of up to 9 mm in the pterygoid process. Pterygoid implants are a viable option and if their main advantage is to decrease the prosthetic distal cantilever [25].

- Zone V/mandibular alveolar buttress: As in the maxilla, in the mandibular alveolar process we can use axial implants, short implants ≤8 mm and tilted implants with a mandible interforaminal anchorage as described in the “All on 4” technique. Subperiosteal custom implants are currently a new line of implementation with promising results. These custom implants generally obtain their retention in this buttress with monocortical screws [26].

- Zone VI/mandibular basal buttress: The basal mandibular buttress is a zone that offers a cortical bone which allows a primary stabilization when it is reached. This area has been used in severe bone atrophy, in oncological resections or after regenerative procedures in blocks. Currently there are various bone anchoring options such as the use of zygomatic mandibular implants, trefoil technique (Trefoil™) and bicortical implants (Strategic Implant®) that have offered adequate and salvage results in full arch rehabilitation treatment [27–29].

In general, full arch rehabilitation treatments with osseointegrated implants combine multiple techniques; regenerative and skeletal anchoring. The advantage of using skeletal anchors is that it allows a greater probability of immediate loading, a lower biological cost by not performing multiple regenerative procedures, less time in the treatment phases with a comparable global cost. The main disadvantages of using skeletal anchors include a higher learning curve, need for sedation or general anesthesia, and special surgical equipment that in most cases is available from commercial companies.

4. From analog to digital implantology

4.1 Computer guide treatment

Technological advances in conventional medicine and implantology offer resources in the diagnosis and treatment of full arch rehabilitation with osseointegrated implants. The digitization of clinical cases thanks to computed tomography and the buccal scanner allow the elaboration of surgical guides which restrict movements in the 3 planes of space. Although some studies confirm that there is no statistically significant difference in digital versus analog procedures, the digitization process in implantology can help avoid human errors and injury to anatomical structures, help to determine a drilling sequence with a greater probability of primary stability, reduce the Surgical times and improve the perceptions of patients by having a modern treatment [30].

When we perform computer-guided planning and see that regenerative procedures around implants are not required, flap-free surgery allows for greater patient comfort, recovery, and acceptance of treatment (**Figure 3**).

4.2 Computer-assisted dynamic navigation

Computer-assisted dynamic navigation has been commonly employed in medicine, recently been implemented for dental implant surgery. The dynamic navigation uses optical motion technology to see the implant placement in real time, this helps to perform a flapless surgery and gives the surgeon the confidence of knowing that the implant placement is adequate. However, dynamic navigation is a recent practice that has a high learning curve in addition to requiring specialized medical equipment [31, 32].

4.3 Biomodels in 3D

Stereolithography is a solid three-dimensional prototype obtained through the processing of data obtained from computed tomography or magnetic resonance imaging. In recent years, stereolithographic manufacturing has made great strides in the quality, resolution, and precision of manufactured parts and is becoming increasingly important in medicine and surgery.

Surgical simulation on a 3D biomodel makes it possible to consider measurements, positions and emergencies of the implants on the prosthetic arch. In addition, its usefulness in the placement of long implants with skeletal anchors allows the surgeon to be prepared for the surgical procedure and minimizes the possibilities of errors, favoring the results of the treatment [33] (**Figure 4A**).

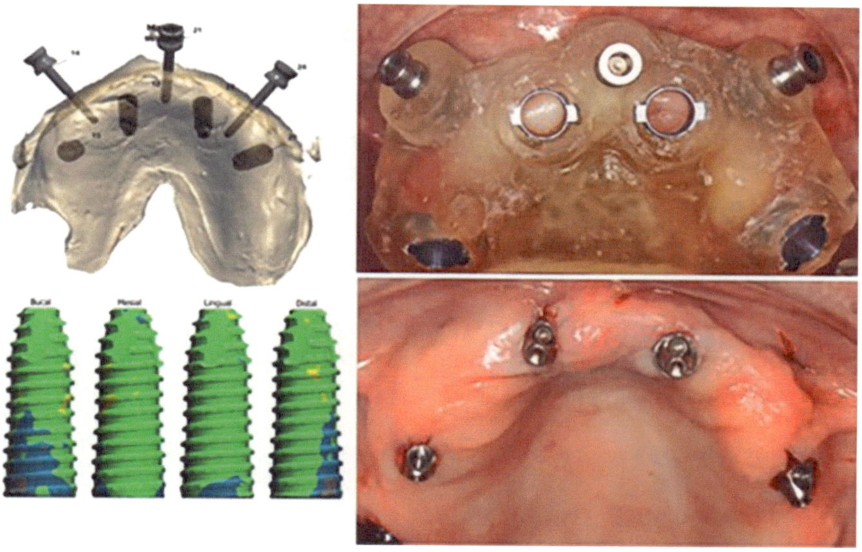

Figure 3.
Computer-guided surgery by means of tomography, scanner and plan (dental system® 3Shape and DIO implants). In this case, flapless surgery was performed.

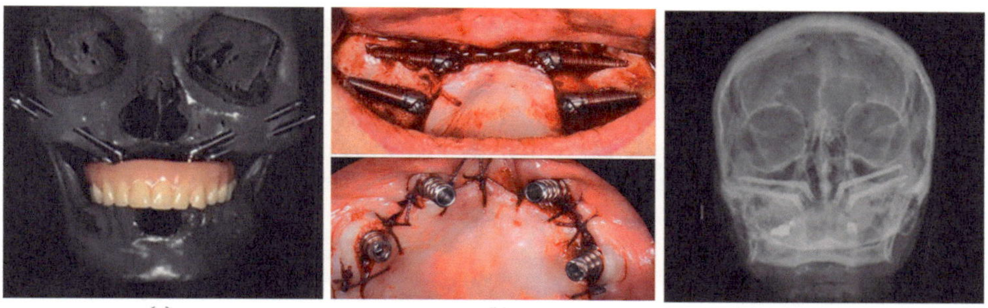

(a) (b) (c)

Figure 4.
A. Simulated surgery of Quadzygoma treatment on a biomodel in ABS (acrylonitrile butadiene styrene) with adaptation of an immediate retained prosthesis to temporary abaument. B and C. clinical application of Quadzygoma treatment (NeoArch – Neodent®).

5. Full arch rehabilitation in maxilla

5.1 Treatment of mild–moderate maxillary alveolar resorption

The maxilla is a paired bone located in the middle third of the face. In its upper part is the orbital cavity, in its middle part the nasal cavity and in its lower part the oral cavity. Towards the oral cavity, there is the alveolar process, which houses the maxillary dental formula and is the main area affected by edentulism. Although the maxillary bone is voluminous, it is quite light due to the presence of the maxillary sinus. A cavity that is part of the respiratory system through which air passes, is heated, humidified and filtered to pass into the respiratory tract. In general, in the treatment of mild maxillary alveolar resorption, it is not necessary to lift the maxillary sinus membrane, allowing the placement of axial implants. If bone resorption is moderate, consideration should be given to regenerative procedures, sinus lift, or placement of tilted implants [34].

The choice of implants will depend on bone availability and prosthetic planning. Although there is no statistically significant variation when choosing narrows versus regular platform implants, we prefer implant placement greater than 4.0 millimeters in diameter in full arch treatment [35]. This has several reasons. Mainly the thickness of the implant walls and prosthetic solutions such as angled abutments available for implants of this diameter or greater.

An important consideration during planning and implantation is that the implants are prosthetically guided achieving a polygonal emergence towards the prosthetic arch. Once the implantation is achieved, an adequate wound closure must be carried out and the patient should be offered immediate rehabilitation with which the healing process will continue.

5.2 Treatment of severe maxillary alveolar resorption

The rehabilitation of a patient with severe maxillary atrophy represents a significant challenge for the surgeon and the prosthetist. Often these patients have undergone multiple treatments that have not been able to meet their demands and their mentality regarding the treatment is expectant. In addition to this, patients with severe maxillary atrophy have suffered a total collapse of all their stomaognathic structures, suffering an aging of the face with loss of self-esteem, esthetics and function.

To achieve a successful rehabilitative treatment, we must consider all our therapeutic options and have an anatomical knowledge of the possible anchor points for the placement of osseointegrated implants. During planning, we must evaluate the advantages and disadvantages of regenerative treatment of lost bone versus using long implants with remote skeletal anchors. Sometimes, regenerating the bone with grafts and membranes entails a higher biological and economic cost for the rehabilitative treatment or could increase the times for the definitive rehabilitation.

When conventional implants are an unfeasible option due to the degree of maxillary atrophy or when multiple regenerative treatments must be performed prior to implantation, anchors with long implants in the buttresses have solved this situation. Zygomatic implants are a suitable option. Arch treatments can be performed on 4 zygomatic implants, two on each side or in combination with conventional implants. Zygomatic implants offer adequate insertion torque and can be used as a rescue when conditions are not ideal with conventional implants [36]. Posterior tilted implants, tuberosity implants and pterygopalatine implants are posterior implants that have reduced the distal cantiliever of the prosthesis and support the biomechanical demands of rehabilitation (**Figure 4B** and **C**) [37].

6. Full arch rehabilitation in jaw

The mandible is an odd bone located in the lower third of the face and is shaped like a horseshoe. It is the largest bone in the face and the only one that moves thanks to the insertion of multiple muscles that participate in chewing. Unlike the maxilla, the mandible has a more corticalized bone, which in most cases allows immediate screw loading. The main anatomical structures of importance include the inferior alveolar nerve, the mental nerve, the insertion of the mylohyoid muscle and the floor of the mouth [38].

6.1 Treatment of jaw alveolar resorption

The rehabilitation of posterior regions and edentulous arches with mild atrophy, still allows the placement of implants of at least 8 mm or more in the posterior sector without compromising important anatomical structures such as the inferior alveolar nerve (IAN). In these cases, the biomicanic demands with the placement of 4 to 6 implants in the jaw allow adequate rehabilitation with screws [39].

When alveolar atrophy is moderate or severe, implants cannot be placed without invading the inferior alveolar nerve (IAN). In this situation, therapeutic options include regeneration of the lost alveolar bone, lateralization of the inferior alveolar nerve, placement of short implants < 8 mm and the placement of tilted implants anterior to the mental nerve in the All-on-4® concept [40].

Although the minimum number of implants required for a screw-retained prosthesis is 4, recently it has been described in jaws with severe atrophy the placement of up to 3 bicortical implants in the chin region in a Trefoil ™ concept with good results [41].

In general, the conventional surgical technique includes elevation of a full thickness flap to visualize the bone to the extent where the dental implants will be placed. If the residual bone crest shows irregularities, a bone plasty must be performed until a plateau is achieved and the implantation can be carried out according to the drilling sequence for each commercial company. When planning tilted implants anterior to the mental nerve (30° to 45°), it is essential to preserve the mental nerve and its labial branch to avoid neurosensory alterations of the lower lip. After carrying out the implantation of the desired number of implants, the hermetic closure of the wound is essential to avoid dehiscences and achieve a healing by first intention (**Figure 5**) [42].

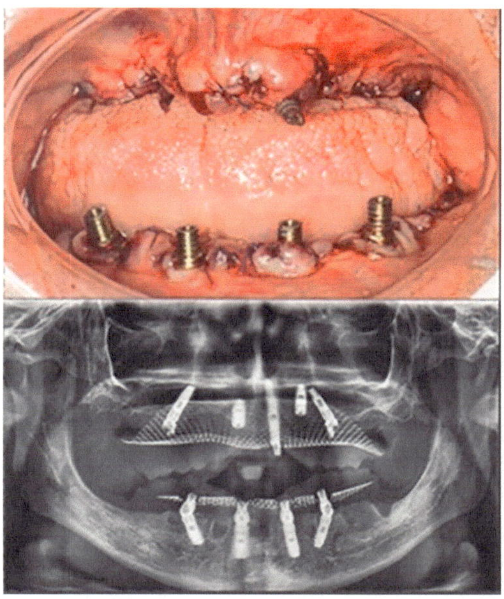

Figure 5.
Clinical and radiographic photograph of maxillary rehabilitation on 5 submerged implants (2 phases) and mandibular rehabilitation on 4 implants with immediate loading (1 phase).

7. Prosthetic considerations: Immediate and definitive prosthesis

7.1 Immediate prosthesis

For the adaptation of an immediate postsurgical prosthesis we will have multiple options that depend on the primary stability of the implants (greater than 35 N), the biotype and bone quality, the thickness of the cortices around the implants and the patient's commitment to comply precise indications such as diet and hygiene [43].

When the previous conditions mentioned are unfavorable, we can leave the implants submerged with covers screws, another option is to offer the patient a conventional removable total prosthesis retained to the implants by means of healing abutments. This favors certain retention and adaptation to the patient while the implants are not loaded during their osseointegration phase (2-phase protocol). When conditions allow an immediate screwed and supported load on the implants (1-phase protocol), this same conventional total prosthesis can be reduced from the flanks, the palate and/or the floor of the mouth to achieve a horseshoe shape, subsequently with a The acrylic relining is mechanically retained to the implants by means of temporarys abauments.

7.2 Definitive prosthesis

The long-term success of our prosthetic treatment depends on an adequate diagnosis and the detection of possible clinical difficulties before treatment. The planning of esthetic and functional prostheses requires the analysis of additional parameters such as smile height, lip sizes, permanence or absence of nasal and labial support given by the pre-maxilla, interocclusal and inter-arch space, functional demands, etc. For full arch reconstruction with dental implants there are several alternatives that we mention below:

- Implant-supported fixed prostheses (ISFPs): When there is an adequate interocclusal distance and the volume of hard and soft tissues has been maintained, fixed prostheses with implants allow a total reconstruction of the teeth with a natural emergence of the gingiva of the patient. Typically, these types of dentures are retained to the implants in a metal/ceramic material by means of a castable abutment (UCLA Abutment) [44].

- Implant-retained overdentures (IODs): Overdentures are total and removable dentures, but with an anchorage system. Overdentures mean fewer implants (2 to 4 per jaw). in older patients, they improve hygiene by being removable, compared to conventional complete dentures (CCDs), they significantly increase patient satisfaction, dental function and quality of life [45].

- Hybrid prosthesis: In addition to rehabilitating missing teeth, a hybrid prosthesis simulates part of the soft tissues. This type of prosthesis requires a minimum distance of 12 to 15 millimeters between the arch and esthetic parameters such as the height of the smile and the exposure of the lower teeth should be evaluated in more detail [46]. Cantilever length is also an important parameter that is to be evaluated when deciding to fabricate implant supported acrylic screw-retained hybrid prosthesis to minimize the risk of framework fracture. The researchers suggested a mandibular extension between 15 and 20 mm to minimize the risk of framework

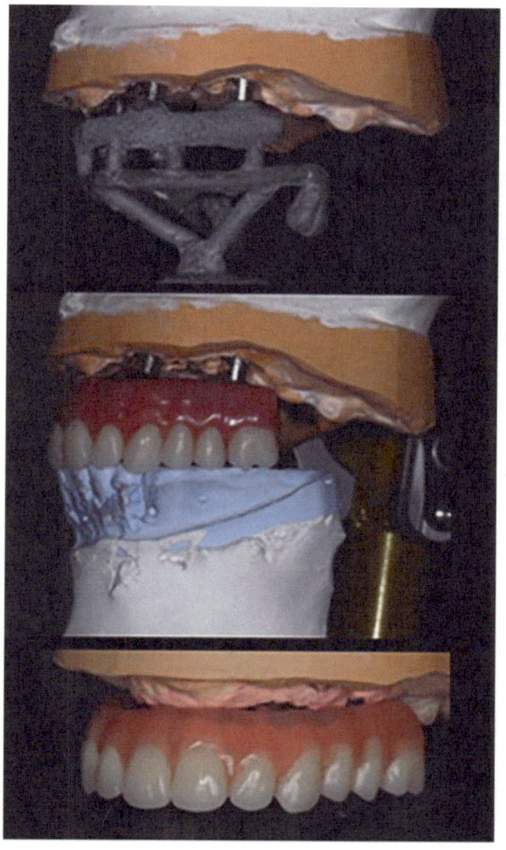

Figure 6.
Workflow for fabrication of hybrid metal-acrylic prosthesis.

fracture. Other authors recommended a cantilever length of 1.5 or 2 times of the anterior/posterior curve of the implants. Hybrid dentures are generally made of acrylic resin and metal or metal and porcelain (**Figure 6**) [47].

8. Complications

Full arch rehabilitation treatments with dental implants can have complications and failures. In general, complications may be related to the patient's systemic compromise, increased functional demand, surgical technique, post-operative care, design and type of prosthesis, etc. The overall success rate for dental implants is between 90–100% according to the study [48].

The most frequent prosthetic complications after the placement of an implant-supported prosthesis are: mucositis, loosening or fracture of the abutment screw or prosthetic components, and fracture of the acrylic or porcelain structure. Although most complications resolve favorably in follow-up appointments, it is essential to establish an adequate surgical and prosthetic management protocol to achieve predictable and successful long-term results [49, 50].

9. Where are we going

Medical and technological advances in medicine applied to current implantology have made it possible to have new rehabilitative treatments. Currently, the diagnosis of the edentulous patient, the design of the rehabilitation and the computer-guided surgery, allow the use of customized implants for full-arch rehabilitation. These devices are generally made of titanium and have a treated surface that allows osseointegration. In addition, they use skeletal anchors in the aforementioned abutments so that they have multiple fixations that work together to rehabilitate a complete dental arch. Currently, although their costs are high, they are accessible for very specific cases (**Figure** 7).

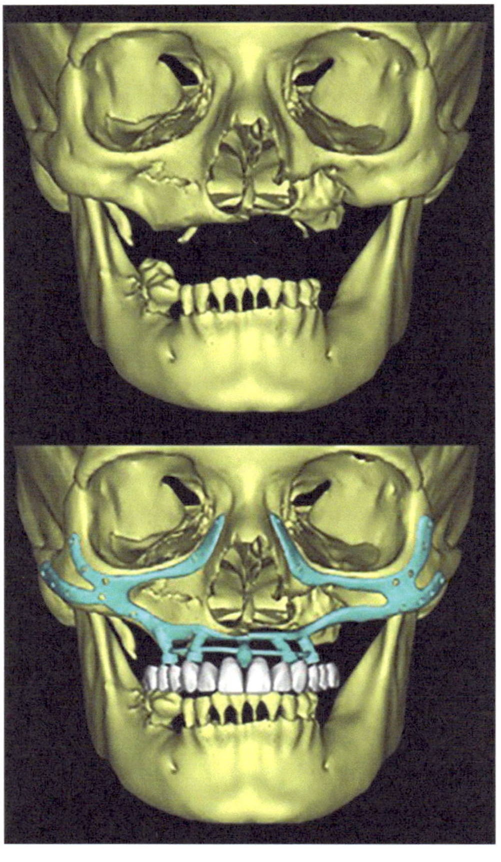

Figure 7.
Planning of a customized prosthesis in grade IV titanium for full-arch rehabilitation after tumor resection in an oncological patient.

10. Conclusions

Based on the current literature, full-arch fixed prostheses supported by a combination of axial implants, angled and placed in the different skeletal anchor points (buttress implant concept) can be considered a predictable and successful treatment modality for prosthetic rehabilitation of edentulous patients.

Acknowledgements

There are no acknowledgments to declare.

Conflict of interest

There are no conflicts of interest to declare.

Ethical approval

Institutional approval was not required. All cases were operated on by the author. All images are original and the author's own.

Author details

Leandro Díez-Suárez
National Cancer Institute and National Autonomous University of Mexico (UNAM), Mexico City, Mexico

*Address all correspondence to: ledisuar@gmail.com

References

[1] Ali Z, Baker SR, Shahrbaf S, Martin N, Vettore MV. Oral health-related quality of life after prosthodontic treatment for patients with partial edentulism: A systematic review and meta-analysis. J Prosthet Dent. 2019 Jan;121(1):59-68.e3. DOI:10.1016/j.prosdent.2018.03.003. Epub 2018 Jul 10.

[2] Laney, W. (2017). Glossary of Oral and Maxillofacial Implants. The International Journal of Oral & Maxillofacial Implants, 32(4), Gi–G200. DOI:10.11607/jomi.2017.4.gomi.

[3] Block MS. Dental implants: The last 100 years. J Oral Maxillofac Surg. 2018 Jan;76(1):11-26. DOI:10.1016/j.joms.2017.08.045.

[4] Pjetursson BE, Lang NP. Prosthetic treatment planning on the basis of scientific evidence. J Oral Rehabil. 2008 Jan;35 Suppl 1:72-79. DOI:10.1111/j.1365-2842.2007.01824.x.

[5] Araújo MG, Silva CO, Misawa M, Sukekava F. Alveolar socket healing: what can we learn? Periodontol 2000. 2015 Jun;68(1):122-34. DOI:10.1111/prd.12082.

[6] Seibert JS. Reconstruction of deformed, partially edentulous ridges, using full thickness onlay grafts. Part I. technique and wound healing. Compend Contin Educ Dent. 1983 Sep-Oct;4(5):437-453.

[7] Cawood JI, Howell RA. A classification of the edentulous jaws. Int J Oral Maxillofac Surg. 1988 Aug;17(4):232-236. DOI:10.1016/s0901-5027(88)80047-x.

[8] Bhochhibhoya A, Rana SB, Sharma R, Khapung A. Impact of sociodemographic factors, duration of edentulism, and medical comorbidities on the mental attitudes of individuals with complete edentulism. J Prosthet Dent. 2021 May 18:S0022-3913(21)00217-1. DOI:10.1016/j.prosdent.2021.04.007.

[9] Strassburger C, Kerschbaum T, Heydecke G. Influence of implant and conventional prostheses on satisfaction and quality of life: A literature review. Part 2: Qualitative analysis and evaluation of the studies. Int J Prosthodont. 2006 Jul-Aug;19(4):339-348.

[10] Mori G, Kobayashi T, Ito T, Yajima Y. Implant-supported prostheses in patient with Sjögren's syndrome: Clinical report with 3-year follow-up. Bull Tokyo Dent Coll. 2018;59(3):201-206. DOI:10.2209/tdcpublication.2017-0036.

[11] Almeida D, Vianna K, Arriaga P, Moraschini V. Dental implants in Sjögren's syndrome patients: A systematic review. PLoS One. 2017;12(12):e0189507. Published 2017 Dec 14. DOI:10.1371/journal.pone.0189507.

[12] Gómez-Pedraza A, González-Cardín V, Díez-Suárez L, Herrera-Villalva M. Maxillofacial rehabilitation with Zygomatic implants in an oncologic patient: A case report. J Oral Maxillofac Surg. 2020 Apr;78(4):547-556. DOI:10.1016/j.joms.2019.10.006.

[13] Javed F, Al-Hezaimi K, Al-Rasheed A, Almas K, Romanos GE. Implant survival rate after oral cancer therapy: A review. Oral Oncol. 2010 Dec;46(12):854-859. DOI:10.1016/j.oraloncology.2010.10.004.

[14] Kovács AF. Influence of chemotherapy on endosteal implant survival and success in oral cancer patients. Int J Oral Maxillofac Surg. 2001

Apr;30(2):144-147. DOI:10.1054/ijom.2000.0023.

[15] Gupta A, Rathee S, Suman T, Ahire M, Madhav S, Chauhan MS. Nicotine, the predictor of success or failure of dental implants: A retrospective study. Contemp Clin Dent. 2018 Oct-Dec;9(4):597-600. DOI:10.4103/ccd.ccd_597_18.

[16] Sicilia A, Cuesta S, Coma G, Arregui I, Guisasola C, Ruiz E, Maestro A. Titanium allergy in dental implant patients: A clinical study on 1500 consecutive patients. Clin Oral Implants Res. 2008 Aug;19(8):823-835. DOI:10.1111/j.1600-0501.2008.01544.x.

[17] Siddiqi A, Payne AGT, De Silva RK, Duncan WJ. Titanium allergy: Could it affect dental implant integration? Clin Oral Implants Res. 2011 Jul;22(7):673-680. DOI:10.1111/j.1600-0501.2010.02081.x.

[18] de Sousa CA, Lemos CAA, Santiago-Júnior JF, Faverani LP, Pellizzer EP. Bone augmentation using autogenous bone versus biomaterial in the posterior region of atrophic mandibles: A systematic review and meta-analysis. J Dent. 2018 Sep;76:1-8. DOI:10.1016/j.jdent.2018.06.014.

[19] Bianchi B, Ferri A, Ferrari S, Copelli C, Boni P, Sesenna E. Iliac crest free flap for maxillary reconstruction. J Oral Maxillofac Surg. 2010 Nov;68(11):2706-2713. DOI:10.1016/j.joms.2010.01.008.

[20] Tran DT, Gay IC, Diaz-Rodriguez J, Parthasarathy K, Weltman R, Friedman L. Survival of dental implants placed in grafted and nongrafted bone: A retrospective study in a university setting. Int J Oral Maxillofac Implants. 2016 Mar-Apr;31(2):310-317. DOI:10.11607/jomi.4681.

[21] Soto-Penaloza D, Zaragozí-Alonso R, Penarrocha-Diago M, Penarrocha-Diago M. The all-on-four treatment concept: Systematic review. J Clin Exp Dent. 2017 Mar 1;9(3):e474-e488. DOI:10.4317/jced.53613.

[22] Laney WR. Glossary of Oral and Maxillofacial Implants. Int J Oral Maxillofac Implants. 2017 Jul/Aug;32(4):Gi-G200. DOI:10.11607/jomi.2017.4.gomi.

[23] Branemark P. Surgery Fixture Installation: Zygomaticus Fixture Clinical Procedures. 1st ed. Gotemburgo, Suecia: Nobel Bio-care, AB; 1998.

[24] Tulasne JF. Implant treatment of missing posterior dentition. In: Albrektson T, Zarb G, editors. The Branemark Osseointegrated Implant. Chicago: Quintessence; 1989. p. 103-115.

[25] Araujo RZ, Santiago Júnior JF, Cardoso CL, Benites Condezo AF, Moreira Júnior R, Curi MM. Clinical outcomes of pterygoid implants: Systematic review and meta-analysis. J Craniomaxillofac Surg. 2019 Apr;47(4):651-660. DOI:10.1016/j.jcms.2019.01.030.

[26] Mangano C, Bianchi A, Mangano FG, Dana J, Colombo M, Solop I, Admakin O. Custom-made 3D printed subperiosteal titanium implants for the prosthetic restoration of the atrophic posterior mandible of elderly patients: a case series. 3D Print Med. 2020 Jan 8;6(1):1. DOI:10.1186/s41205-019-0055-x.

[27] Muñoz R, Gajos G, Bladimir J, Carvajal D, Luis A, Del Valle Speranza G. Protocol for mandibular reconstruction with zygomatic implants (zygomatic mandibular implant). Oral Maxillofac Surg. 2018 Mar;22(1):39-44. DOI:10.1007/s10006-017-0664-8.

[28] Borgonovo AE, Galbiati SLM, Re D. Trefoil system for the treatment of mandibular Edentulism: A case report with 30 months follow-up. Case Rep Dent. 2020 Oct 17;2020:8845649. DOI:10.1155/2020/8845649.

[29] Lazarov A. Immediate functional loading: Results for the concept of the strategic implant®. Ann Maxillofac Surg. 2019 Jan-Jun;9(1):78-88. DOI:10.4103/ams.ams_250_18.

[30] Papaspyridakos P, Vazouras K, Chen YW, Kotina E, Natto Z, Kang K, Chochlidakis K. Digital vs conventional implant impressions: A systematic review and meta-analysis. J Prosthodont. 2020 Oct;29(8):660-678. DOI:10.1111/jopr.13211.

[31] Kasten, B., Arastu, A., & Panchal, N. (2018). Dental implant surgery: From conventional to guided to navigated approach. Current Oral Health Reports, 5(2), 140-146. DOI:10.1007/s40496-018-0182-2.

[32] Ewers R, et al. Computer aided navigation in dental implantology: 7 years of clinical experience. J Oral Maxillofac Surg. 2004;62:32-334.

[33] Raman R, Bashir R. Stereolithographic 3D bioprinting for biomedical applications. In: Essentials of 3D Biofabrication and Translation. Elsevier Inc.; 2015. pp. 89-121. DOI:10.1016/B978-0-12-800972-7/00006-2.

[34] Mertens C, Steveling HG. Implant-supported fixed prostheses in the edentulous maxilla: 8-year prospective results. Clin Oral Implants Res. 2011 May;22(5):464-472. DOI:10.1111/j.1600-0501.2010.02028.x.

[35] Moreira de Melo EJ Jr, Francischone CE. Three-dimensional finite element analysis of two angled narrow-diameter implant designs for an all-on-4 prosthesis. J Prosthet Dent. 2020 Oct;124(4):477-484. DOI:10.1016/j.prosdent.2019.09.015.

[36] Bedrossian E. Rescue implant concept: The expanded use of the zygoma implant in the graftless solutions. Oral Maxillofac Surg Clin North Am. 2011 May;23(2):257-276, vi. DOI:10.1016/j.coms.2011.01.009.

[37] Curi MM, Cardoso CL, Ribeiro Kde C. Retrospective study of pterygoid implants in the atrophic posterior maxilla: Implant and prosthesis survival rates up to 3 years. Int J Oral Maxillofac Implants. 2015 Mar-Apr;30(2):378-383. DOI:10.11607/jomi.3665.

[38] Genç T, Duruel O, Kutlu HB, Dursun E, Karabulut E, Tözüm TF. Evaluation of anatomical structures and variations in the maxilla and the mandible before dental implant treatment. Dent Med Probl. 2018 Jul-Sep;55(3):233-240. DOI:10.17219/dmp/94303.

[39] Soto-Penaloza D, Zaragozí-Alonso R, Penarrocha-Diago M, Penarrocha-Diago M. The all-on-four treatment concept: Systematic review. J Clin Exp Dent. 2017 Mar 1;9(3):e474-e488. DOI:10.4317/jced.53613.

[40] Abayev, Boris, and Gintaras Juodzbalys. "Inferior alveolar nerve lateralization and transposition for dental implant placement. Part I: A systematic review of surgical techniques." Journal of oral & maxillofacial research vol. 6,1 e2. 30 Mar. 2015, DOI:10.5037/jomr.2014.6102.

[41] Rozov RA, Trezubov VN, Gerasimov AB, Kopylov MV, Azarin GS. Klinicheskii analiz blizhaishikh i otdalennykh rezul'tatov primeneniya

implantatsionnogo protezirovaniya «Trefoil» v Rossii [Clinical analysis of the short-term and long-term results of the implant-supported Trefoil dental rehabilitation in Russia]. Stomatologiia (Mosk). 2020;99(5):50-57. Russian. DOI:10.17116/stomat20209905150.

[42] Krennmair S, Weinländer M, Malek M, Forstner T, Krennmair G, Stimmelmayr M. Mandibular full-arch fixed prostheses supported on 4 implants with either axial or tilted distal implants: A 3-year prospective study. Clin Implant Dent Relat Res. 2016 Dec;18(6):1119-1133. DOI:10.1111/cid.12419.

[43] De Bruyn H, Raes S, Ostman PO, Cosyn J. Immediate loading in partially and completely edentulous jaws: a review of the literature with clinical guidelines. Periodontol 2000. 2014 Oct;66(1):153-187. DOI:10.1111/prd.12040.

[44] Bergkvist G, Sahlholm S, Nilner K, Lindh C. Implant-supported fixed prostheses in the edentulous maxilla. A 2-year clinical and radiological follow-up of treatment with non-submerged ITI implants. Clin Oral Implants Res. 2004 Jun;15(3):351-359. DOI:10.1111/j.1600-0501.2004.01017.x.

[45] Harris D, Höfer S, O'Boyle CA, Sheridan S, Marley J, Benington IC, Clifford T, Houston F, O'Connell B. A comparison of implant-retained mandibular overdentures and conventional dentures on quality of life in edentulous patients: A randomized, prospective, within-subject controlled clinical trial. Clin Oral Implants Res. 2013 Jan;24(1):96-103. DOI:10.1111/j.1600-0501.2011.02368.x.

[46] Oh SH, Kim Y, Park JY, Jung YJ, Kim SK, Park SY. Comparison of fixed implant-supported prostheses, removable implant-supported prostheses, and complete dentures: Patient satisfaction and oral health-related quality of life. Clin Oral Implants Res. 2016 Feb;27(2):e31-e37. DOI:10.1111/clr.12514.

[47] Egilmez F, Ergun G, Cekic-Nagas I, Bozkaya S. Implant-supported hybrid prosthesis: Conventional treatment method for borderline cases. Eur J Dent. 2015;9(3):442-448. DOI:10.4103/1305-7456.163324.

[48] Lin WS, Eckert SE. Clinical performance of intentionally tilted implants versus axially positioned implants: A systematic review. Clin Oral Implants Res. 2018 Oct;29 Suppl 16:78-105. DOI:10.1111/clr.13294.

[49] Ülkü SZ, Acun Kaya F, Uysal E, Gulsun B. Clinical evaluation of complications in implant-supported dentures: A 4-year retrospective study. Med Sci Monit. 2017 Dec 27;23:6137-6143. DOI:10.12659/msm.907840.

[50] Real-Osuna J, Almendros-Marqués N, Gay-Escoda C. Prevalence of complications after the oral rehabilitation with implant-supported hybrid prostheses. Med Oral Patol Oral Cir Bucal. 2012 Jan 1;17(1):e116-e121. DOI:10.4317/medoral.17099.

Chapter 16

Implant-Retained Maxillary and Mandibular Overdentures - A Solution for Completely Edentulous Patients

Dubravka Knezović Zlatarić, Robert Ćelić and Hrvoje Pezo

Abstract

The main goal of modern removable prosthodontics is to restore the normal appearance, function, esthetics and speech in each completely edentulous patient. However, if all teeth are missing in a patient, it becomes very complicated to achieve it using traditional protocols. Therefore, implants were introduced into removable prosthodontics to ensure better retention and stability of the conventional dentures. In case of a large amount of bone missing in the jaw it is necessary to ensure the functioning of the dentures constructing various additional stabilizing and retentive prosthodontic solutions on the osseointegrated implants. Numerous types of attachment systems have been used recently for relating implant-retained overdentures to underlying implants: basically splinting (various bar shape designs) and non-splinting attachments (various ball type attachment, magnet attachment, telescopic coping systems). Indications for their use depend on the surgical and prosthodontic factors such as the number and position of the implants, the amount of free intermaxillary space and the type and size of the overdentures. Different indications, types of the overdentures and the attachment systems will be discussed in this chapter.

Keywords: edentulous patient, implant-retained overdenture, bar shape attachment, ball type attachment, telescopic coping attachment, retention, stability

1. Introduction

Edentulism is defined as an irreversible condition in the patient's mouth and the "final marker of disease burden for oral health" [1, 2]. It is still one of the major problems among older adults globally, regardless of its declining incidence. The prevalence of complete edentulism varies among different countries all around the world since it depends on numerous factors such as education, economic and social situations, lifestyle, oral and general health knowledge and views, and attitudes to dental care [3, 4]. The rate of edentulism tends to vary not only among different countries but among different regions within a country too, with wealthier, more industrialized provinces tending to have lower rates than others [5]. A large number of studies confirm the close relationship between edentulism and age and gender of the patients, their educational and income level, activities of daily living, social isolation and poor self-experienced health [6, 7]. These findings should be recognized at the national level of each country and used to create preventive measures identifying older people who are in need of oral care.

2. Aging - tooth loss - bone loss

Edentulous patients are in need of wearing some kind of prosthodontic replacement to establish lost oral function caused by tooth loss. It occurs because of biologic disease processes and age-related changes, such as dental caries, trauma, periodontal conditions and diseases, as well as poor oral hygiene and oral cancer [8, 9]. Total tooth loss is not only reflected in patients' inability to chew and speak but to their social behavior and self-image and it has a complex and multidimensional impact on oral health related and general quality of life [10, 11].

A large number of studies have already proven that bone loss represents an ongoing process following tooth loss [12, 13], affecting the mandible four times more than the maxilla [14]. This particularly affects the patients who become completely edentulous and creates a large problem for their future maintenance (**Figure 1**).

For the purpose of better understanding of the existing conditions, analysis of the edentulous jaws, easier diagnosis and therapy determination the American College of Prosthodontists (ACP) has developed a classification system for complete edentulism helping prosthodontists determine appropriate treatments for their edentulous patients [15]. This classification consists of four categories, the first representing an uncomplicated clinical situation with ideal or minimally compromised bone height, inter-jaw relationship, residual ridge morphology and muscle attachments and the fourth, representing the most complex and severely compromised oral conditions significantly negatively affecting the prosthodontic outcome [16].

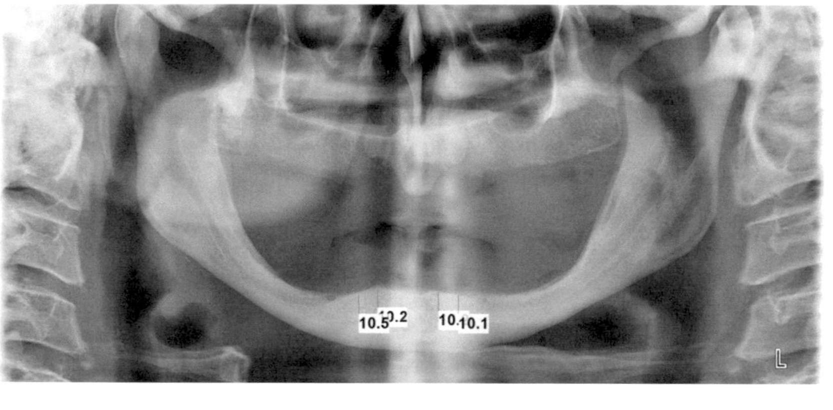

Figure 1.
Current condition of the edentulous maxilla and mandible caused by years of toothlessness. The height of the frontal mandibular bone has been measured to evaluate the possibility of implant placement.

3. Prosthodontic solutions in completely edentulous patients

Toothless residual alveolar ridges in edentulous patients imply the construction of retentive and stable conventional complete dentures [17]. Unfortunately, this can only be achieved in favorable oral conditions that mostly apply to the satisfactory edentulous ridge form and height affecting stability and retention of the dentures in function [18, 19]. It has already been proved that ill-fitting conventional complete dentures can compromise patient's oral function and therefore cause psychosocial problems and decrease his/her oral health-related quality of life (OHRQoL) [20, 21]. The most often recorded complains among conventional complete denture wearers are pure or fair chewing ability, mostly within the subjects who had lost more than 50% of their estimated original ridge height, correlating the residual ridge resorption with worsening of the complete denture stability during mastication [22, 23].

4. Implant prosthodontics

In the last few decades, implants have been increasingly introduced in prosthodontics to replace patient's tooth/teeth lost for several reasons including trauma, caries, and periodontal disease as one of the main causes of edentulism occurring in the elderly population [24]. The loss of single, several or even all the teeth in the jaws can be compensated by placing one or more implants and constructing fixed or removable prosthodontic restorations on them [25–30].

A large number of risk factors related to the implant-prosthodontic therapy are listed in the literature, both at the level of implants as well as of implant prosthodontic restorations [31–34]. It has already been proved in many studies that poorer bone quality and lack of bone volume may be the one of the main reasons of implant failure [35]. Therefore, numerous classifications assisting the therapist in determination of the proper implant-prosthodontic therapy have been suggested for assessment of the degree of atrophy of edentulous jaws, among which the classification system for jaw bone shape and quality proposed by Lekholm and Zarb in 1985 is very often used [36]. One of the major problems in elderly population certainly is the lack and poorer quality of bone structure (Lekholm and Zarb quality 3 or 4 and quantity C, D, or E), especially in the distal part of the alveolar ridges, offering a great challenge for the placement of multiple implants or immediate implant loading and fixed implant prosthodontic constructions [37, 38]. Therefore, in these patients, having compromised bone conditions, implant-retained overdentures may be the best solution [39].

5. McGill consensus statement on overdentures

With an increase of the life expectancy in the following years an increased number of completely edentulous patients will visit dental offices [40]. With a higher standards of their life quality they will expect the same level of standards in prosthodontic treatments demanding improvement in the oral health quality of life, too [40]. With conventional complete dentures relying upon resorbed residual bone ridges of maxilla and mandible and overlying mucosal soft tissues satisfactory retention and stability of the dentures is usually not possible to achieve. Therefore, it is up to the prosthodontics to find new solutions to this issue.

In May 2002, at McGill University in Montreal, Canada, prosthodontic symposium was held where numerous relevant experts who worked in the field of removable prosthodontics stated that the current available evidence suggested the restoration of the completely edentulous mandible using conventional complete denture is no longer the first choice in prosthodontic treatments and instead it should be a two-implant overdenture, regardless of the type of attachment system used (bar, ball or magnet) [41, 42]. According to the available literature patients find mandibular implant-retained overdentures to be superior over conventional ones in retention, ability to chew and speak, comfort, and satisfaction and in oral health related quality of life [43–46]. In April 2009. In York, UK a further consensus statement created by members of British Society for the Study of Prosthetic dentistry Council was released highlighting that uptake by dentists of implants for completely edentulous patients has still been rather slow [47].

As it is stated in the Consensus Statement, the solution in completely edentulous patient should be maxillary conventional complete denture and mandibular two implant-retained overdenture and this therapy presents a minimum standard that should be sufficient for the most patients, taking into account patient comfort and satisfaction, costs and both clinical and dental laboratory time [41, 47]. According to the Statement, placement of only two implants increases the total cost of the treatment, but it is still low enough (in comparison to the multiple implant-prosthodontic restorations) to be affordable to most edentulous patients [41].

6. Prosthodontic indications and advantages for implant supported overdenture in completely edentulous patients

A large number of completely edentulous patients wearing conventional complete dentures are dissatisfied with their prosthodontic restorations [48]. Therefore, implant-retained overdentures were introduced to fulfill a need for maximum support

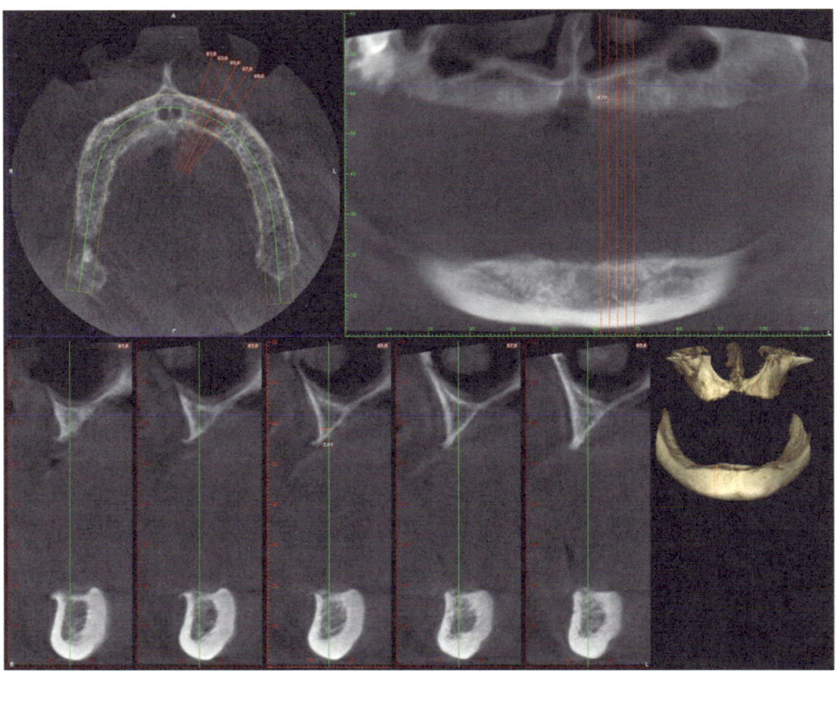

Figure 2.
Three-dimensional measurement of maxillary bone in completely edentulous patient. Notice the extreme resorption of the whole maxillary residual arch.

in edentulous dental arches together with the desire to improve esthetic appearance [49]. Consequently, they are indicated in patients suffering from severe morphological destruction of denture supporting regions with significant loss of denture retention and stability (**Figures 2** and **3**), those with poor oral muscular coordination and low

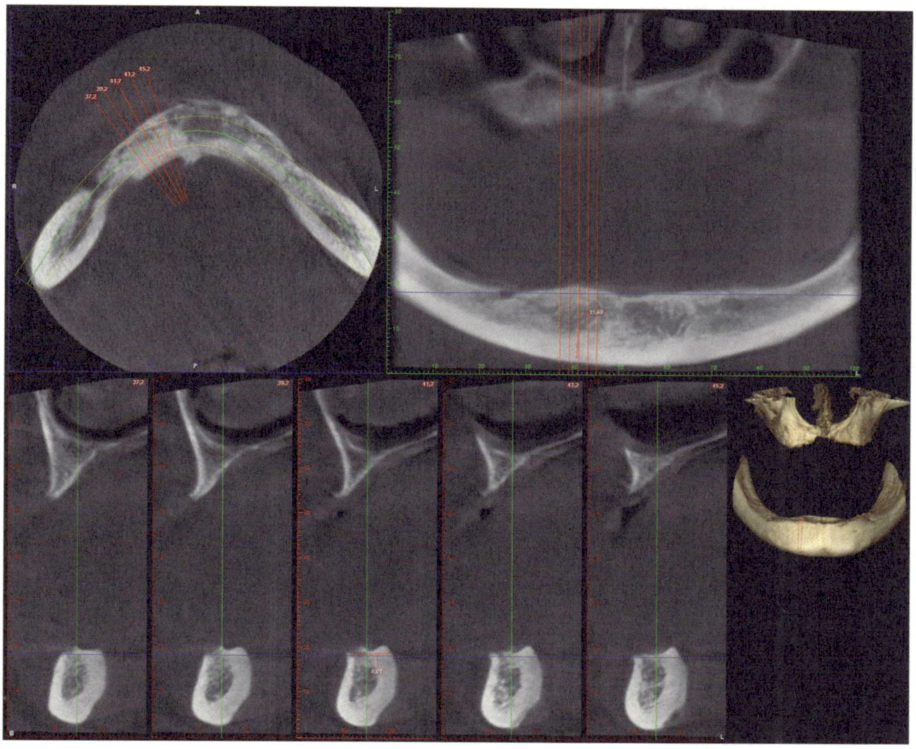

Figure 3.
Three-dimensional measurement of mandibular bone in completely edentulous patient. The resorption of the mandibular residual arch is not so progressive, therefore the placement of 4 implants in the frontal region is indicated.

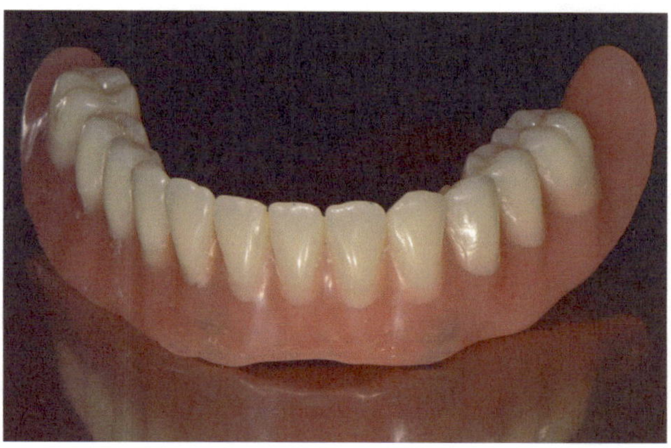

Figure 4.
Vestibular view of 2 implant-retained mandibular overdenture.

tolerance of soft underlying tissues, having parafunctional habits increasing soreness and instability of the conventional restorations or severe gag reflexes [50].

This type of removable prosthodontic rehabilitation is also strongly recommended in patients with unrealistic conventional prosthodontic expectations and those having psychological problems in wearing removable dentures, even when adequate retention and stability are present in the function [50].

This type of implant-prosthodontic rehabilitation offers several advantages such as need for less implants resulting in lower component costs and less expensive treatments for the patient, easy handling and home care maintenance, achieving extremely high level of facial esthetics by labial acrylic flanges and denture teeth replacing missing bone structure and avoiding parafunctions by removing dentures at night (**Figures 4** and 5).

The results of the trial reported in Feine et al. and Grandmont et al. suggested that many patients having the chance to compare both fixed and removable

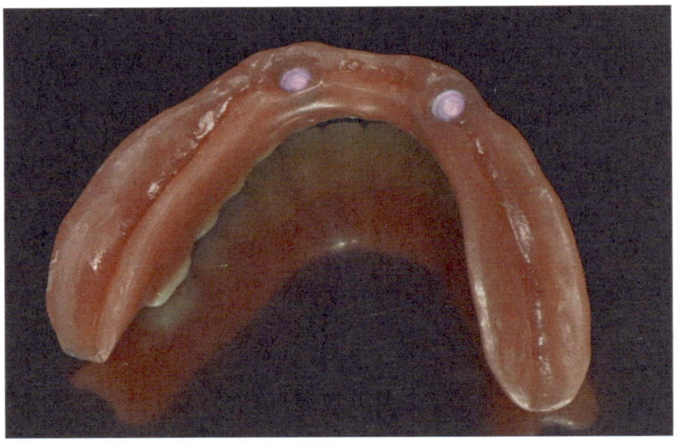

Figure 5.
Oral view of 2 implant-retained mandibular overdenture.

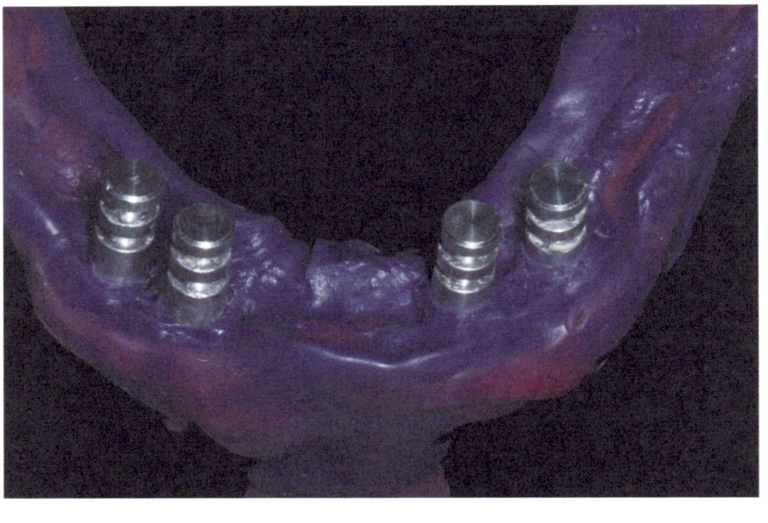

Figure 6.
Individual tray, functional imporession and laboratory analogs for 4 implant-retained mandibular overdenture.

implant-supported mandibular prostheses considered removable types to be a first class treatment [51, 52]. Half of the primarily older individuals monitored in this trial preferred removable over fixed prostheses for easier cleaning and ability to take them out during the night, but reported to be less efficient for chewing [51, 52]. Therefore, this finding should be used by clinicians when choosing the most appropriate type of dentures in completely edentulous patients, too.

It is also important to mention that both clinical and dental laboratory procedures when fabricating implant-retained maxillary and mandibular overdentures do not differ significantly from the conventional on, with the exception of the use of implant transfers, laboratory analogs and individually adjusted trays (**Figures 6–8**).

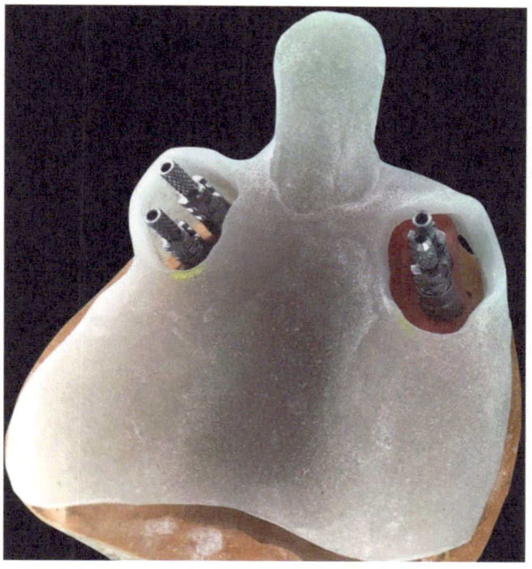

Figure 7.
Open acrylic individual tray and implant transfers ready for impression.

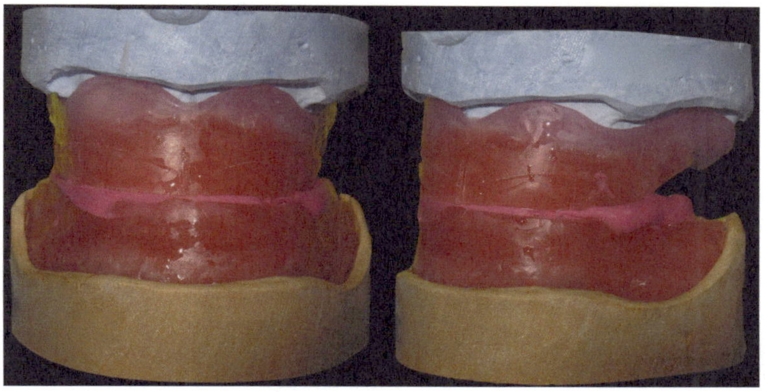

Figure 8.
Both vertical and horizontal dimension registration of the future maxillary conventional and 4 implant-retained mandibular overdenture using wax rims.

7. Number of implants in implant-retained overdentures

Implant-retained overdentures are usually indicated in completely edentulous cases with mild to severe bone resorption in certain regions and therefore go with reduced number of implants. The minimum number of implants needed for an over denture is still in debate.

According to the literature in case of maxillary overdenture with both implant and soft tissue support four to six implants are needed for retention and stability [53–55]. In case of four implants reduction in palatal plate of the denture is reported and recommended (**Figures 9** and **10**) [56, 57].

There are many reports in literature on two implant-retained overdentures in maxilla, too, but it is still the subject of debates (**Figure 11**).

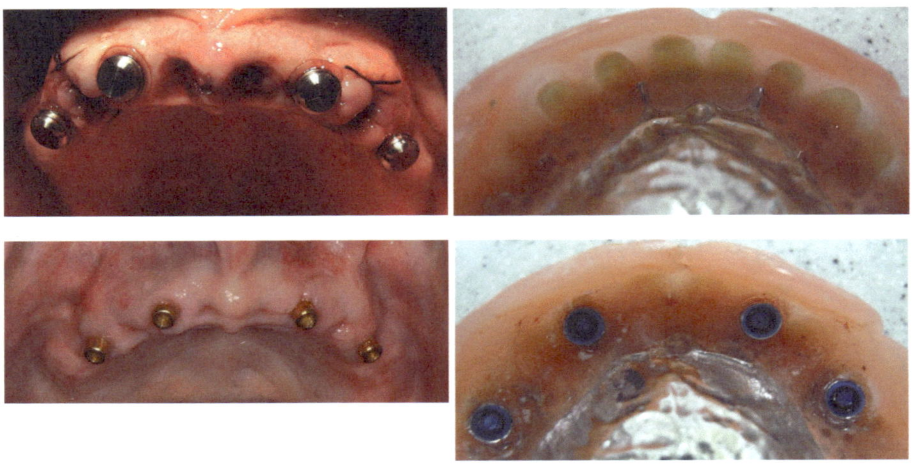

Figure 9.
Four dental implants in maxilla. Clinical procedure of adjusting locators in 4 implant-retained maxillary overdenture.

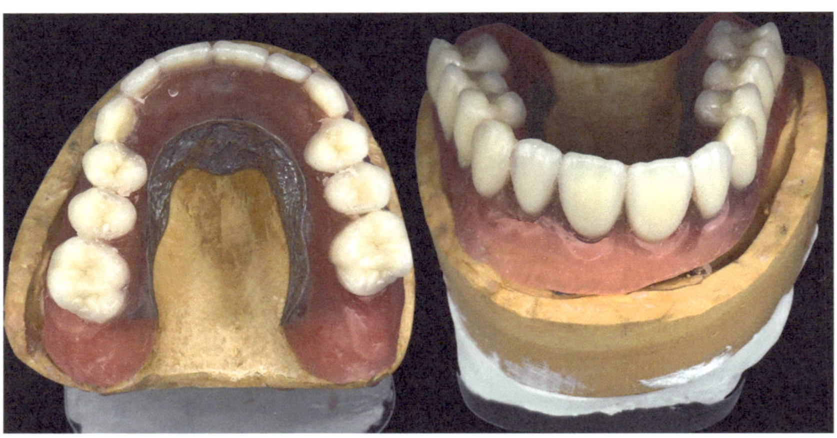

Figure 10.
Distal reduction of the 4 implant-retained maxillary overdenture palatal plate.

DOI: http://dx.doi.org/10.5772/intechopen.99575

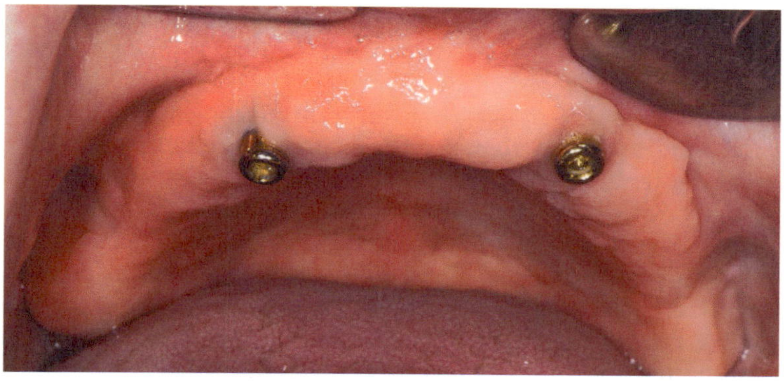

Figure 11.
Clinical check-up of the patient five years following the placement of two implants in maxilla and delivery of the 2 implant-retained maxillary overdenture.

Klemetti et al. concluded that using only two implants in the maxilla did not compromise the dentures longevity or patient satisfaction when compared with four implant overdentures on one hand, but many authors claim that this design of implant-retained overdenture may result in a hinging movement and cause discomfort [58–60].

In mandible, in case of overdenture with both implant and soft tissue support, two implants supported overdenture or single implant retained overdenture is also advisable [61–64].

8. Types of attachment systems on implant-retained overdentures

According to The McGill Consensus Statement on overdentures mandibular two-implant overdentures (**Figure 12**) are considered to be the first choice standard of care for edentulous patients regardless of the type of attachment system used [41].

Numerous types of attachment systems supporting implant overdentures have been developed over years, such as bars, balls, magnets, different cylindrical attachments etc., made of different materials, according to different concepts and designs [65–71].

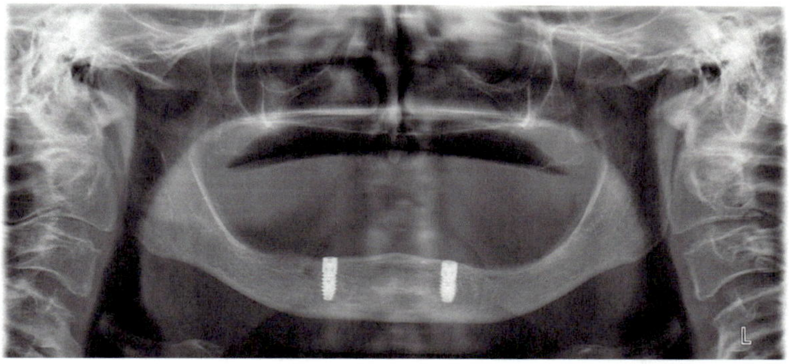

Figure 12.
Standard implant-prosthodontic procedure in completely edentulous patient according to the McGilly consensus.

Of the previously listed systems, only bars require mechanically constructed splinting of the implants and the need to connect them via rigid construction or not is still being discussed.

Both splinted and unsplinted overdenture implant attachment systems have unique advantages and disadvantages. Although different in construction, it seems that both systems achieve similar results with regard to marginal bone loss, prosthetic complications and implant survival rate [72]. A systematic research, carried out from 2000. to 2018., investigated the influence of splinted vs. unsplinted designs for 4 implants retained maxillary overdentures in terms of the outcome assessed in implant survival, prosthodontic longevity and patients' satisfaction. The results revealed no influence of the overdenture design on survival rates of both implants and dentures, as well as on patients' satisfaction with implant survival rate higher than 97%, overdenture survival rate of 100% and patients' satisfaction scores higher than 4.5 (on a 1 to 5 Likert scale) for general satisfaction, chewing ability, denture stabilization, esthetic results and speech [73].

Location of the implants in the edentulous jaw serving for the retention and stability of the overdenture as well as each edentulous arch shape highly influence the stress concentration and distribution around the implants and denture bearing area [74, 75].

If it is about splinted overdenture implant attachment systems using bars made from different materials polyetheretherketone (PEEK), titanium and Co-Cr alloys) the question of designing additional distal cantilever arises. Numerous authors confirmed that, if used, the length of the cantilevel should not exceed the anteroposterior span length, with most commonly mentioned length from 7 to 12 mm (**Figure 13**) [76, 77].

Although it has already been proven that cantilevering of the bars in this type of implant prosthodontic restoration may increase bone loss around supporting implants, especially around the implant adjacent to cantilever, without cantilevers there is less retention and stability of the dentures in the function [78–80]. However, not only does the cantilever and its length cause the problems with loss of bone structure around the implants, but increase in bar height can increase stress levels on the peri-implant crestal bone, too [81].

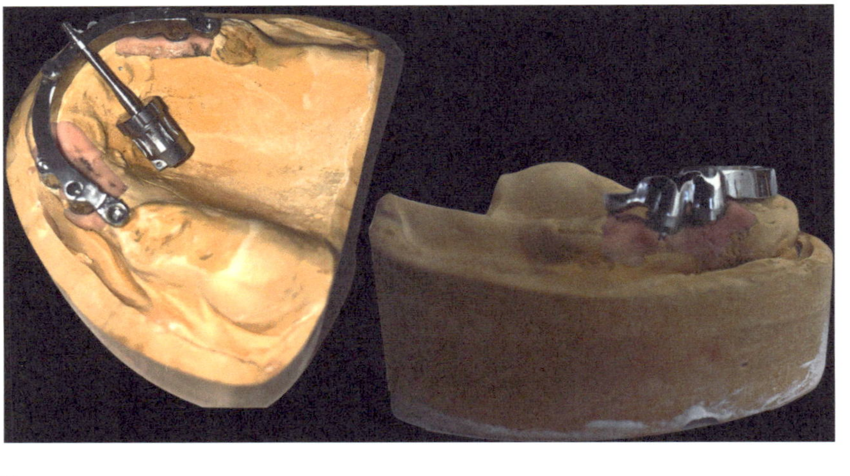

Figure 13.
Splinted 4 implant-retained maxillary overdenture with short distal cantilevers.

From the technical point of view, unsplinted overdenture implant attachment systems such as Locators, balls or magnets are much easier to construct, provide more prosthodontic space and require up to 1 cm vertical space for the attachments (**Figures 14–16**) [82, 83].

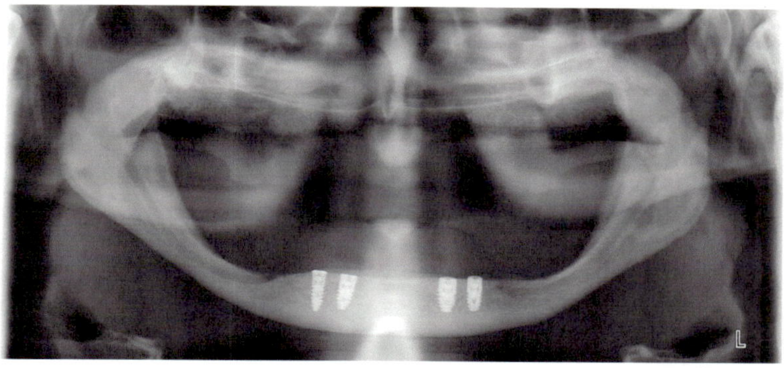

Figure 14.
Radiological assessment of implant osseointegration prior to the delivery of 4 implant-retained mandibular overdenture.

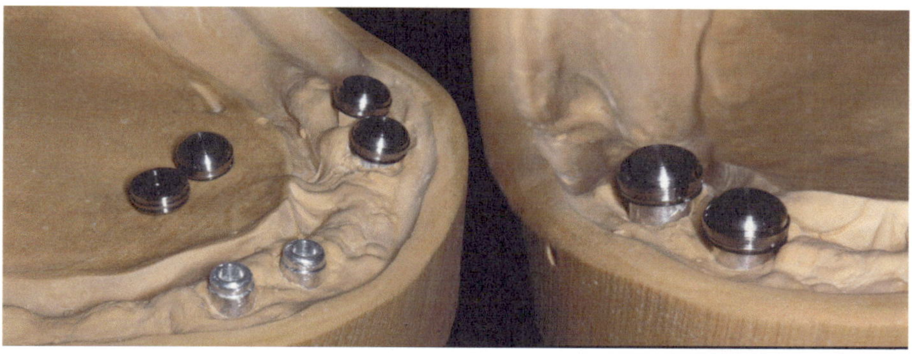

Figure 15.
Stone casts with laboratory analogs indicating the position of the locators in the edenetulous mandible.

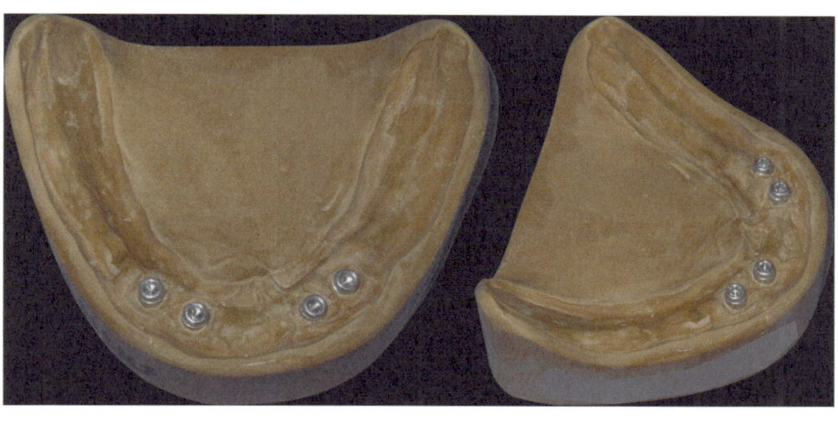

Figure 16.
Titanium housings on the laboratory analogs.

9. Prosthodontic maintenance of different implant-retained overdentures

Prosthetic complications with implant-retained overdentures are unavoidable and are mostly mechanical [84]. Compared with conventional complete dentures there is a higher rate of repair and replacement of this type of dentures, mostly regarding their design and type of the attachment system [84].

In cases where implant retained overdenture is not reinforced by the metal framework higher rate of acrylic fractures must be expected, especially in the cases where the patrix size of the attachment system is relatively too large [85].

Different attachment systems require different care. It has been proven that rigid bars connecting 4 implants show lower incidence rate of maintenance such as clip activation or resolving the fracture, than resilient system such as round bars most likely because of its inability to rotate around the fulcrum line during the function [86]. The data also demonstrates an increase in prosthodontic maintenance for ball attachments related to the wear or fracture of the ball head or need for activation of the ball matrix or relining of the denture [87, 88].

Numerous authors reported different types of matrix repairs, too, such as clip fractures or clip activation in the period of 5 years, most commonly in the first year [89, 90].

Furthermore, the longevity of the implant retained overdenture depends on maintaining oral and denture hygiene, as well as frequency of use. It is clear that simpler constructions, away from mucosa, are easier to maintain and clean, such as balls and locators in comparison to the bars, especially if they are in the close relationship with the mucosa [91]. Nocturnal use of this type of dentures has also showed higher

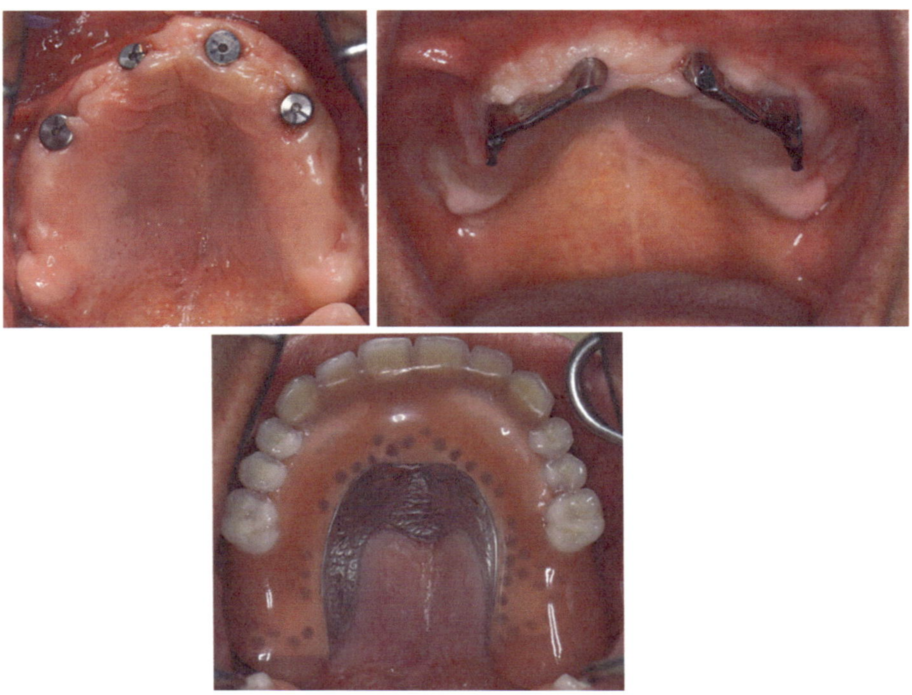

Figure 17.
4 implant-retained maxillary overdenture follow-up protocol.

incidence of stomatitis due to the excellent retention, less saliva produced and more bacteria to develop in that environment [92].

It is necessary to emphasize that the prosthodontic complications can be reduced to an expected level if a close follow-up protocol is applied (**Figures 17** and **18**).

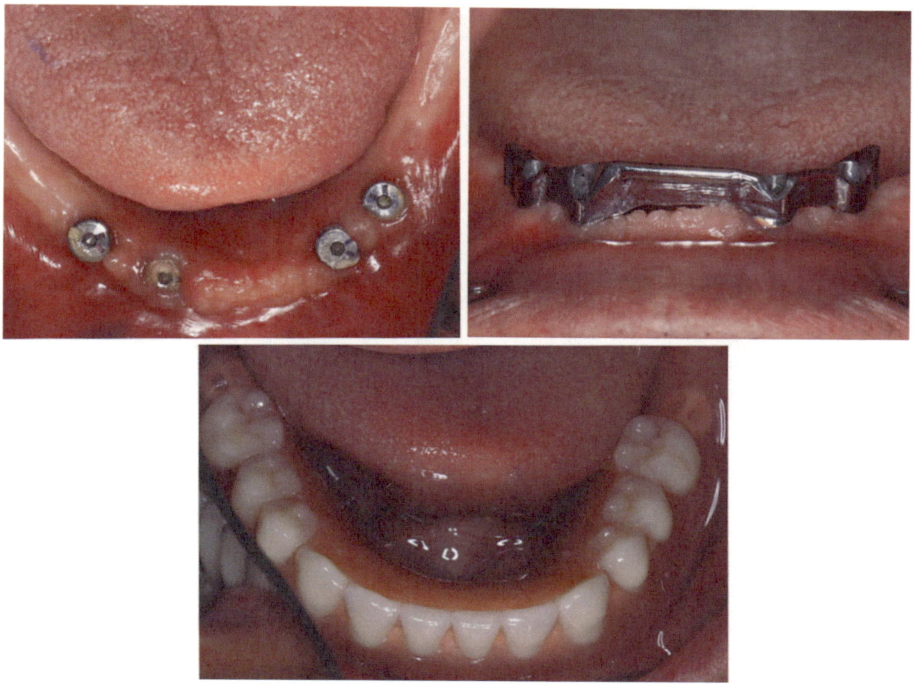

Figure 18.
4 implant-retained mandibular overdenture follow-up protocol.

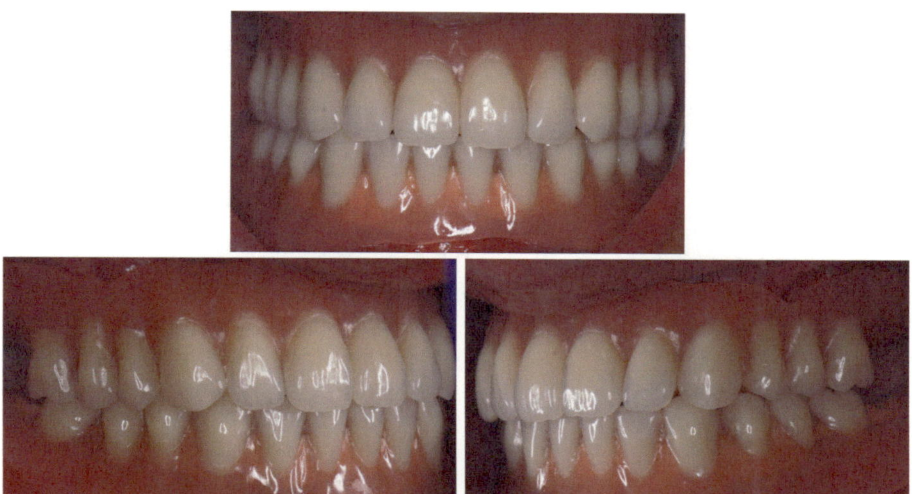

Figure 19.
Appearance of 4 implant-retained maxillary and mandibular overdentures - frontal and both lateral views.

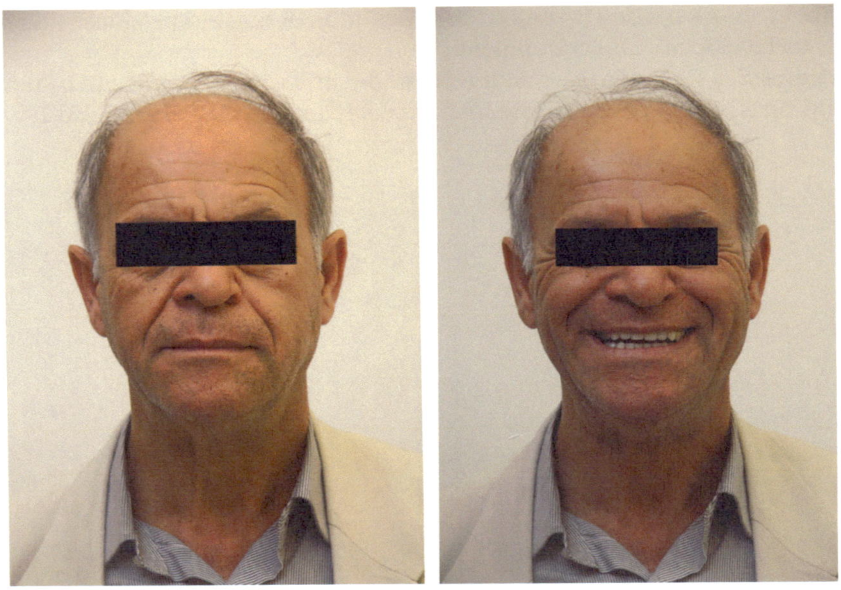

Figure 20.
Portrait view of the patient with 4 implant-retained maxillary and mandibular overdentures in occlusion and in smile.

We must also not forget that ultimate goal of producing implant-retained overdentures is patient's satisfaction not only with the esthetics but also with the long-term function of the removable prosthodontic restoration (**Figures 19** and **20**).

10. Conclusion

Implant-retained overdentures are very attractive implant-prosthodontic treatment because of its relative simplicity in construction and design, easy handling, minimal invasiveness and lower costs. They are particularly suitable to maintain facial support and achieve higher level of esthetics with denture acrylic material when moderate to extreme alveolar ridge resorption is present in patient's mouth, mainly in the older population. It is very important to emphasize that the implant-retained overdentures are supported by both implants and denture underlying soft tissue and therefore fewer implants are requested compared to the prosthodontic restorations supported only by implants.

This type of overdenture is usually connected with two or four implants, depending on which jaw is involved and on quality and quantity of the residual bone structure. These implants are mainly placed within the alveolar bone on the opposite sides of the completely edentulous arch and connected to the complete denture using different correspondent coupling units placed on the tissue surface of the prosthodontic restoration. When implant and denture attachments are appropriately connected, the complete denture is held in position over the denture bearing area and both implants and mucosa provide support, retention and stability in function. The main advantage of this type of implant-prosthodontic solution over fixed one is that the implant-retained overdenture can be easily removed and cleaned (easy access to both the denture and the implants' abutments) and therefore provides better oral hygiene and may affect greater longevity of the restoration itself.

The results of this systematic review indicate the superiority of implant-retained overdentures when compared to conventional complete dentures in fully edentulous patients suffering from moderate to severe alveolar bone resorption with regards to efficacy, patients' satisfaction and quality of their life.

Notes

All the cases presented in this chapter were patients from Dental Polyclinic Ars Salutaris, Zagreb, Croatia, and the laboratory work was done in Naturaldent dental laboratory, Zagreb, Croatia.

Author details

Dubravka Knezović Zlatarić[1]*, Robert Ćelić[1] and Hrvoje Pezo[2]

1 Department of Removable Prosthodontics, School of Dental Medicine, University of Zagreb, Zagreb, Croatia

2 Dental Polyclinic Ars Salutaris, Zagreb, Croatia

*Address all correspondence to: knezovic@sfzg.hr

References

[1] Cunha-Cruz J, Hujoel PP, Nadanovsky P. Secular trends in socio-economic disparities in edentulism: USA, 1972-2001. *J Dent Res.* 2007;86 (2):131-6. DOI: 10.1177/154405910708600205.

[2] Emami E, de Souza RF, Kabawat M, Feine JS. The impact of edentulism on oral and general health. Int J Dent. 2013;2013:498305. DOI: 10.1155/2013/498305.

[3] Müller F, Naharro M, Carlsson GE. What are the prevalence and incidence of tooth loss in the adult and elderly population in Europe? *Clin Oral Implants Res.* 2007;18 Suppl 3:2-14. DOI: 10.1111/j.1600-0501.2007.01459.x.

[4] Douglass CW, Shih A, Ostry L. Will there be a need for complete dentures in the United States in 2020? *J Prosthet Dent. 20*02;87(1):5-8. DOI: 10.1067/mpr.2002.121203.

[5] Kailembo A, Preet R, Stewart Williams J. Common risk factors and edentulism in adults, aged 50 years and over, in China, Ghana, India and South Africa: results from the WHO Study on global AGEing and adult health (SAGE). BMC Oral Health. 2016;27;17(1):29. doi: 10.1186/s12903-016-0256-2.

[6] Olofsson H, Ulander EL, Gustafson Y, Hörnsten C. Association between socioeconomic and health factors and edentulism in people aged 65 and older - a population-based survey. Scand J Public Health. 2018;46(7):690-8. DOI: 10.1177/1403494817717406.

[7] Roberto LL, Crespo TS, Monteiro-Junior RS, Martins AMEBL, De Paula AMB, Ferreira EF, et al. Sociodemographic determinants of edentulism in the elderly population: A systematic review and meta-analysis. Gerodontology. 2019;36(4):325-37. DOI: 10.1111/ger.12430.

[8] Lee DJ, Saponaro PC. Management of Edentulous Patients. Dent Clin North Am. 2019;63(2):249-61. DOI: 10.1016/j.cden.2018.11.006.

[9] Balic A. Biology Explaining Tooth Repair and Regeneration: A Mini-Review. Gerontology. 2018;64(4):382-88. DOI: 10.1159/000486592.

[10] Peyron MA, Woda A, Bourdiol P, Hennequin M. Age-related changes in mastication. J Oral Rehabil. 2017;44(4):299-312. DOI: 10.1111/joor.12478.

[11] Alves AC, Cavalcanti RV, Calderon PS, Pernambuco L, Alchieri JC. Quality of life related to complete denture. Acta Odontol Latinoam. 2018;31(2):91-6.

[12] Lombardi T, Bernardello F, Berton F, Porrelli D, Rapani A, Camurri Piloni A, et al. Efficacy of Alveolar Ridge Preservation after Maxillary Molar Extraction in Reducing Crestal Bone Resorption and Sinus Pneumatization: A Multicenter Prospective Case-Control Study. Biomed Res Int. 2018;2018:9352130. DOI: 10.1155/2018/9352130.

[13] Rahim-Wöstefeld S, El Sayed N, Weber D, Kaltschmitt J, Bäumer A, El-Sayed S, et al. Tooth-related factors for tooth loss 20 years after active periodontal therapy-A partially prospective study. J Clin Periodontol. 2020;47(10):1227-36. doi: 10.1111/jcpe.13348.

[14] Tallgren A. The continuing reduction of the residual alveolar ridges in complete denture wearers: a mixed-longitudinal

study covering 25 years. J Prosthet Dent. 1972; 27(2):120-32.

[15] McGarry TJ, Nimmo A, Skiba JF, Ahlstrom RH, Smith CR, Koumjian JH. Classification system for complete edentulism. The American College of Prosthodontics. J Prosthodont. 1999;8(1):27-39. DOI: 10.1111/j.1532-849x.1999.tb00005.x.

[16] Mazurat RD, Mazurat NM. Communicating complexity: using a diagnostic classification system for edentulous patients. J Can Dent Assoc. 2003;69(8):511-4.

[17] Fitzpatrick B. Standard of care for the edentulous mandible: a systematic review. J Prosthet Dent. 2006;95(1):71-8. DOI: 10.1016/j.prosdent.2005.11.007.

[18] Yamaga E, Sato Y, Minakuchi S. A structural equation model relating oral condition, denture quality, chewing ability, satisfaction, and oral health-related quality of life in complete denture wearers. J Dent. 2013;41(8):710-7. DOI: 10.1016/j.jdent.2013.05.015.

[19] Canger EM, Celenk P. Radiographic evaluation of alveolar ridge heights of dentate and edentulous patients. Gerodontology. 2012;29(1):17-23. DOI: 10.1111/j.1741-2358.2010.00391.x.

[20] Teng CJ, Lin SC, Chen JH, Chen Y, Kuo HC, Ho PS. The association between denture self-satisfaction rates and OHRQoL - a follow-up study. BMC Oral Health. 2020;20(1):140. DOI: 10.1186/s12903-020-01119-1.

[21] Yamamoto S, Shiga H. Masticatory performance and oral health-related quality of life before and after complete denture treatment. J Prosthodont Res. 2018;62(3):370-4. DOI: 10.1016/j.jpor.2018.01.006.

[22] Närhi TO, Ettinger RL, Lam EW. Radiographic findings, ridge resorption, and subjective complaints of complete denture patients. Int J Prosthodont. 1997;10(2):183-9.

[23] Karesvuo P, Gursoy UK, Pussinen PJ, Suominen AL, Huumonen S, Vesti E, et al. Alveolar bone loss associated with age-related macular degeneration in males. J Periodontol. 2013;84(1):58-67. DOI: 10.1902/jop.2012.110643.

[24] Clark D, Levin L. In the dental implant era, why do we still bother saving teeth? Dent Traumatol. 2019;35(6):368-75. DOI: 10.1111/edt.12492.

[25] Hebel K, Gajjar R, Hofstede T. Single-tooth replacement: bridge vs. implant-supported restoration. J Can Dent Assoc. 2000 Sep;66(8):435-8.

[26] Pjetursson BE, Heimisdottir K. Dental implants - are they better than natural teeth? Eur J Oral Sci. 2018;126 Suppl 1:81-7. DOI: 10.1111/eos.12543.

[27] Ravidà A, Tattan M, Askar H, Barootchi S, Tavelli L, Wang HL. Comparison of three different types of implant-supported fixed dental prostheses: A long-term retrospective study of clinical outcomes and cost-effectiveness. Clin Oral Implants Res. 2019;30(4):295-305. DOI: 10.1111/clr.13415.

[28] Chan MH, Holmes C. Contemporary "All-on-4" concept. Dent Clin North Am. 2015;59(2):421-70. DOI: 10.1016/j.cden.2014.12.001.

[29] Sadowsky SJ, Zitzmann NU. Protocols for the Maxillary Implant Overdenture: A Systematic Review. Int J Oral Maxillofac Implants. 2016;31 Suppl:s182-91. DOI: 10.11607/jomi.16suppl.g5.2.

[30] Chen KW, Lin TM, Liu PR, Ramp LC, Lin HJ, Wu CT, Pan YH. An analysis of the implant-supported overdenture in the edentulous mandible. J Oral Rehabil. 2013;40(1):43-50. DOI: 10.1111/joor.12010.

[31] Borba M, Deluiz D, Lourenço EJV, Oliveira L, Tannure PN. Risk factors for implant failure: a retrospective study in an educational institution using GEE analyses. Braz Oral Res. 2017;31:e69. DOI: 10.1590/1807-3107BOR-2017.vol31.0069.

[32] Ramanauskaite A, Becker J, Sader R, Schwarz F. Anatomic factors as contributing risk factors in implant therapy. Periodontol 2000. 2019;81(1):64-75. DOI: 10.1111/prd.12284.

[33] Salvi GE, Brägger U. Mechanical and technical risks in implant therapy. Int J Oral Maxillofac Implants. 2009;24 Suppl:69-85.

[34] Goodacre CJ, Bernal G, Rungcharassaeng K, Kan JY. Clinical complications with implants and implant prostheses. J Prosthet Dent. 2003;90(2):121-32. DOI: 10.1016/S0022-3913(03)00212-9.

[35] Chrcanovic BR, Albrektsson T, Wennerberg A. Bone Quality and Quantity and Dental Implant Failure: A Systematic Review and Meta-analysis. Int J Prosthodont. 2017;30(3):219-37. DOI: 10.11607/ijp.5142.

[36] Juodzbalys G, Kubilius M. Clinical and radiological classification of the jawbone anatomy in endosseous dental implant treatment. J Oral Maxillofac Res. 2013;4(2):e2. DOI: 10.5037/jomr.2013.4202.

[37] Thor A, Ekstrand K, Baer RA, Toljanic JA. Three-year follow-up of immediately loaded implants in the edentulous atrophic maxilla: a study in patients with poor bone quantity and quality. Int J Oral Maxillofac Implants. 2014;29(3):642-9. DOI: 10.11607/jomi.3163.

[38] Bryant SR, Zarb GA. Outcomes of implant prosthodontic treatment in older adults. J Can Dent Assoc. 2002;68(2):97-102.

[39] Mericske-Stern R. Treatment outcomes with implant-supported overdentures: clinical considerations. J Prosthet Dent. 1998;79(1):66-73. DOI: 10.1016/s0022-3913(98)70196-9.

[40] Melescanu Imre M, Marin M, Preoteasa E, Tancu AM, Preoteasa CT. Two implant overdenture--the first alternative treatment for patients with complete edentulous mandible. J Med Life. 2011;4(2):207-9.

[41] Feine JS, Carlsson GE, Awad MA, Chehade A, Duncan WJ, Gizani S, et al. The McGill consensus statement on overdentures. Mandibular two-implant overdentures as first choice standard of care for edentulous patients. Montreal, Quebec, May 24-25, 2002. Int J Oral Maxillofac Implants. 2002;17(4):601-2.

[42] White GS. Treatment of the edentulous patient. Oral maxillofac Surg Clin North Am. 2015;27(2):265-72. DOI: 10.1016/j.coms.2015.01.005.

[43] Possebon APDR, Schuster AJ, Bielemann AM, Porto BL, Boscato N, Faot F. Evaluation of Bite Force and Masticatory Performance: Complete Denture vs Mandibular Overdenture Users. Braz Dent J. 2020;31(4):399-403. DOI: 10.1590/0103-6440202003525.

[44] Boven GC, Raghoebar GM, Vissink A, Meijer HJ. Improving masticatory performance, bite force, nutritional state and patient's satisfaction

with implant overdentures: a systematic review of the literature. J Oral Rehabil. 2015;42(3):220-33. DOI: 10.1111/joor.12241.

[45] Awad MA, Rashid F, Feine JS; Overdenture Effectiveness Study Team Consortium. The effect of mandibular 2-implant overdentures on oral health-related quality of life: an international multicentre study. Clin Oral Implants Res. 2014;25(1):46-51. DOI: 10.1111/clr.12205.

[46] Kutkut A, Bertoli E, Frazer R, Pinto-Sinai G, Fuentealba Hidalgo R, Studts J. A systematic review of studies comparing conventional complete denture and implant retained overdenture. J Prosthodont Res. 2018;62(1):1-9. DOI: 10.1016/j.jpor.2017.06.004.

[47] Thomason JM, Kelly SA, Bendkowski A, Ellis JS. Two implant retained overdentures--a review of the literature supporting the McGill and York consensus statements. J Dent. 2012;40(1):22-34. DOI: 10.1016/j.jdent.2011.08.017.

[48] Allen PF, McMillan AS. The impact of tooth loss in a denture wearing population: an assessment using the Oral Health Impact Profile. Community Dent Health. 1999;16(3):176-80.

[49] Bergendal T, Engquist B. Implant-supported overdentures: a longitudinal prospective study. Int J Oral Maxillofac Implants. 1998;13(2):253-62.

[50] Rasmussen RA. The Branemark System of Oral Reconstruction: A Clinical Atlas. St. Louis: Ishiyaku EuroAmerica, Inc.;1992.

[51] Feine JS, de Grandmont P, Boudrias P, Brien N, LaMarche C, Taché R, et al. Within-subject comparisons of implant-supported mandibular prostheses: choice of prosthesis. J Dent Res. 1994;73(5):1105-11. DOI: 10.1177/00220345940730051301.

[52] de Grandmont P, Feine JS, Taché R, Boudrias P, Donohue WB, Tanguay R, et al. Within-subject comparisons of implant-supported mandibular prostheses: psychometric evaluation. J Dent Res. 1994;73(5):1096-104. DOI: 10.1177/00220345940730051201.

[53] Misch C. Dental Implant Prosthetics. 2nd ed. Amsterdam: Elsevier; 2014.

[54] Mericske-Stern R, Oetterli M, Kiener P, Mericske E. A follow-up study of maxillary implants supporting an overdenture: clinical and radiographic results. Int J Oral Maxillofac Implants. 2002;17(5):678-86.

[55] Di Francesco F, De Marco G, Capcha EB, Lanza A, Cristache CM, Vernal R, et al. Patient satisfaction and survival of maxillary overdentures supported by four or six splinted implants: a systematic review with meta-analysis. BMC Oral Health. 2021;21(1):247. doi: 10.1186/s12903-021-01572-6.

[56] Di Francesco F, De Marco G, Gironi Carnevale UA, Lanza M, Lanza A. The number of implants required to support a maxillary overdenture: a systematic review and meta-analysis. J Prosthodont Res. 2019;63(1):15-24. DOI: 10.1016/j.jpor.2018.08.006.

[57] Hegazy SA, El Mekawy N, Emera RMK. Impact of implants number and attachment type on the peri-implant stresses and retention of palateless implant-retained overdenture. Ind J Dent Res. 2020;31(3):414-9. DOI: 10.4103/ijdr.IJDR_772_18.

[58] Klemetti E. Is there a certain number of implants needed to retain an

overdenture? J Oral Rehabil. 2008;35 Suppl 1:80-4. DOI: 10.1111/j.1365-2842.2007.01825.x.

[59] Mericske-Stern RD, Taylor TD, Belser U. Management of the edentulous patient. Clin Oral Implants Res. 2000;11 Suppl 1:108-25.

[60] Kiener P, Oetterli M, Mericske E, Mericske-Stern R. Effectiveness of maxillary overdentures supported by implants: maintenance and prosthetic complications. Int J Prosthodont. 2001;14(2):133-40.

[61] Shah K, Yilmaz B, McGlumphy E. Fabrication of a Mandibular Implant-Supported Overdenture with a New Attachment System: A Review of Current Attachment Systems. Int J Prosthodont. 2017;30(3):245-7. DOI: 10.11607/ijp.5068.

[62] Liu W, Zhang X, Qing H, Wang J. Effect of LOCATOR attachments with different retentive forces on the stability of 2-implant-retained mandibular overdenture. J Prosthet Dent. 2020;124(2):224-9. DOI: 10.1016/j.prosdent.2019.09.005.

[63] Nogueira TE, Dias DR, Leles CR. Mandibular complete denture versus single-implant overdenture: a systematic review of patient-reported outcomes. J Oral Rehabil. 2017;44(12):1004-6. DOI: 10.1111/joor.12550.

[64] Mahoorkar S, Bhat S, Kant R. Single implant supported mandibular overdenture: A literature review. J Indian Prosthodont Soc. 2016;16(1):75-82. DOI: 10.4103/0972-4052.164881.

[65] Kern JS, Kern T, Wolfart S, Heussen N. A systematic review and meta-analysis of removable and fixed implant-supported prostheses in edentulous jaws: post-loading implant loss. Clin Oral Implants Res. 2016;27(2):174-95. DOI: 10.1111/clr.12531.

[66] Payne AG, Alsabeeha NH, Atieh MA, Esposito M, Ma S, Anas El-Wegoud M. Interventions for replacing missing teeth: attachment systems for implant overdentures in edentulous jaws. Cochrane Database Syst Rev 2018;10(10):CD008001. DOI: 10.1002/14651858.CD008001.pub2.

[67] Matthys C, Vervaeke S, Besseler J, Doornewaard R, Dierens M, De Bruyn H. Five years follow-up of mandibular 2-implant overdentures on locator or ball abutments: Implant results, patient-related outcome, and prosthetic aftercare. Clin Implant Dent Relat Res. 2019;21(5):835-44. DOI: 10.1111/cid.12840.

[68] Takahashi T, Gonda T, Tomita A, Maeda Y. Effect of Attachment Type on Implant Strain in Maxillary Implant Overdentures: Comparison of Ball, Locator, and Magnet Attachments. Part 2: Palateless Dentures. Int J Oral Maxillofac Implants. 2018;33(2):357-64. DOI: 10.11607/jomi.6157.

[69] Ceruti P, Bryant SR, Lee JH, MacEntee MI. Magnet-retained implant-supported overdentures: review and 1-year clinical report. J Can Dent Assoc. 2010;76:a52.

[70] Boven GC, Meijer HJA, Vissink A, Raghoebar GM. Maxillary implant overdentures retained by use of bars or locator attachments: 1-year findings from a randomized controlled trial. J Prosthodont Res. 2020;64(1):26-33. DOI: 10.1016/j.jpor.2019.04.013.

[71] Pisani M, Bedos C, da Silva CHL, Fromentin O, de Albuquerque RF Jr. A Qualitative Study on Patients' Perceptions of Two Types of Attachments for Implant Overdentures. J

Oral Implantol. 2017;43(6):476-81. DOI: 10.1563/aaid-joi-D-17-00166.

[72] Leão RS, Moraes SLD, Vasconcelos BCE, Lemos CAA, Pellizzer EP. Splinted and unsplinted overdenture attachment systems: A systematic review and meta-analysis. J Oral Rehabil. 2018;45(8):647-56. doi: 10.1111/joor.12651.

[73] Di Francesco F, De Marco G, Sommella A, Lanza A. Splinting vs Not Splinting Four Implants Supporting a Maxillary Overdenture: A Systematic Review. Int J Prosthodont. 2019;32(6):509-18. DOI: 10.11607/ijp.6333.

[74] de Almeida EO, Rocha EP, Freitas AC Jr, Freitas MM Jr. Finite element stress analysis of edentulous mandibles with different bone types supporting multiple-implant superstructures. Int J Oral Maxillofac Implants. 2010;25(6):1108-14.

[75] de Almeida EO, Rocha EP, Assunção WG, Júnior AC, Anchieta RB. Cortical bone stress distribution in mandibles with different configurations restored with prefabricated bar-prosthesis protocol: a three-dimensional finite-element analysis. J Prosthodont. 2011;20(1):29-34. DOI: 10.1111/j.1532-849X.2010.00656.x.

[76] Semper W, Heberer S, Nelson K. Retrospective analysis of bar-retained dentures with cantilever extension: marginal bone level changes around dental implants over time. Int J Oral Maxillofac Implants. 2010; 25(2): 385-93.

[77] Elsyad MA, Al-Mahdy YF, Salloum MG, Elsaih EA. The effect of cantilevered bar length on strain around two implants supporting a mandibular overdenture. Int J Oral Maxillofac Implants. 2013; 28(3):e143-50.DOI: 10.11607/jomi.2467.

[78] Bilhan H, Mumcu E, Arat S. The comparison of marginal bone loss around mandibular overdenture-supporting implants with two different attachment types in a loading period of 36 months. Gerodontology. 2011;28(1):49-57. DOI: 10.1111/j.1741-2358.2009.00334.x.

[79] Sadowsky SJ, Caputo AA. Effect of anchorage systems and extension base contact on load transfer with mandibular implant-retained overdentures. J Prosthet Dent. 2000;84(3):327-34.

[80] Ebadian B, Mosharraf R , Khodaeian N. Effect of cantilever length on stress distribution around implants in mandibular overdentures supported by two and three implants. Eur J Dent. 2016;10(3):333-40. DOI: 10.4103/1305-7456.184152.

[81] Joshi S, Kumar S, Jain S, Aggarwal R, Choudhary S, Reddy NK. 3D Finite Element Analysis to Assess the Stress Distribution Pattern in Mandibular Implant-supported Overdenture with Different Bar Heights. J Contemp Dent Pract. 2019;20(7):794-800.

[82] Ionescu C, Gălbinaşu BM, Manolea H, Pătraşcu I. Implant overdenture and Locator system in edentulous patient with severely resorbed mandible - a case report. Rom J Morphol Embryol. 2014;55 Suppl 2:693-6.

[83] Assaf A, Daas M, Boittin A, Eid N, Postaire M. Prosthetic maintenance of different mandibular implant overdentures: A systematic review. J Prosthet Dent. 2017;118(2):144-52.e5. DOI: 10.1016/j.prosdent.2016.10.037.

[84] Osman RB, Payne AG, Ma S. Prosthodontic maintenance of maxillary implant overdentures: a systematic

literature review. Int J Prosthodont. 2012;25(4):381-91.

[85] Osman RB, Ma S. Prosthodontic maintenance of overdentures on zirconia implants: 1-year results of a randomized controlled trial. Int J Prosthodont. 2014;27(5):461-8. DOI: 10.11607/ijp.3626.

[86] Krennmair G, Krainhöfner M, Piehslinger E. The influence of bar design (round versus milled bar) on prosthodontic maintenance of mandibular overdentures supported by 4 implants: a 5-year prospective study. Int J Prosthodont. 2008;21(6):514-20.

[87] Cakarer S, Can T, Yaltirik M, Keskin C. Complications associated with the ball, bar and Locator attachments for implant-supported overdentures. Med Oral Patol Oral Cir Bucal. 2011;16(7):e953-9. DOI: 10.4317/medoral.17312.

[88] ELsyad MA, Errabti HM, Mustafa AZ. Mandibular Denture Base Deformation with Locator and Ball Attachments of Implant-Retained Overdentures. J Prosthodont. 2016;25(8):656-64. DOI: 10.1111/jopr.12356.

[89] Payne AG, Solomons YF. Mandibular implant-supported overdentures: a prospective evaluation of the burden of prosthodontic maintenance with 3 different attachment systems. Int J Prosthodont. 2000;13(3):246-53.

[90] Watson RM, Jemt T, Chai J, Harnett J, Heath MR, Hutton JE, Johns RB, Lithner B, McKenna S, McNamara DC, Naert I, Taylor R. Prosthodontic treatment, patient response, and the need for maintenance of complete implant-supported overdentures: an appraisal of 5 years of prospective study. Int J Prosthodont. 1997;10(4):345-54.

[91] Park JH, Shin SW, Lee JY. Bar versus ball attachments for maxillary four-implant retained overdentures: A randomized controlled trial. Clin Oral Implants Res. 2019;30(11):1076-84. DOI: 10.1111/clr.13521.

[92] Naert I, Gizani S, van Steenberghe D. Rigidly splinted implants in the resorbed maxilla to retain a hinging overdenture: a series of clinical reports for up to 4 years. J Prosthet Dent. 1998;79(2):156-64. DOI: 10.1016/s0022-3913(98)70210-0.

Chapter 17

Strategic Implants under Existing Partial Removable Dentures, Why, How Many, and Which Type?

Ahmad Al Jaghsi

Abstract

Inserting strategic implants under existing removable partial dentures requires a comprehensive understanding of removable prosthodontic basics and possible designs, as well as a thorough understanding of implant therapy. Prior to the widespread adoption of implants as standard prosthetic therapy, remaining roots were preserved and used to minimize bone resorption under the removable denture. Root-supported overdentures become less common after the overwhelming clinical studies that emphasize dental implants' reliability and high success and survival rate. Fixed prostheses cannot be used to treat a severely decreased dentition unless a significant number of implants can be inserted, sufficient bone quantity and quality are available, and the patients can afford the treatment. On the other hand, using strategic implants under existing RPD upgrades the design to a more favorable support type. It improves patient satisfaction with the RPD in speaking, chewing, retention, stability, and RPD support. This improvement could be reached earlier if the patient received immediate loading. Strategic implants can also improve chewing ability, stabilize the occlusion, increase bite force and improve patient oral health-related quality of life. Moreover, better distribution of occlusal forces that may reduce bone resorption may be gained. Furthermore, strategic implants can improve comfort, confidence, and esthetics by reducing the RPD size and removing the retainers from the esthetic zone.

Keywords: strategic implants, mini-implants, immediate loading, delayed loading, removable partial dentures, implant-assisted removable partial dentures, patient satisfaction

1. Introduction

Dental implant service is a life-changing treatment modality for many patients. Giving our patients a fixed restoration is a very rewarding procedure, especially if the patients have difficulties: gage reflex, bulky prostheses, lack in retention, stability, or support. Unfortunately, this is not applicable for all patients, especially patients who cannot afford multiple implants or bone grafting. By considering the strategic implants under the existing removable partial denture (RPD), we make implant treatment simple and affordable for more patients.

The removable partial denture (RPD) is the dental prostheses that the patient, who suffers the absence of some but not all the natural teeth, can readily insert and remove from his/her mouth. The prostheses restore the missing teeth as well as the gingiva and the missing bone if needed. Removable partial dentures (RPDs) are indicated for patients with a long edentulous span, too long for a fixed prosthesis. The RPD is indicated for a patient with no posterior abutment to support a fixed prosthesis, and the cantilever bridge is contraindicated. Also, it is preferred if excessive alveolar bone loss is encountered, especially in the esthetic zone. Those patients who are not indicated for bone grafting or unable to afford the costly treatment are good candidates for the removable denture (RD). The acrylic flang is a good approach to compensate for the bone and soft tissue deficiency within a short fabrication time and a less aggressive approach. Moreover, this treatment option allows the patient to remove his prostheses for easier intraoral access, subsequently, better oral hygiene. The RD enables the dentist to repair or adjust the prostheses easily.

On the other hand, RD is less secure with limited retention and stability than fixed prostheses. RD metal clasp may compromise the final esthetic result. It may act as a gum stripper and accelerate alveolar bone resorption. These drawbacks in the RD can be managed by upgrading the RD using strategic implants, which are "the implants that change the prosthetic support type to a more favorable configuration" [1].

In this chapter the folllowing points is going to be discussed:

1. Classification as a systematic approach for communication and planning:
    - Kennedy classification system
    - Steffel classification and modified Steffel classification
    - Implant-Corrected Kennedy (ICK) Classification System for Partially Edentulous Arches
    - Strategic mini dental implants (MDI) and standard dental implant (SDI) under existing RPD, how many implant?
    - The abutment prosthetic value
2. Immediate and delayed restoration/loading, what is the difference?
3. Why strategic implant?
4. Mini-implant-assisted removable partial denture
5. Conclusion

2. Classification as a systematic approach for communication and planning

A classification is a systematic approach in which the items or units are categories in groups or subgroups according to specific criteria. This approach facilitates the discussion regarding the most suitable treatment options, eases the communication between the dentist and the technician. The classification also allows for visualization and differentiation between the RPD support types: tooth-supported, tooth tissue-supported, tissue-supported, implant-supported, implant tissue-supported, and implant tooth-supported.

2.1 Kennedy classification system

In 1925 Dr. Edward Kennedy introduced his approach of categorizing partially edentulous arches into four classes. He categorized the partially edentulous arches in a way that considered the edentulous area position in the arch and if it was surrounded with teeth or not. This approach was beneficial in visualizing the cases and reaching the decisions regarding the RPD designs.

The following is the Kennedy classification:

Class I: Edentulous free-end areas located on both sides (bilateral), posterior to the remaining teeth (**Figure 1**).

Class II: Edentulous free-end area located on one side (unilateral), posterior to the remaining teeth (**Figure 2**).

Class III: Edentulous bounded area with natural teeth remaining both anterior and posterior to it (**Figure 3**). The area is located on one side (unilateral).

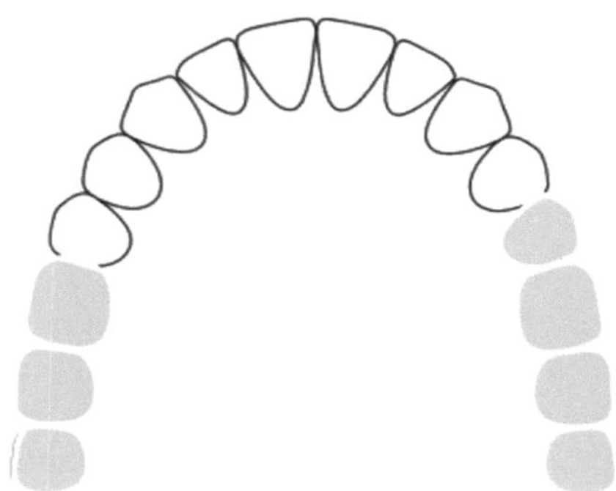

Figure 1.
Class I maxillary arch.

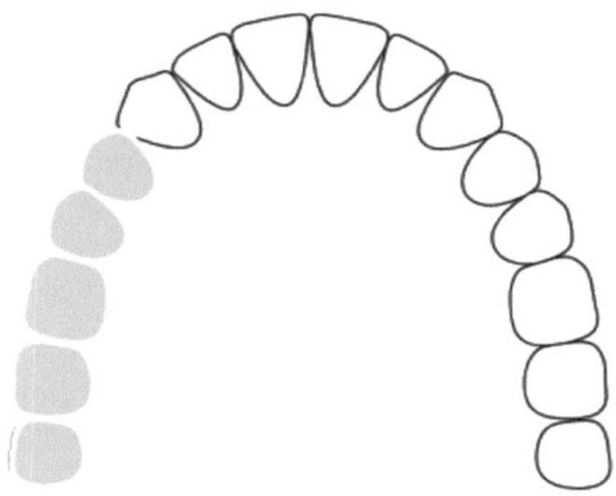

Figure 2.
Class II maxillary arch.

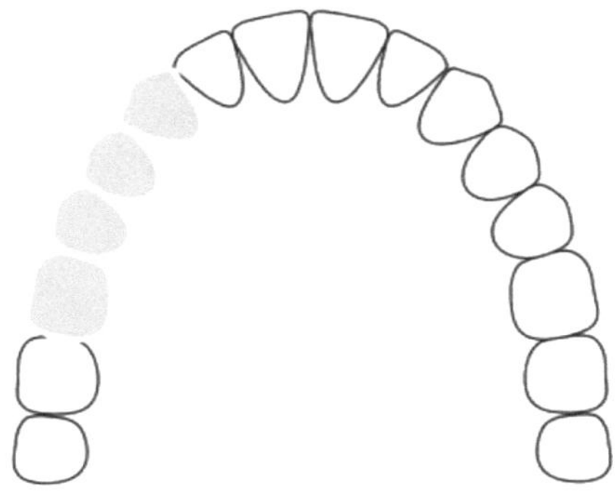

Figure 3.
Class III maxillary arch.

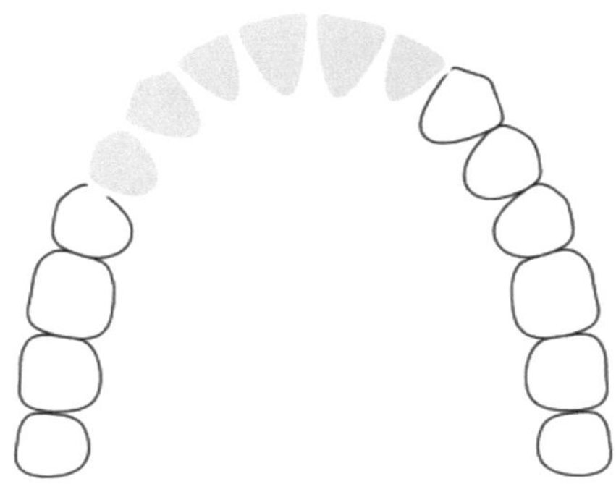

Figure 4.
Class IV maxillary arch.

Class IV: Edentulous bounded area with natural teeth remaining posterior to it. The area is located anteriorly and crossing the mid-line (**Figure 4**).

In 1965 Applegate's added eight rules to the classification. The rules can be summarized by the following: The categorization (classification) is always determined by the most posterior edentulous region (or regions). Any additional edentulous area (other than those that define the categorization) is considered a modification (**Figures 6** and 7). If the teeth posterior to the edentulous area are not used to support the RPD, the edentulous area is classified as a free end (**Figures** 5 and 7), and vice versa (**Figures 6** and 7). If the posterior free end edentulous region is not going to receive artificial teeth, it will not be considered in the classification (**Figures 6–8**), and vice versa. Putting the design and the structure of the RPD into consideration is a cornerstone in giving the correct RPD classification. Subsequently, the classification will be the start point making the best clinical decision regarding the number and the position of strategic implants under the RPD.

2.2 Steffel classification

In 1962 Steffel described six support possibilities that can be encountered in RPD [2]. He labeled the classification categories from A to F based on the fulcrum, and the number and distribution of the abutments, **Figure 9**. The fulcrum line is a hypothetical line formed between abutments, teeth or implants. The RPD may rotate somewhat around the fulcrum during function.

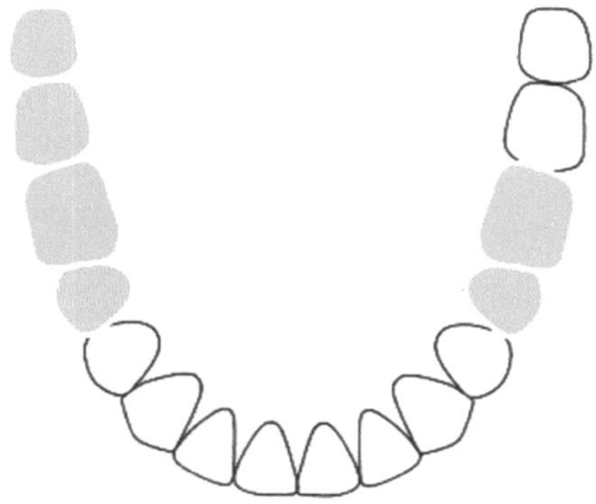

Figure 5.
No rest is going to be costructed on # 38 or 37 → the arch has two free end areas → Class I mandibular arch.

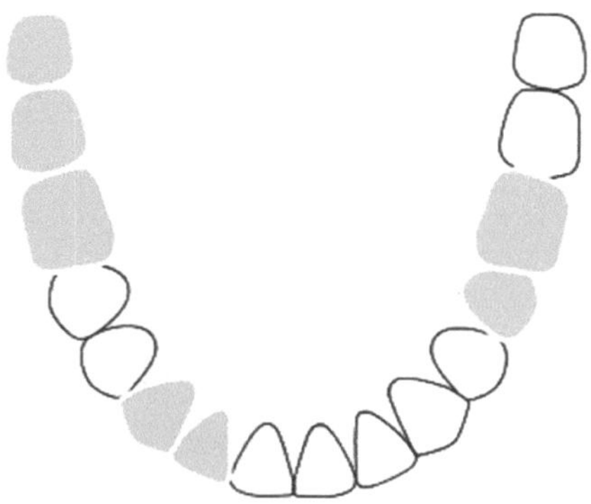

Figure 6.
Direct retainer is going to be constructed on 37. No artificial teeth is going to replace 46, 47 or 48 → no free end → Class III mod 1 mandibular arch.

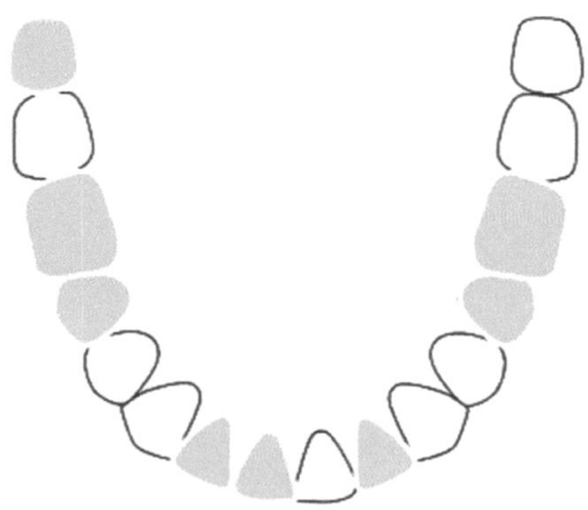

Figure 7.
No artificial teeth is going to replace, 48. Direct retainer is going to be constructed on 37 but not on 47 → one free end → Class II mod 3 mandibular arch.

In this chapter, we suggest a modification to this classification to simplify the communication and decision-making regarding the strategic implant under the existing RPD. In the modification, B, C, and D will be labeled together.

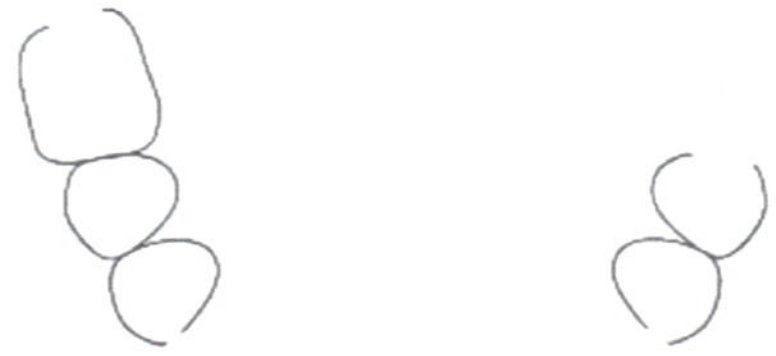

Figure 8.
No artificial teeth is going to replace, 38, 37, 36, 47 or 48. Class IV mandibular arch.

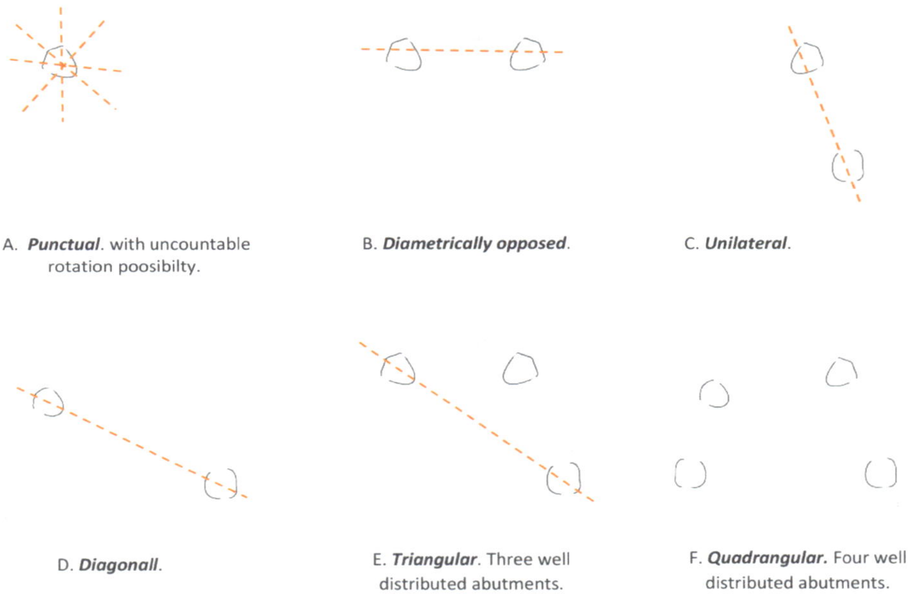

Figure 9.
Steffel classification.

The following is the *modified Steffel classification:*

- Punctual-support, only one abutment.
- Linear-support, two abutments; separated with edentulous area or at least one tooth.
- Triangular-support, three well-distributed abutments; separated with edentulous area or at least one tooth. One of the abutments should be on the opposite quadrant.
- Quadrangular-support, two well-distributed abutments on every quadrant.

Providing the patient with a stable prosthesis is a crucial target for the dentist. However, the RPD is not rigidly attached to the intraoral hard (teeth) and soft (mucosa) tissues, which have different levels of compressibility and mobility. Subsequently, the chewing and occlusal forces may generate different levels of tissue stress and prosthesis mobility. Both (stress and mobility) should be within the physiological level and cause no harm or trauma. Achieving this critical goal depends on the clinician's understanding of the biomechanics and the different design solutions. The RPD design should consider the unique nature of each clinical case and counter the expected RPD movement in response to loading. The design also should minimize the potentially destructive forces that may affect the supporting tissues; teeth, mucosa, and bone. That can be achieved by avoiding a long lever system, good selection for the RPD supporting elements, and wide symmetrical distribution of the functional forces [3, 4]. Many of the previous points (if not all) can be achieved (fully or partially) by delivering an RPD with quadrangular-support type.

According to the modified Steffel classification, there are four types of prosthetic support: punctual, linear, triangular, and quadrangular. The RPD support improves gradually as the classification change from I to IV. Classification IV provides the best support to the RPD with the highest resistance of rotation. The strategic implant aims to change the prosthetic support type to a more favorable configuration. *Delivering an RPD with a better support type can be considered the start point in a multifactorial process for deciding the number, type, and position of strategic implants.*

2.3 Implant-corrected kennedy (ICK) classification system for partially edentulous arches

One of the simple classification systems for RPD supported with implants or implants and natural teeth is Implant-Corrected Kennedy (ICK) classification system for partially edentulous arches by Al-Johany et al. [5]. The ICK is based on the Kennedy classification system and the Applegate eight rules (Applegate–Kennedy system) [6]. According to the ICK classification system coding guidelines, the Kennedy classification comes first, followed by the number of modification spaces (Applegate rules). Finally, round brackets enclose # followed by the implant's or implants' position will be added, **Figures 10–18**.

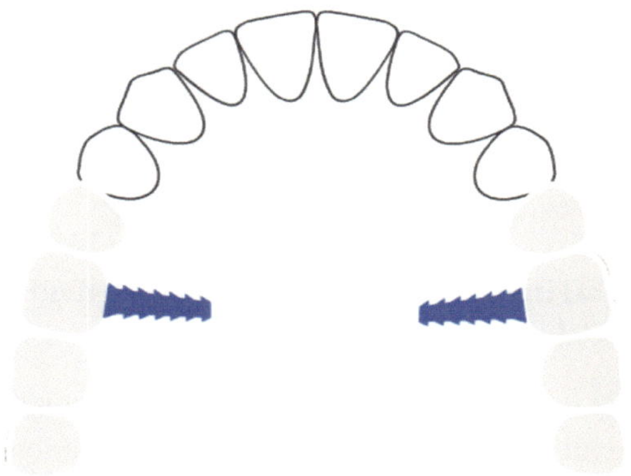

Figure 10.
ICK I (# 25).

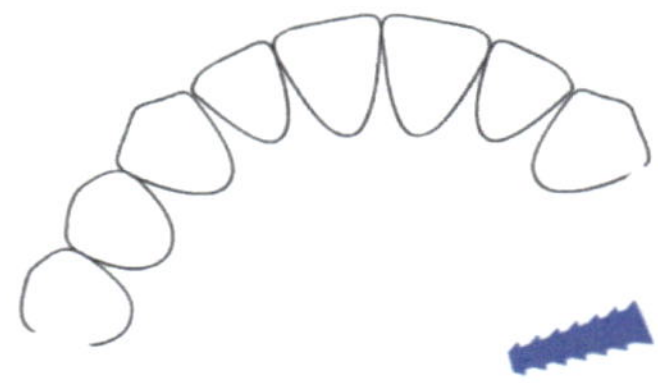

Figure 11.
ICK II mod 2 (# 33, 36). Direct retainer is going to be constructed on 28.

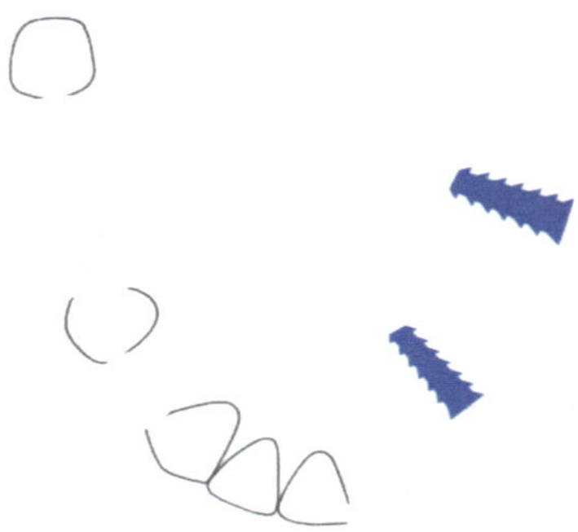

Figure 12.
ICK II mod 3 (# 13, 23). Direct retainer is going to be constructed on 28.

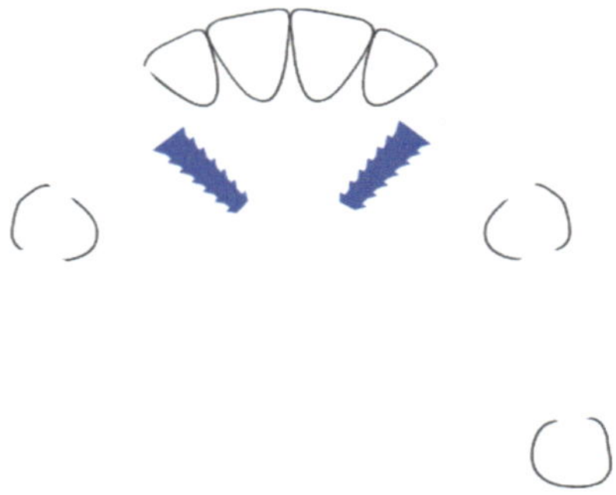

Figure 13.
ICK II mod 1 (# 16, 13, 23).

2.4 Strategic mini dental implants (MDI) and standard dental implant (SDI) under existing RPD, how many implant?

Meeting our patient's expectations is a priority. That cannot be reached if the dentist did not provide the patient with a full straightforward clarification for the treatment plan. The clarification should cover the advantages, disadvantages, risks, time, cost, and alternatives. The explanation should be done in a way that helps both the patient first and the dentist second to reach the decision that best matches the patients' needs, health

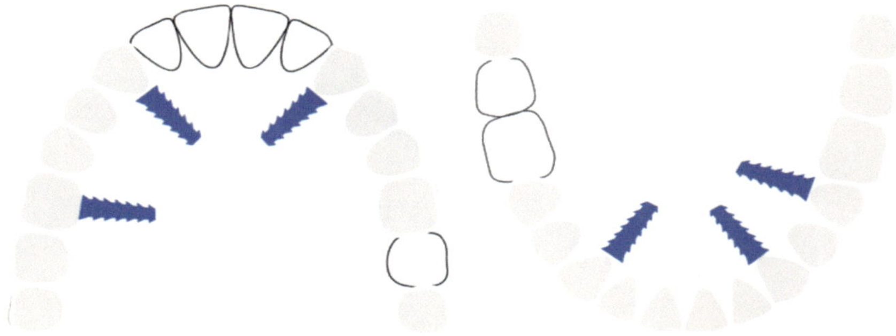

Figure 14.
ICK II (# 35, 33, 43).

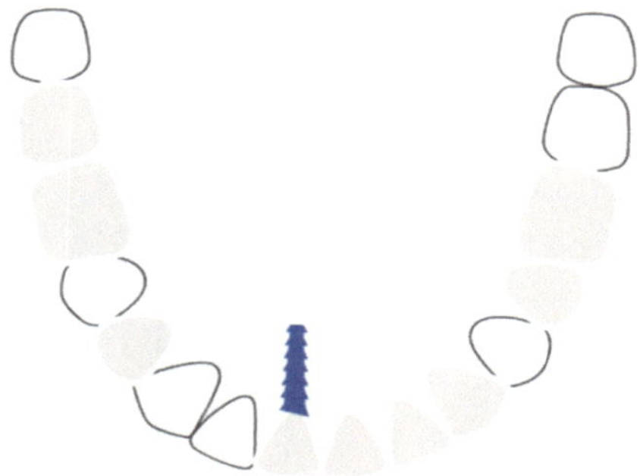

Figure 15.
ICK III mod 3 (# 41).

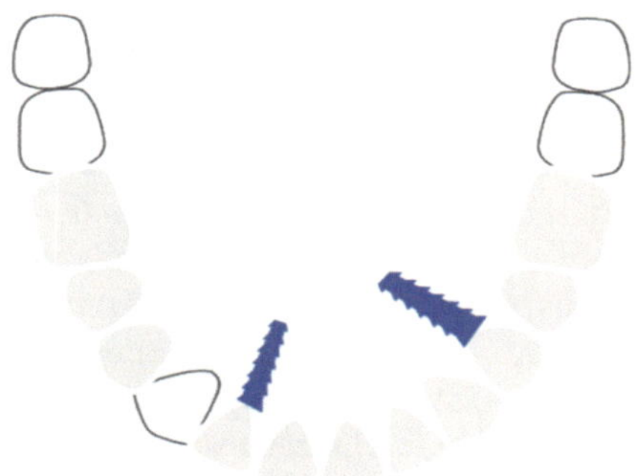

Figure 16.
ICK III mod 1 (# 34, 42).

status, and financial ability, as well as respect the patient's chief complaint and consideration. Generally speaking, teeth-implant- or implant-supported removable dentures reduce (and in many cases eliminate) traditional denture problems [1, 7–9]. It helps the dentist widen his options to meet the patient's needs and expectations by inserting one or few implants in strategic positions, but how many implants?

The needed number of mini dental implants (MDIs) or standard dental implants (SDIs) under existing RPD is a multifactorial process (see paragraph 2.5) and taken on the quadrant level. To give the patient an RPD with acceptable retention, stability,

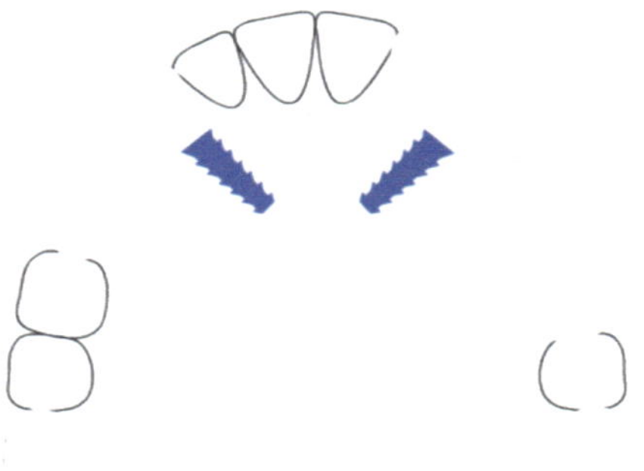

Figure 17.
ICK III mod 1 (# 13, 23).

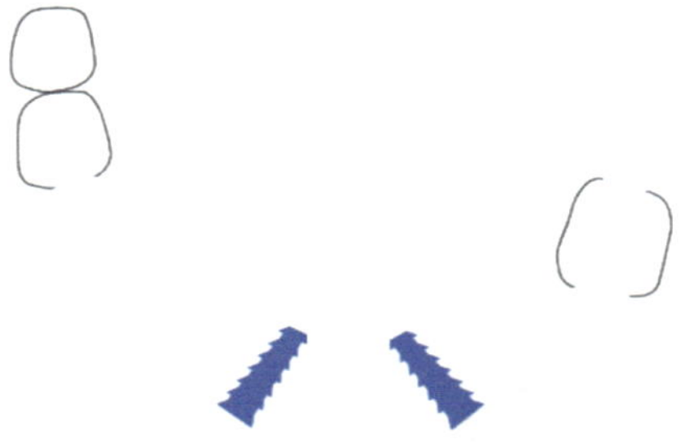

Figure 18.
ICK IV (# 33, 43). Direct retainers are going to be constructed on 36 and 47. No artificial teeth are going to replace 37 or 38.

and support, the abutments should be well distributed. Two abutments on every quadrant in symmetrical position as possible are needed. On every quadrant, the sum of the abutments prosthetic value should be ≥2, **Table 1** and **Figure 19**. *The abutment prosthetic value is defined as the importance of the tooth or implant from a specific prosthodontic point of view,* (see paragraph 2.5). The availability of several abutments on both sides allows a wide distribution of stress, improving bilateral stabilization, support, and stability [2]. Many studies reported the positive impact of more abutments and wide distribution [10–13]. Although putting two implants in the lower edentulous jaw is widely accepted in the literature,[14] achieving a quadrangular-support type needs at least two MDIs or two SDIs in every quadrant. In the edentulous upper jaw, which generally has less bone density than the lower jaw,[15] two SDIs or three MDIs in every quadrant are needed [16].

For partially edentulous patients, the abutments can be implants or natural teeth and should be well-distributed with a sum of the prosthetic value ≥2 on quadrant level.

Deciding the number of the strategic implants can be started with Table 1, but it will be finished after a comprehensive evaluation of the case, see paragraph 2.5.

2.5 The abutment prosthetic value

In the course of formulating the prosthodontic plan, not all teeth or abutments have the same prosthetic value. The prosthetic value stands for the importance of the tooth

		The abutments prosthetic value
Teeth	Upper or lower incisor or lateral incisor	0–0.5*
	Upper or lower canine	1.3**
	Upper or lower premolar or molar	1***
MDI	Upper MDI	0.5–0.7****
	lower MDI	1
SDI	Upper Standard Implant	1
	Lower Standard Implant	1

**The numbers represent the prosthetic value if abutment rest is planned; if not, the value will be 0.*
***If the four natural anterior abutment teeth are missing (11, 12, 13, 14), strategic implant/s is recommended even if all posterior teeth are available, and vice versa.*
****If there is no space (edentulous area or at least one natural tooth) between the abutment teeth, the prosthetic value will decrease to 0.5 for each abutment.*
*****Bone quality impacts the MDI prosthetic value.*

Table 1.
The prosthetic value of the available teeth and the planned MDIs and SDIs. The recommendations are on the quadrant level.

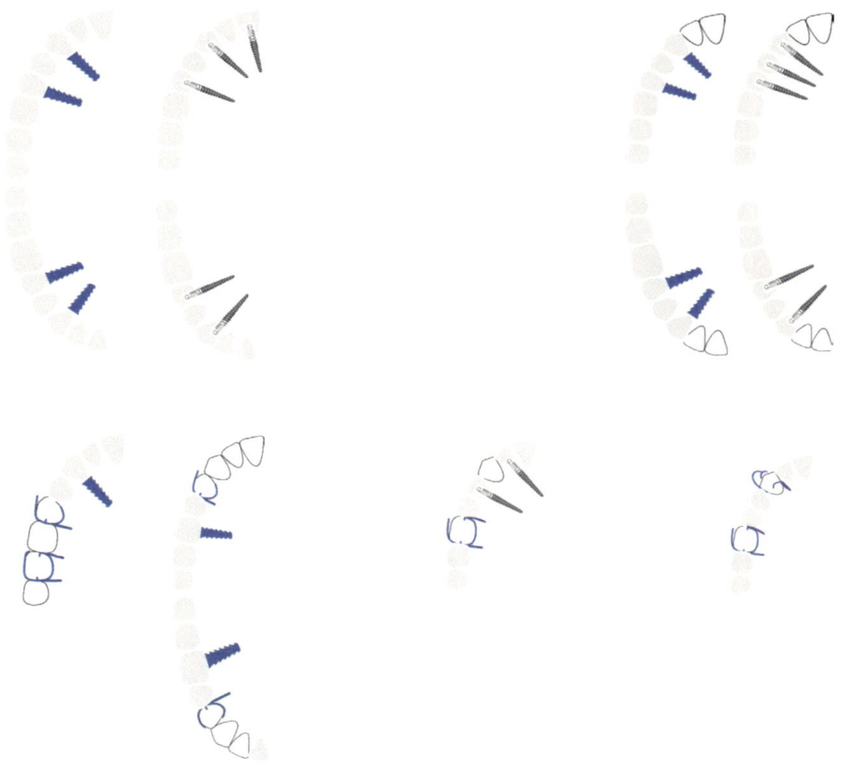

Figure 19.
(A1 upper jaw and A2 lower jaw to G1 upper jaw): The recommended number of strategic standard implants (SDIs) or mini dental implants (MDIs) under existing RPD.

or implant from a specific prosthodontic point of view. The last first molar (#36) in **Figure 20** has a very high prosthetic value than the lateral incisor #32. Extracting #36 shifts the treatment modality (if an implant is not feasible) from fixed partial denture to

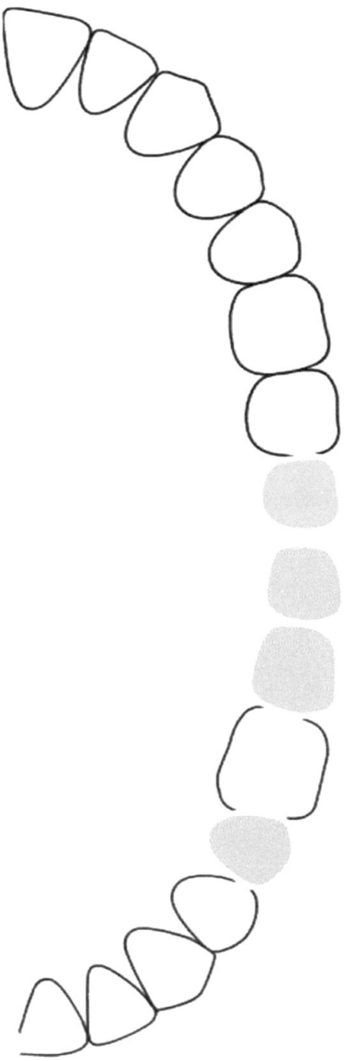

Figure 20.
The #36 has a very high prosthetic value because the extracting change the treatment modality (if implant is not feasible) from fixed partial denture to removable partial denture.

removable partial denture. Suppose the dentist changes his prosthodontic point of view by selecting RPD as a treatment modality. In that case, the prosthetic value of #36 will be reduced a little for this specific treatment modality. However, the prosthetic value for the same tooth (#36, **Figure 20**) and the same treatment modality (RPD) will be very high if the patient has a knife-edge thin, sensitive mucosa. Usually, this type of patient can tolerate tooth-tooth-supported RPD better than tooth tissue-supported RPD. Therefore, it can be concluded that: *estimating the prosthetic value of an abutment is a multifactorial assessment*. This estimation includes the intraoral, extraoral, and general health status and many other factors like esthetics.

The hidden #23 MDI under the saddle (**Figure 21**) has a very high esthetic value as it helps the dentist avoid metal clasp in the esthetic zone. In some cases,

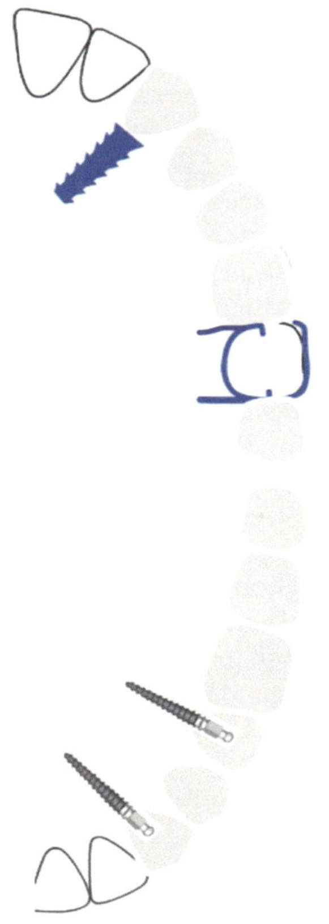

Figure 21.
The SDI #23 and MDI #33 have very high esthetic value as they help the dentist avoiding anterior metal clasps. #27 and MDI 35 have relatively high prosthetic value as they shift the RPD from tooth tissue supported to more implant tooth-supprted or implat implant-supported RPD.

strategic implants enable the dentist to reduce or remove the flange to achieve a better esthetic result by reducing lip protrusion. In other cases, it gives the dentist the ability to minimize the RPD size (palate, **Figure 24**) and increase patient acceptance.

The prosthetic value (importance) for each abutment is estimated according to **Table 1** and mainly the following points: [11, 12, 17, 18].

- Periodontal status, mobility, and bone level around the abutment.
- Crown-root ratio.
- Tooth vitality, size of the defect (caries), size, and type of the restoration.
- The shape and number of the abutment roots.
- Occlusion, parafunctional activity and opposite jaw status: natural teeth, implant, fixed partial denture, complete denture, or partial denture.

3. Immediate and delayed restoration/loading, what is the difference?

In 1981 Albrektsson et al. suggested a protocol in which the implants are left to heal in situ for at least 3 to 4 months without loading [19]. He considered the non-loading phase a crucial period to achieve successful osseointegration and avoid fibrous tissue formation between the implant surface and the bone. On the other hand, many clinical studies proved that immediate restoration, immediate loading, or early loading are acceptable treatment modalities [20, 21]. These studies were in response to the social and psychological needs of many patients. The immediate or early treatment modalities aim to reduce the overall recovery time between the surgical intervention and the insertion of the final restoration. These approaches are known as immediate restoration protocol, immediate loading protocol, and early loading protocol.

Patients typically are uncomfortable and, in many cases, refuse to stay without their RPD for a long time, especially if it restores a lot of missing teeth or teeth in the esthetic zone. The immediate protocols can reduce the patient concerns related to the final restoration by reducing the waiting period. In some cases, a temporary restoration is immediately delivered to give the patient a hint on the form, size, and position (in some cases, the shade) of the final restoration. Moreover, the second surgical intervention can be averted through immediate protocols. To achieve a good success rate in this treatment modality, a good understanding of the topic, terminology, limitation, and biology is essential. These topics will be discussed in other chapters, but it is crucial to clarify a few terms.

The loading can be classified into four categories:

- Conventional loading: The implants are left without loading for around two to three months.

- Delayed loading: If the loading on the implant is applied after the conventional loading time, it is classified as delayed. That can be indicated if the tissue needs more healing time, such as external sinus lift with bone grafting. In such cases, the final restoration and implant loading may be applied after six to nine months.

- Early loading: The implant is loaded by placing dental restoration in contact with opposing dentition at any time after one week but within two months after implant insertion.

- Immediate loading: The dental restoration is inserted intraorally and placed in contact with opposing dentition within one week after the surgical intervention.

The timing of dental restoration can also be categorized to:

- Conventional restoration in which the implant is left without temporary or final restoration for around two to three months.

- Immediate restoration: The temporary or final restoration is placed within one week after surgical intervention.

- Early restoration: The temporary or final restoration is placed any time after one week but within two months after implant insertion.

- Delayed restoration: If the dental restoration is placed intraorally after the conventional loading time, the restoration is classified as delayed restoration.

According to the previous classifications, the dentist has different types of intervention. For example, he can go for immediate restoration with conventional loading or implement early restoration with delayed loading.

In the case of the strategic implant under existing RPD, there are seven scenarios: immediate restoration with one of the four loading types, or early restoration with early, conventional, or delayed loading. The decision regarding the best approach is multifactorial: age, esthetic expectations, oral hygiene level, bone quality and quantity, and treatment expenses. According to the 2018 census supported by the International Team for Implantology (ITI), the most critical factors that may impact the loading protocol selection are patient-related factors, especially patient's general health, implant primary stability (ISQ), bone grafting, the size and shape of the implant, and the doctor skills and experience [22]. Moreover, the ITI tried to unify the two classifications (loading and restoration timing) to make it less complicated for the clinician and easier for the researchers to perform clinical studies and compare their results. They described four protocols:

a. Immediate loading: Within one week after implant placement, dental implants are linked to a prosthesis in occlusion with the opposing arch.

b. Immediate restoration: Within one week after implant placement, dental implants are linked to the dental restoration and are kept out of occlusion.

c. Early loading: Between one week and two months following implant placement, dental implants are linked to the prosthesis.

d. Conventional loading: dental implants are linked to the prosthesis after two months of implantation.

4. Why strategic implant?

Improving dental treatment output by using implants to enhance the functional performance of the complete denture is a well-known approach in prosthodontics. The McGill Consensus Statement stated that the first option in treating the lower jaw edentulous patient should be two implants retained overdenture and not lower jaw conventional complete denture (CD) [23]. Overwhelming scientific evidence supports the statement [23]. The evidence emphasized the superiority of two implants retained overdenture treatment modality on the conventional CD in many aspects, such as patients' chewing efficiency, positive modification in patients' diet, patients' satisfaction with the CD stability, retention, and comfort as well as quality of life [23]. Although a lot of scientific evidence highlighted the positive impact of inserting implants under existing RPD, no similar Consensus Statement is available regarding implant-retained or implant-assisted removable partial denture [24–26].

Not all patients are suitable for implant-supported fixed dental prostheses. For example, many patients are unwilling to have an extra surgical intervention (bone grafting, sinus lifting, bone splitting, or expansion). Other patients are not suitable for such intervention because they are medically compromised or do not have adequate financial flexibility. As an alternative to inserting multiple implants, the dentist can improve the quality of the prosthodontic treatment by changing the support type of the RPD to the quadrangular-support type. The improvement can be achieved by inserting one/two standard implants or one/two/three mini-implants per quadrant to reach a symmetrical quadrangular-support type. The prostheses will be tooth implant-supported RPD instead of tooth tissue-supported RPD. This prosthodontic approach is affordable to many patients.

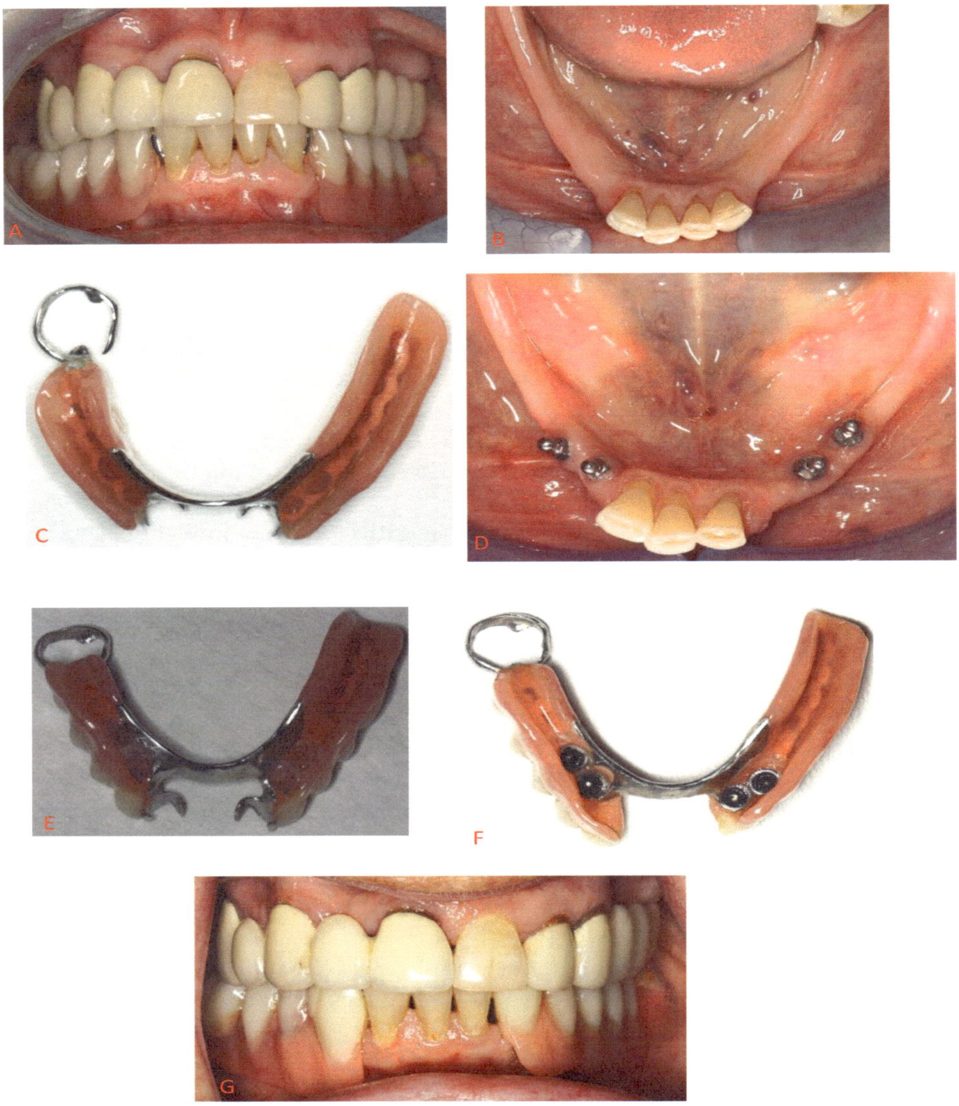

Figure 22.
Upgrading the existing clasp retained lower RPD by inserting strategic mini-implants, immediate restoration with immediate loading/soft material. A- Intraoral image with lower RPD before implantation. B- Partial edentulous lower jaw before implantation. C- Tissue surface of the RPD before implantation. D- Four strategic mini-implants in the interforaminal region, tooth 32 was extracted. E- Tissue surface of the RPD after implantation, soft relining in the areas opposing the implants' head. F- Tissue surface of the RPD after 4 months, the matrix pick-up (housings). G- Intraoral image with lower RPD after the housing, clasps in esthetic zone were removed.

The strategic implant is "the implant that can change the prosthetic support type to a more favorable configuration" [1]. It is a reliable way of treatment with an implant survival rate of 91.7–100% [4]. Also, it can support both the RPD and the other abutments effectively. In two clinical studies with 2 and 3 years follow-up, the survival rate of the natural teeth abutments was 100% [9, 24].

Moreover, it can improve the survival rate of the RPD. The 10-year survival rate of RPDs; clasp-retained removable partial dentures, conical crown-retained dentures, or a combination of conical crown and clasp-retained dentures is 71.3% [27]. On the other hand, clinical studies with observation periods between 1 and 12.2 years reported survival rates of 90–100% for the implant-assisted removable partial denture prostheses [7, 28–31]. This remarked difference in the survival rate plays an essential role in formulating the prosthodontic plan.

Many clinical studies have shown that implant placement in strategic locations under an existing RPD can enhance chewing efficiency, dental health-related quality of life, and patient satisfaction with speaking and eating, as well as RPD retention, stability, and support [1, 8, 32]. Above that, it gives the dentist the ability to reduce the tissue coverage and reduce the size of the RPD, which can positively impact the patient's acceptance of the RPD, especially if he suffers hyperactive gag reflex, **Figure 24**. Also, it can improve the final esthetic result by avoiding the traditional metal clasp, **Figures 19** and **22**.

Unfortunately, inserting a standard implant under the existing RPD is not always feasible. The patient may have a very narrow bone that prevents inserting a standard implant without bone grafting. A procedure that is not suitable or acceptable by some patients. In this case, mini-implants can be considered a good alternative, **Figures 22** and **25** [1, 8, 16].

5. Mini-implant-assisted removable partial denture

In 1976, the U.S. Food and Drug Administration (FDA) approved the 3 mm root-form dental implant. With time, dental implants proved to be a predictable and reliable prosthodontic treatment modality with a high success rate [33–35]. After 21 years, the approval was cleared for implants less than 3 mm. The approval widens the spectrum of the patients treated with dental implants, particularly the cases with reduced bone width.

In literature, there is no standardization regarding the terminology of dental implant diameter [36]. For example, some authors considered the implants with diameters from 1.8 to 2.9 mm as small implants; others call them mini-implants [37]. Some authors defined the mini-implant as the implant with 2.2 mm [38]. Al-Johany et al. proposed a classification scheme and used four terms: Extra-narrow <3.0 mm, Narrow ≥3.0 mm to <3.75 mm, Standard 3.75 mm to <5 mm, and Wide ≥5 mm [36]. In this text, we will follow the lead of Resnik et al. and Schiegnitz et al. by considering the mini-implant as the implant with a diameter < 3.0 and the narrow-diameter implant as the implant with a diameter ≤ 3.5 [25, 37]. This implant type is mainly used in heavily atrophic jaws but with sufficient bone height. The mini-implant gives the dentist the ability to avoid bone augmentation procedure, which is considered a time and cost-consuming surgical intervention. Avoiding additional surgical procedures can reduce morbidity and possible complications such as nerve trauma, hemorrhage, postoperative pain, or infection [25]. The infection may lead to the failure of bone grafting [25]. Above that, it is less invasive than the standard implant as it requires a smaller implant bed and no flap in a considerable number of cases [26]. Therefore, it is more appropriate for the compromised or elderly patients. Moreover, it is cost-effective and affordable. On the other hand, the small diameter of the implant may create a shear load to the crestal bone. That may increase the risk of bone resorption [37, 39]. Narrow -implant has been linked to biomechanical risk factors as implant fatigue or fracture, particularly when used in the canine area where high occlusal loads are applied or in parafunctional habits patients [40].

A systematic review and meta-analysis reported that mini-implants (diameter < 3.0 mm) performed substantially worse than standard diameter implants with survival rates of 94.7 ± 5% [25]. However, narrow implants with a diameter (3–3.5 mm) have a better survival rate of 97.7 ± 2.3% [25]. Therefore, some

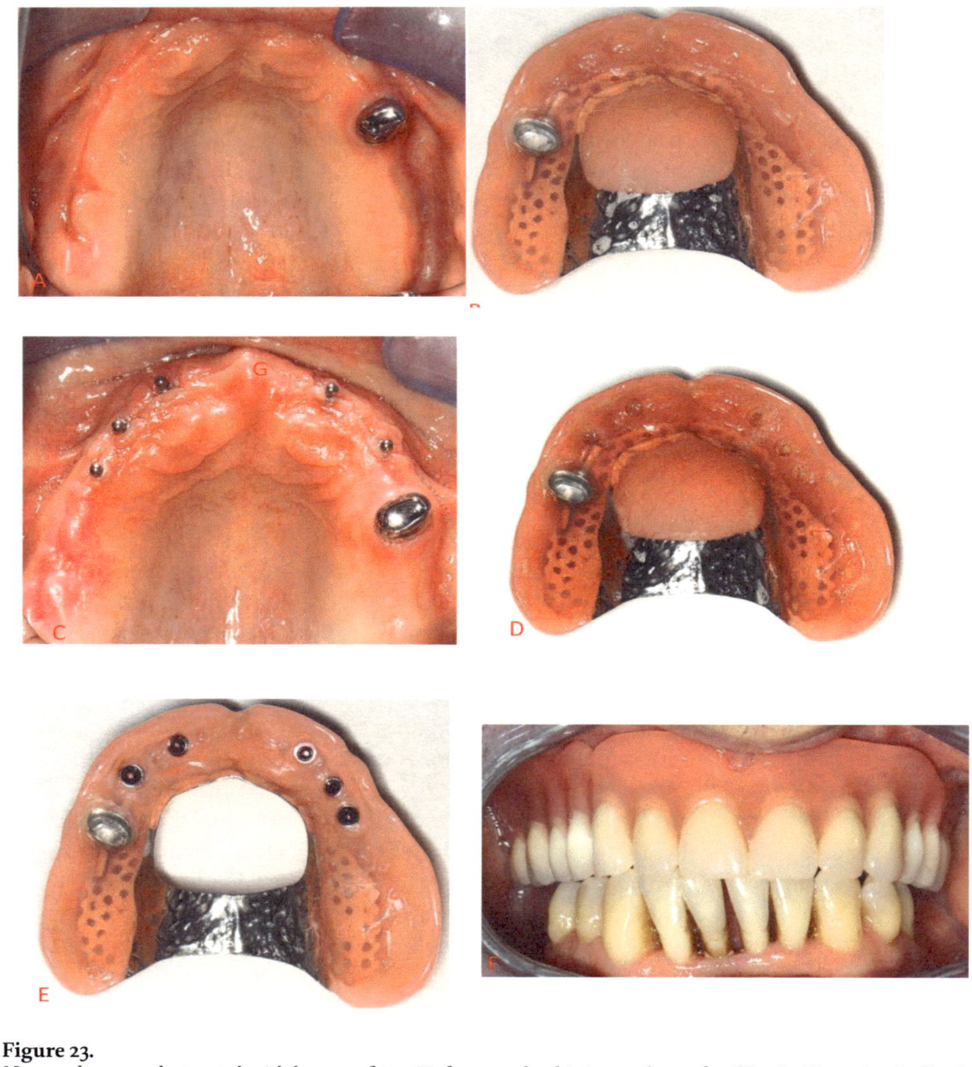

Figure 23.
Narrow bone can be treated with bone grafting. Unfortunately, this is not always feasible. A- Biomechanically, the narrow implant is not always the best approach, see paragraph 5. B- Osteoplasty is used to insert a wider implant by increasing the bone width, which will impact the crown-implant ratio negatively and may place the implant near vital anatomical structure. C- One-piece mini-implant with ball attachment and preferable crown-implant ratio can be used to stabilize a complete removable denture or partial removable denture.

researchers believe the best approach for a thin bone is bone augmentation [37]. If this is not feasible, narrow implant, osteoplasty and standard implant, or one-piece mini-implant with ball attachment and removable denture can be considered, **Figure 23**.

The small diameter implant is used to replace missing individual teeth in the anterior region, lower and upper jaw [41, 42]. Mini-implant is used as an orthodontic implant or transitional or provisional implant to support interim prostheses during the healing period after extensive implantations or augmentations and bone grafting [43]. The one-piece mini-implant with ball attachment is used as assisting / anchoring element under the removable denture [1]. Strategic min-implant under existing RPD and CD proved to be a reliable and straightforward approach [1, 8, 44]. New studies reported that the one-piece mini-implant with ball attachment has a significant advantage on the final prosthodontic treatment [1, 8].

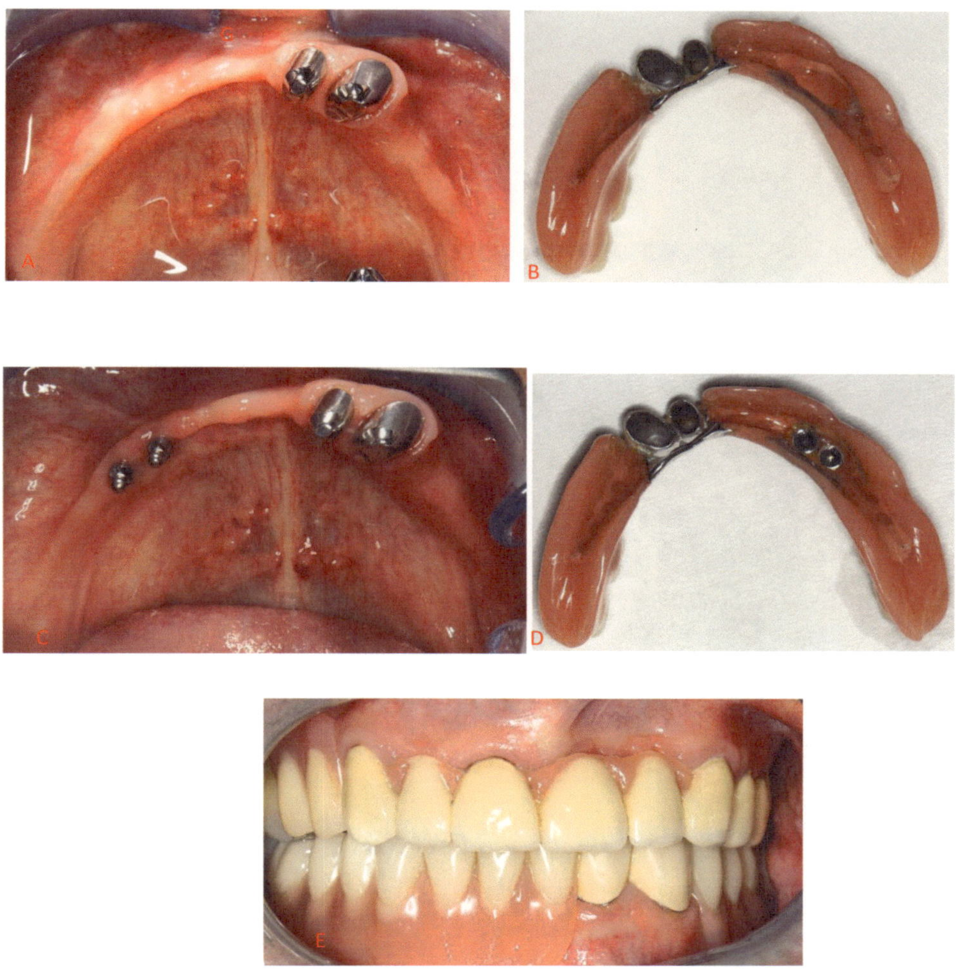

Figure 24.
Upgrading the existing double crown retained upper RPD by inserting strategic mini-implants, immediate restoration, and delayed loading. A- Partial edentulous upper jaw before implantation. B- Tissue surface of the RPD before implantation. C- Five strategic mini-implants. D- Tissue surface of the RPD after implantation, recesses (empty notches) against the mini-implants. E- Tissue surface of the RPD after 4 months, the matrix pick-up (housings). The palate coverage was reduced. F- Intraoral image with the RPD after the housing.

The one-piece implant mimics nature by having a solid unibody structure with no microgaps between the implant and the abutment. As a result, the possible biological complication (bone resorption) and structural flaw are reduced. Also, the flap or flapless single-stage surgery allows the dentist to implement immediate loading or immediate restoration [42]. Moreover, delayed loading is possible by preparing a recess against the mini-implant in the RPD's tissue surface. The treatment protocol can be conventional or delayed loading. However, the recess (cavity) distorts the fit of the RPD's, **Figure 24**.

On the other hand, if the mini-implants are inserted in a healthy, not compromised patent with insertion torque ≥35 Ncm, immediate loading can be considered.

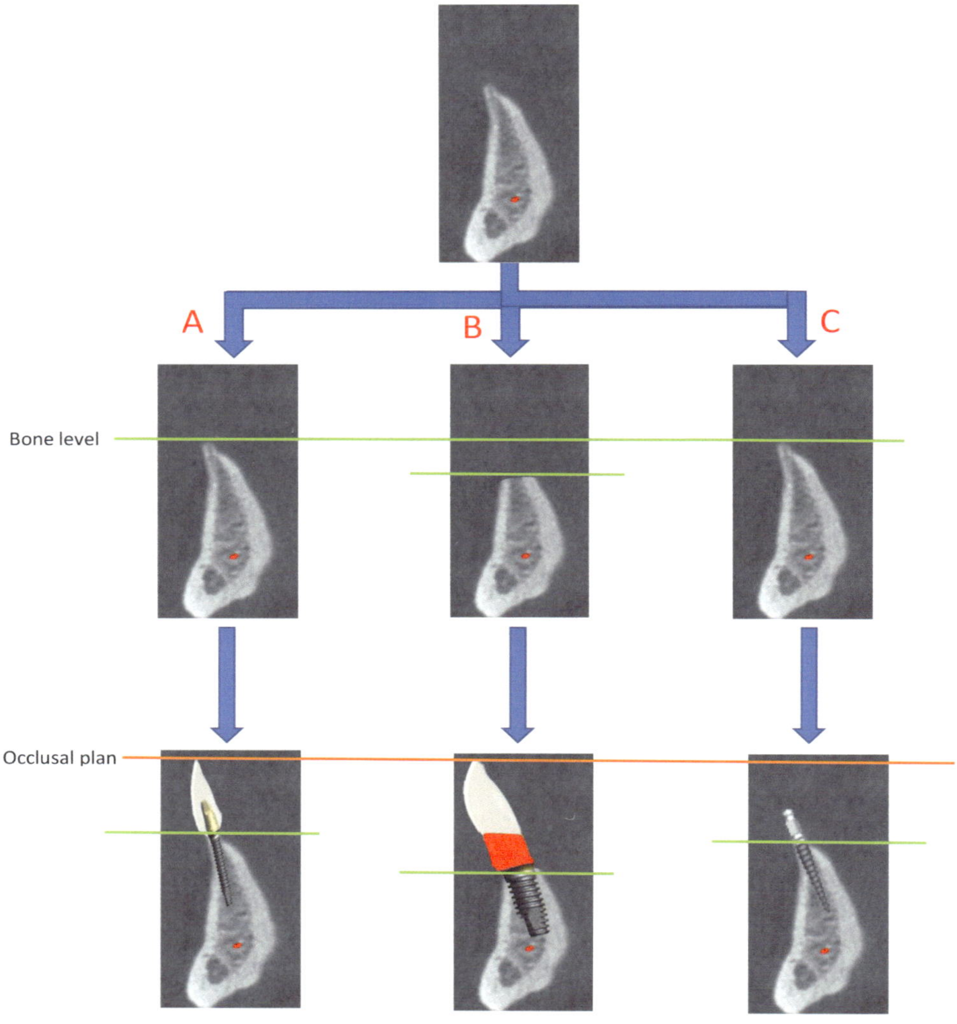

Figure 25.
Upgrading the existing double crown retained lower RPD by inserting strategic mini-implants, immediate restoration and immediate loading. A- Partial edentulous lower jaw before implantation. B- Tissue surface of the RPD before implantation. C- Two strategic mini-implants. D- Tissue surface of the RPD after implantation, the matrix pick-up (housings) inserted in the same implantation session. E- Intraoral image with the RPD in place after implantation.

The immediate restoration with immediate loading can be implemented through one of two forms:

- immediate loading using soft relining material, **Figure 22**.
- immediate loading using the matrix pick-up (housings), **Figure 25**.

After implantation, soft relining material can restore the fit of the RPD, ease tissue pressure, and give the patient a secure feeling because the relining material encircles the implant head and minimizes RPD rocking. If all mini-implants have a high insertion torque, the patient can receive the final restoration with matrix pick-up (housings). Subsequently, no additional session for adjusting the RPD is needed. In this approach, the patient can directly feel and recognize the significant improvement in the RPD in many domains especially, retention, support stability, and chewing [1, 8].

Studies proved that inserting strategic implants under existing RPD improves patient satisfaction on short- and medium-term follow-up (3-years) [1, 43]. The improvement can be explained by the symmetrical distribution of the abutments and the increased number of the rests/abutments [1, 17]. Gorai S, et al. study reported a correlation between the rests number and denture usage [17].

6. Conclusion

To sum it up, using strategic implants under existing RPD upgrade the design to more favorable support type and improve patient satisfaction with the RPD on several domains like speaking, chewing, retention, stability, and support of the RPD. This improvement could be reached earlier if the patient received immediate loading [1].

In many cases, after putting into consideration the patient's main complaint, expectation, desire, general health, intraoral/extraoral findings, evaluating the risks (do no harm) and the benefits of bone grafting and several implants, the dentist is able to provide his patient with one or few strategic standard or mini-implants that can satisfy the patients' needs *without overtreatment* "Less is more".

Strategic implants can also improve chewing ability, stabilize the occlusion, increase bite force and improve patient oral health-related quality of life. Moreover, better distribution of occlusal forces that may reduce bone resorption may be gained. Furthermore, strategic implants can improve comfort, confidence, and esthetics by reducing the RPD size and removing metal clasps from the esthetic zone.

Author details

Ahmad Al Jaghsi[1,2,3]

1 Department of Restorative Dentistry, College of Dentistry, Ajman University, UAE

2 Department of Prosthodontics, Gerodontology and Dental Materials, Greifswald University, Germany

3 Center of Medical and Bio-Allied Health Sciences Research, Ajman University, Ajman, United Arab Emirates

*Address all correspondence to: aljaghsi@ajman.ac.ae

References

[1] Al Jaghsi A, Heinemann F, Biffar R, Mundt T: **Immediate versus delayed loading of strategic mini-implants under existing removable partial dentures: patient satisfaction in a multi-center randomized clinical trial.** *Clin Oral Investig* 2021, **25**(1):255-264.

[2] Steffel VL: **Planning removable partial dentures.** *Journal of Prosthetic Dentistry* 1962, **12**(3):524-535.

[3] Alan B. Carr DMDMS, David T. Brown DDSMS: **McCracken's Removable Partial Prosthodontics**: Elsevier Health Sciences; 2015.

[4] Bassetti RG, Bassetti MA, Kuttenberger J: **Implant-Assisted Removable Partial Denture Prostheses: A Critical Review of Selected Literature.** *Int J Prosthodont* 2018, **31**(3):287-302.

[5] Al-Johany SS, Andres C: **ICK classification system for partially edentulous arches.** *J Prosthodont* 2008, **17**(6):502-507.

[6] Applegate OC: **Essentials of Removable Partial Denture Prosthesis**: W.B. Saunders Company; 1965.

[7] Bernhart G, Koob A, Schmitter M, Gabbert O, Stober T, Rammelsberg P: **Clinical success of implant-supported and tooth–implant-supported double crown-retained dentures.** *Clinical Oral Investigations* 2012, **16**(4):1031-1037.

[8] Mundt T, Schwahn C, Heinemann F, Schimmel M, Lucas C, Al Jaghsi A: **Stabilizing Removable Partial Dentures by Immediate or Delayed Loading of Mini-implants: Chewing Efficiency in a Randomized Controlled Clinical Trial.** *Int J Oral Maxillofac Implants* 2020, **35**(1):178-186.

[9] Krennmair G, Krainhöfner M, Waldenberger O, Piehslinger E: **Dental implants as strategic supplementary abutments for implant-tooth-supported telescopic crown-retained maxillary dentures: a retrospective follow-up study for up to 9 years.** *Int J Prosthodont* 2007, **20**(6):617-622.

[10] Igarashi Y, Goto T: **Ten-year follow-up study of conical crown-retained dentures.** *Int J Prosthodont* 1997, **10**(2):149-155.

[11] Yoshino K, Ito K, Kuroda M, Sugihara N: **Survival rate of removable partial dentures with complete arch reconstruction using double crowns: a retrospective study.** *Clin Oral Investig* 2020, **24**(4):1543-1549.

[12] Tada S, Ikebe K, Matsuda K, Maeda Y: **Multifactorial risk assessment for survival of abutments of removable partial dentures based on practice-based longitudinal study.** *J Dent* 2013, **41**(12):1175-1180.

[13] Tada S, Allen PF, Ikebe K, Zheng H, Shintani A, Maeda Y: **The Impact of the Crown-Root Ratio on Survival of Abutment Teeth for Dentures.** *J Dent Res* 2015, **94**(9 Suppl):220S–225S.

[14] Bornstein MM, Al-Nawas B, Kuchler U, Tahmaseb A: **Consensus statements and recommended clinical procedures regarding contemporary surgical and radiographic techniques in implant dentistry.** *Int J Oral Maxillofac Implants* 2014, **29 Suppl**:78-82.

[15] Gulsahi A, Paksoy CS, Ozden S, Kucuk NO, Cebeci ARI, Genc Y: **Assessment of bone mineral density in the jaws and its relationship to radiomorphometric indices.**

Dentomaxillofac Radiol 2010, **39**(5):284-289.

[16] Mundt T, Al Jaghsi A, Schwahn B, Hilgert J, Lucas C, Biffar R, Schwahn C, Heinemann F: **Immediate versus delayed loading of strategic mini dental implants for the stabilization of partial removable dental prostheses: a patient cluster randomized, parallel-group 3-year trial**. *BMC Oral Health* 2016, **17**(1):30.

[17] Gorai S, Koyama S, Chiba T, Ogawa T, Hatori K, Sasaki K: **[Multivariate analysis of factors affecting the status of wearing removable partial dentures]**. *Nihon Hotetsu Shika Gakkai Zasshi* 2008, **52**(2):126-134.

[18] Rosenstiel SF, Land MF: **Contemporary Fixed Prosthodontics - E-Book**: Elsevier Health Sciences; 2015.

[19] Albrektsson T, Brånemark PI, Hansson HA, Lindström J: **Osseointegrated titanium implants. Requirements for ensuring a long-lasting, direct bone-to-implant anchorage in man**. *Acta Orthop Scand* 1981, **52**(2):155-170.

[20] Joshi N, Joshi M, Angadi P: **Immediate loading of dental implants: review of the literature**. *J Long Term Eff Med Implants* 2011, **21**(4):269-279.

[21] Liu W, Cai H, Zhang J, Wang J, Sui L: **Effects of immediate and delayed loading protocols on marginal bone loss around implants in unsplinted mandibular implant-retained overdentures: a systematic review and meta-analysis.** *BMC Oral Health* 2021, **21**(1):122.

[22] Morton D, Gallucci G, Lin WS, Pjetursson B, Polido W, Roehling S, Sailer I, Aghaloo T, Albera H, Bohner L *et al*: **Group 2 ITI Consensus Report: Prosthodontics and implant dentistry**. *Clin Oral Implants Res* 2018, **29 Suppl 16**:215-223.

[23] Feine JS, Carlsson GE, Awad MA, Chehade A, Duncan WJ, Gizani S, Head T, Heydecke G, Lund JP, MacEntee M *et al*: **The McGill consensus statement on overdentures. Mandibular two-implant overdentures as first choice standard of care for edentulous patients**. *Gerodontology* 2002, **19**(1):3-4.

[24] Bernhart G, Koob A, Schmitter M, Gabbert O, Stober T, Rammelsberg P: **Clinical success of implant-supported and tooth-implant-supported double crown-retained dentures**. *Clin Oral Investig* 2012, **16**(4):1031-1037.

[25] Schiegnitz E, Al-Nawas B: **Narrow-diameter implants: A systematic review and meta-analysis**. *Clin Oral Implants Res* 2018, **29 Suppl 16**:21-40.

[26] Sendax VD: **Mini Dental Implants: Principles and Practice**: Elsevier Health Sciences; 2012.

[27] Wagner B, Kern M: **Clinical evaluation of removable partial dentures 10 years after insertion: success rates, hygienic problems, and technical failures**. *Clin Oral Investig* 2000, **4**(2):74-80.

[28] Hug S, Mantokoudis D, Mericske-Stern R: **Clinical evaluation of 3 overdenture concepts with tooth roots and implants: 2-year results**. *Int J Prosthodont* 2006, **19**(3):236-243.

[29] Kaufmann R, Friedli M, Hug S, Mericske-Stern R: **Removable dentures with implant support in strategic positions followed for up to 8 years**. *Int J Prosthodont* 2009, **22**(3):233-241; discussion 242.

[30] Payne AG, Tawse-Smith A, Wismeijer D, De Silva RK, Ma S:

Multicentre prospective evaluation of implant-assisted mandibular removable partial dentures: surgical and prosthodontic outcomes. *Clin Oral Implants Res* 2017, **28**(1):116-125.

[31] Rinke S, Ziebolz D, Ratka-Krüger P, Frisch E: **Clinical Outcome of Double Crown-Retained Mandibular Removable Dentures Supported by a Combination of Residual Teeth and Strategic Implants.** *J Prosthodont* 2015, **24**(5):358-365.

[32] Gonçalves TM, Campos CH, Garcia RC: **Implant retention and support for distal extension partial removable dental prostheses: satisfaction outcomes.** *J Prosthet Dent* 2014, **112**(2):334-339.

[33] Al-Nawas B, Kämmerer PW, Morbach T, Ladwein C, Wegener J, Wagner W: **Ten-year retrospective follow-up study of the TiOblast dental implant.** *Clin Implant Dent Relat Res* 2012, **14**(1):127-134.

[34] Moraschini V, Poubel LA, Ferreira VF, Barboza Edos S: **Evaluation of survival and success rates of dental implants reported in longitudinal studies with a follow-up period of at least 10 years: a systematic review.** *Int J Oral Maxillofac Surg* 2015, **44**(3):377-388.

[35] Schiegnitz E, Al-Nawas B, Tegner A, Sagheb K, Berres M, Kämmerer PW, Wagner W: **Clinical and Radiological Long-Term Outcome of a Tapered Implant System with Special Emphasis on the Influence of Augmentation Procedures.** *Clin Implant Dent Relat Res* 2016, **18**(4):810-820.

[36] Al-Johany SS, Al Amri MD, Alsaeed S, Alalola B: **Dental Implant Length and Diameter: A Proposed Classification Scheme.** *J Prosthodont* 2017, **26**(3):252-260.

[37] Resnik R: **Misch's Contemporary Implant Dentistry**: Elsevier - Health Sciences Division; 2019.

[38] Ertugrul HZ, Pipko DJ: **Measuring mobility of 2 dental implant fixtures of different configurations: an in vitro study.** *Implant Dent* 2006, **15**(3):290-297.

[39] Klein MO, Schiegnitz E, Al-Nawas B: **Systematic review on success of narrow-diameter dental implants.** *Int J Oral Maxillofac Implants* 2014, **29 Suppl**:43-54.

[40] Karl M, Krafft T, Kelly JR: **Fracture of a narrow-diameter roxolid implant: clinical and fractographic considerations.** *Int J Oral Maxillofac Implants* 2014, **29**(5):1193-1196.

[41] Vigolo P, Givani A: **Clinical evaluation of single-tooth mini-implant restorations: a five-year retrospective study.** *J Prosthet Dent* 2000, **84**(1):50-54.

[42] Mazor Z, Steigmann M, Leshem R, Peleg M: **Mini-implants to reconstruct missing teeth in severe ridge deficiency and small interdental space: a 5-year case series.** *Implant Dent* 2004, **13**(4):336-341.

[43] Bidra AS, Almas K: **Mini implants for definitive prosthodontic treatment: a systematic review.** *J Prosthet Dent* 2013, **109**(3):156-164.

[44] Mundt T, Kobrow j, Schwahn C: **Follow-up examination of patients with mini-implants for the stabilization of existing removable partial dentures.** *Deutsche Zahnärztliche Zeitschrift International* 2020, **2**:38-49.